Exploring Bacterial Biofilms

Edited by Sadık Dincer,
Melis Sumengen Ozdenefe
and Hatice Aysun Mercimek Takci

Published in London, United Kingdom

Exploring Bacterial Biofilms
http://dx.doi.org/10.5772/intechopen.1005710
Edited by Sadık Dincer, Melis Sumengen Ozdenefe and Hatice Aysun Mercimek Takci

Contributors
Alaa T. Qumsani, Alisha Javed, Atiye Karadoğan, Aylin Turksever Tetiker, Dilawaiz Khan, Eiichi Osono, Esra Sündüz Yiğittekin, Faryal Gohar, Fatma Azgin, Fuat Bulut, Hafiza Sehrish Kiani, Ivo Ganchev, Jiddu Joseph, Leela Kakithakara Vajravelu, Maheswary Datchanamoorthy, Michael Ikechukwuka Ejafu, Mirza Imran Shehzad, Muhammed Shafeekh Muyyarikkandy, Nimra Irfan, Omodamola Paulina Akinro, Peng Li, Rimpei Morita, Sadik Dinçer, Sai Sristi Panda, Sanya Boby, Shahzar Khan, Shama Zahra, Siqi Yao, Syed Hamza Abbas, Tugba Kilic, W. Richard Thilagaraj

First published in London, United Kingdom, 2025 by IntechOpen
IntechOpen is the global imprint of INTECHOPEN LIMITED, registered in England and Wales, registration number: 11086078, 167-169 Great Portland Street, London, W1W 5PF, United Kingdom

For EU product safety concerns: IN TECH d.o.o., Prolaz Marije Krucifikse Kozulić 3, 51000 Rijeka, Croatia, info@intechopen.com or visit our website at intechopen.com.

British Library Cataloguing-in-Publication Data
A catalogue record for this book is available from the British Library

Exploring Bacterial Biofilms
Edited by Sadık Dincer, Melis Sumengen Ozdenefe and Hatice Aysun Mercimek Takci
p. cm.
Print ISBN 978-0-85466-947-9
Online ISBN 978-0-85466-946-2
eBook (PDF) ISBN 978-0-85466-948-6

Meet the editors

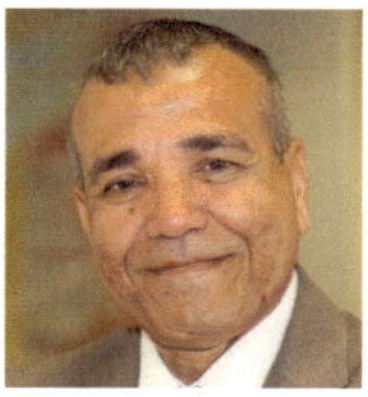

For the past 36 years, Prof. Sadık Dincer has been involved in teaching, research, and academic work at numerous distinguished universities in Turkey. Currently, he is working in the Biology and Biotechnology Departments, Cukurova University, Adana, Turkey. He has published numerous articles in national and international journals, manuscripts, and book chapters. To date, he has trained twenty-six MSc and eleven Ph.D. students. He received the Technology Development Award from the Scientific and Technological Research Council of Turkey (TÜBİTAK) in 2013 and a national study patent in 2019. His research is focused on bacteriology, microbial ecology, and industrial biotechnology.

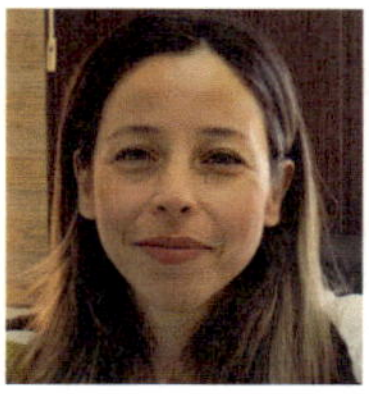

Prof. Dr. Hatice Aysun Mercimek Takci received her M. Sc. and Ph.D. degrees in Biotechnology and Biology from Cukurova University, Turkey, in 2007 and 2011, respectively. Since 2009, she has worked at Kilis 7 Aralik University, Kilis, Turkey. Her teaching interests include Bacteriology, Biotechnology, Enzymology, Microbial Genetics, and Nanotechnology by green synthesis. She has 64 manuscripts published in national and international journals, and her works have been cited 558 times. Her research interests focus on multiple antibiotic and heavy metal resistance in bacteria, quorum sensing inhibition, production and characterization of bacterial enzymes, water remediation by nanoparticles synthesized via a green approach, and aquatic bacterial contamination. Related to these research areas, she has 20 projects supported by the Scientific and Technological Research Council of Turkey (TÜBİTAK) and coordinates scientific research projects.

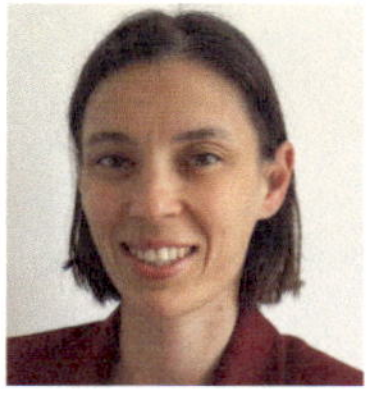

Associate Professor Dr. Melis Sumengen Ozdenefe received her BSc, MSc, and Ph.D. in Biology from Çukurova University, Turkey, in 2009, 2011, and 2014, respectively. During her MSc, she spent six months at Anhalt University, Germany, as an international exchange student and a researcher. She has worked in the Department of Biomedical Engineering at Near East University, Northern Cyprus, since 2014. Her teaching interests include industrial microbiology, bacteriology, biotechnology, enzymology, environmental microbiology, and nanobiotechnology. Her research areas involve enzymes and biosurfactants produced from various bacteria and fungi for industrial applications, the production and characterization of bacterial enzymes and bacteriocins, the antimicrobial and antioxidant activity of various plant structures, multiple antibiotic resistance, heavy metal resistance in Gram-negative bacteria, water quality assessment and green synthesis of nanoparticles with antibacterial activity using plant extracts. Dr. Ozdenefe's works have been published in national and international journals, conferences, congresses, and symposiums, and cited 339 times.

Contents

Preface

Bacterial biofilms are sessile cellular communities that attach to biotic and abiotic surfaces. Cells embedded in an extracellular matrix of highly hydrated polymeric substances (EPS) adopt a "multicellular lifestyle" by self-production. This prevailing microbial lifestyle in ecosystems allows them to survive against extreme living conditions such as humidity, pressure, temperature, extreme pH values, osmotic stress, and antimicrobial chemicals, among others.

Bacteria growing predominantly in a biofilm matrix can persist on any kind of clinical instrument and industrial surface. The presence of biofilms at these unwanted locations triggers infections and diseases, causing water and food contamination. It is estimated to be responsible for up to 75% of microbial infections in humans due to the biofilms harbored on indwelling medical devices. The biofilm-associated critical problems have resulted in the biofouling of membranes, obstruction of equipment, and metal surface corrosion in industrial settings. On the other hand, most laboratory studies indicate that it can be applied in surface/ground water treatment, bioremediation of soils, and biotechnological productions of chemicals.

The aforementioned knowledge and biofilms are the subject of interdisciplinary studies, including analytics, biology, chemistry, medicine, and engineering. So, in this book, topics including the biofilm-producing bacteria, genetic fundamentals of biofilm development, quorum sensing, prevention of biofilm formation, and implications of biofilms in industry will be discussed.

Sadik Dinçer
Cukurova University,
Adana, Turkey

Hatice Aysun Mercimek Takcı
Kilis 7 Aralik University,
Kilis, Turkey

Melis Sumengen Ozdenefe
Near East University,
Nicosia, Turkish Republic of Northern Cyprus

Section 1

Infection, Resistance, Control and Innovative Treatment of Microbial Biofilms

Chapter 1

Biofilm Disinfection in Medical Devices

Eiichi Osono and Rimpei Morita

Abstract

We evaluated the disinfection of biofilms in the fluid piping of dialysis equipment, focusing on *Methylobacterium radiotolerance*. Using a Center for Disease Control and Prevention (CDC) biofilm reactor, we analyzed the disinfection effects of chemical and physical disinfectants based on concentration and reaction time. Sodium hypochlorite showed dose-dependent disinfection, achieving a log reduction value (LRV) of 4 at 1000 ppm in 10 minutes, while lower concentrations also achieved similar values over longer periods, 6 hours. The bactericidal effect of peracetic acid correlated with its concentration, reaching an LRV of 6 within 10 minutes in certain products. Hot water at 80°C for 2 minutes also proved effective. Ozone and hydrogen peroxide were less effective; however, they had the advantage of decomposing quickly and returning to water. This study highlights the importance of daily disinfection to maintain dialysis equipment, providing scientific evidence through cleanliness for a practical approach to sustain patient care.

Keywords: hemodialysis equipment, sodium hypochlorite, peracetic acid, hot water, *Methylobacterium* spp., CDC biofilm reactor, neutralization

1. Introduction

Hemodialysis is a critical treatment for maintaining homeostasis in patients with kidney failure by removing waste products from their bodies. This process involves using a semipermeable membrane to filter and purify blood waste. It is typically conducted three times a week for 4 hours per session, enabling patients to maintain daily activities while sustaining their natural lifespan.

During hemodialysis, blood is exposed to a dialysis fluid—a glucose-added Ringer's solution with pH adjusted using sodium bicarbonate—produced at each treatment facility. Effective microbiological control of hemodialysis systems depends on three key strategies [1]: (1) appropriate system design, (2) proper operation, and (3) regular disinfection. The final cleanliness of dialysis fluid is ensured by filtration through UF membranes; endtoxin retentive filter (ETRF). However, controlling the upstream bioburden requires not only maintaining aseptic handling to prevent contamination [2] but also implementing proper daily disinfection. Otherwise, the function of reusable ETRF can rapidly deteriorate. The disinfection protocols for these systems are outlined in the operation manuals of dialysis equipment, based on standards such as JIS-T0601-2-16 (the Japanese adaptation of IEC standards). These

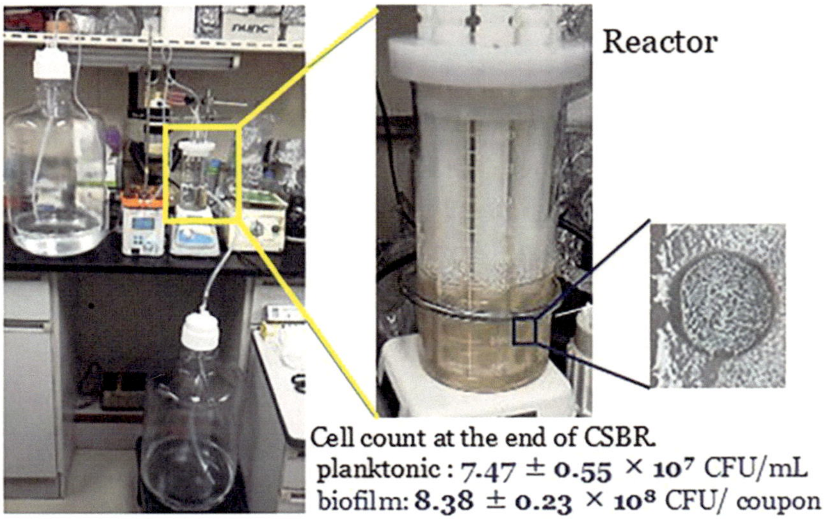

Figure 1.
CDC biofilm reactor. Left: full picture. Center: the reactor, with eight rods in three coupons each, was filled with a 1:10 TSB solution, and after Methylobacterium radiotolerance *suspension was added, the mixture was stirred at 125 rpm at room temperature for 72 hours. A 1:100 TSB solution was then injected continuously for 24 hours at a flow rate of 10.5–11.7 ml/min (Continuous Stirring Biofilm Reactor: CSBR) Right: visible biofilm on a coupon.*

guidelines employ the test microorganism suspension method (TMSM) [3] to verify disinfection efficacy against planktonic bacteria. However, in practice, significant inconsistencies have been observed, with large numbers of bacteria still being isolated from dialysis systems despite adherence to these protocols.

In contrast, the U.S. Environmental Protection Agency (EPA) has adopted the CDC Biofilm Reactor (CDC-BFR; **Figure 1**) as a standard evaluation method for disinfectants targeting biofilms on non-porous hard surfaces [4]. This reactor simulates robust biofilm formation under high shear forces and flow rates, a system known as the continuous stirring biofilm reactor (CSBR) [5]. In this chapter, we examine disinfection strategies for biofilm-forming bacteria, focusing on *Methylobacterium radiotolerans*, an aquatic species commonly found within dialysis equipment [6]. Using the CDC-BFR, we assessed the efficacy of practical disinfection methods, analyzing the effects of disinfectant concentration and exposure time on biofilm removal. Based on these findings, we propose a scientifically validated framework for selecting effective disinfectants for flow piping.

2. Disinfection

2.1 Sodium hypochlorite (NaClO)

Sodium hypochlorite (NaOCl) is one of the most widely used disinfectants in manufacturing systems [7] and is the only disinfectant specified in the operating manuals for dialysis equipment manufactured in Japan. The ionization ratio of hypochlorous acid (HOCl) to hypochlorite ion (ClO^-) varies depending on pH: at pH 5, the ratio is 10:0; at pH 7.5, it is 5:5; and at pH 10.5, it is 0:10. HOCl effectively penetrates bacterial cell membranes, whereas ClO^- cannot enter the cytoplasm unless the membrane is damaged.

When a 6% NaOCl solution (Pulax, Oyarax, Osaka) was diluted to concentrations ranging from 50 to 1000 ppm and tested for its bactericidal effect on planktonic cells using the TMSM [3], complete bacterial inactivation was achieved even at the lowest concentration of 50 ppm (open triangle in **Figure 2**, upper panel) [8]. However, its efficacy against biofilms varied with concentration: the logarithmic reduction value (LRV) was 1.25 (1.14–1.36) at 50 ppm, 2.37 (1.58–3.30) at 200 ppm, and 5.22 (4.68–5.68) at 1000 ppm; this satisfies the European Norm (EN) and U.S. EPA standards for disinfectant efficacy when using the CDC-BFR, achieving a significant reduction within 10 minutes (0.17 hours).

The effect of pH on NaOCl efficacy was also evaluated. At 1000 ppm, alkalization tended to reduce bactericidal activity, but no significant differences were observed under other conditions, possibly due to the cleaning effect of ClO^- in account (**Figure 2**, lower panel). When examining the effect of reaction time at 200 ppm, the LRV exceeded 2 (2.01-2.49) within 10 minutes, increasing to 3.61 (2.94-4.08) after

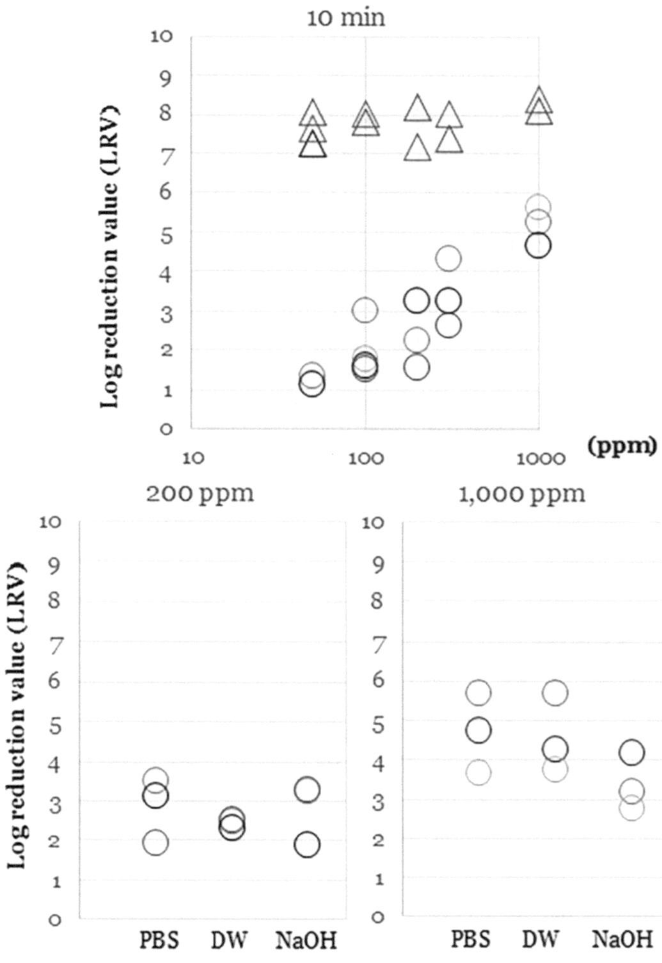

Figure 2.
Effects of NaOCl on planktonic and biofilms of M radiotolerance *prepared with CDC-BFR, reacted for 10 minutes as specified by EPA. Reprinted from Ref. [8]. △: TMSM ○: CDC-BFR. Upper: Effect of concentration. Lower: Effect of pH. The measured pH diluted by PBS/DW/0.01 N NaOH was 8.5/9.7/10.9 at 200 ppm and 9.7/10.4/11.0 at 1000 ppm.*

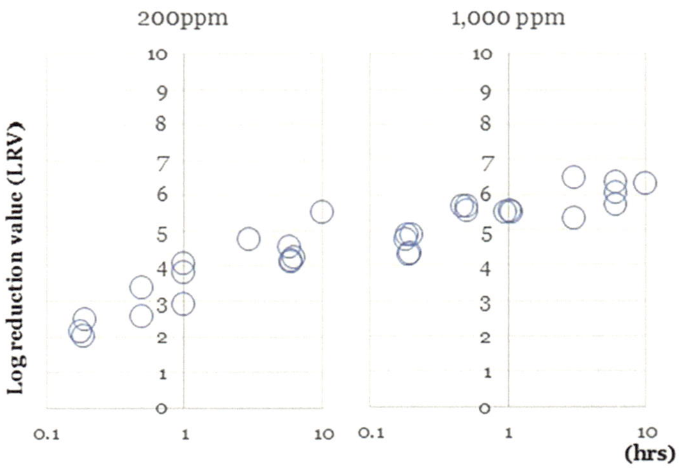

Figure 3.
Effect of reaction time of NaOCl on biofilm of M radiotolerance. *Reprinted from Ref. [8].*

1 hour and 4.27 (4.11-4.54) after 6 hours (**Figure 3**). At 1000 ppm, the LRV exceeded 4 (4.31-4.86) within 10 minutes and increased slightly 5 to 6 (5.53-5.63) after 0.5 hours, but no further improvement was observed with extended exposure times of up to 6 hours. Tests using acidic, low-conductivity, high-purity hypochlorite water (C.L. Fine, Nipro, Osaka) yielded similar results, confirming that both concentration and exposure time significantly influence biofilm disinfection efficacy [9]. However, there is a precaution that it is an acidic formulation with a pH of 5, so it penetrates into the silicone material and takes a long time to flush with care after disinfection [10].

The LRV of biofilms formed using the CDC-BFR increased proportionally with NaOCl concentration (**Figure 2**) and improved with longer exposure times (**Figure 3**), confirming that both concentration and duration are key metrics for quantitative disinfection evaluation. Notably, a NaOCl concentration of 1000 ppm achieves effective disinfection within 10 minutes when the system is properly rinsed, and the concentration is kept stable. Even at a lower concentration of 200 ppm, NaOCl demonstrated strong disinfectant efficacy, highlighting its practicality for maintaining dialysis systems.

2.2 Peracetic acid (PAA)

Peracetic acid (PAA) effectively penetrates bacterial cell membranes and disrupts the outer wall by inactivating enzyme-active sites. This action is mediated by hydroxyl radicals, which specifically target amino acids containing SH groups during the decomposition of PAA [11]. Additionally, hydrogen peroxide (H_2O_2), a component present in PAA formulations, enhances its antimicrobial activity through the generation of reactive oxygen species [12]. The release of oxygen bubbles caused by catalase activity may further contribute to the physical disruption of biofilms. However, PAA is not effective as a peeling agent for encapsulated biofilms, limiting its ability to fully remove them. PAA is synthesized by combining acetic acid and H_2O_2, leading to variations in the concentrations of PAA, acetic acid, and H_2O_2 depending on the formulation.

In the study [13], the pH of 12 PAA-based products diluted as designation ranged from 1.75 to 4.96, and a positive correlation was observed between the concentrations of PAA and H_2O_2 (r = 0.702, p = 0.005). Against planktonic bacteria, all products eradicated bacteria completely within a 10-minute reaction time, regardless of PAA concentration (**Figure 4**, upper panel). However, efficacy against biofilms varied significantly among products, with LRVs (logarithmic reduction values) ranging from 2.47 to 9.40 after a 10-minute reaction under appropriate neutralization conditions. One product designated as a chemical sterilizer, containing 450 ppm of PAA, achieved an LRV of 8.93. The LRV positively correlated with increasing PAA concentration (**Figure 4**, lower-left panel, r = 0.861) and showed a similar, though weaker, trend with H_2O_2 (**Figure 4**, lower-right panel, r = 0.501). However, stepwise multiple regression analysis revealed that the bactericidal effect was primarily driven by PAA (p = 0.011), with H_2O_2 contributing a secondary effect when catalase neutralized it completely. The additive antimicrobial effects of PAA and H_2O_2 suggest distinct mechanisms of action on biofilms. Concentration-dependent changes in LRV were evident when a single PAA product was diluted 100×, 150×, and 300×, corresponding to reductions in PAA concentration to 2/3 and 1/3, respectively (**Figure 5**). At 300× dilution, extending the reaction time to 1 or 3 hours further enhanced biofilm reduction.

Similar time-dependent effects were observed with both PAA and NaOCl products on biofilms. From a clinical perspective, PAA-based products are promising

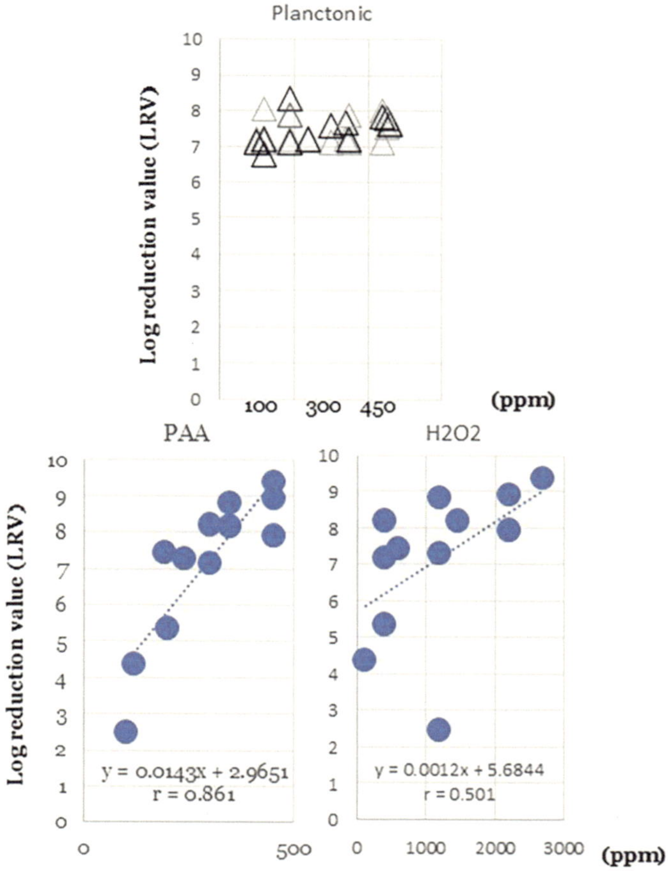

Figure 4.
Effect of PAA concentration on planktonic and biofilms of M radiotolerance *reacted for 10 minutes. Reprinted from Ref. [13]. Upper: Against planktonic cells. △: TMSM. Lower: Against biofilms. Dots are averages of 3 to 6 experiments for each product Left: PAA Right:* H_2O_2.

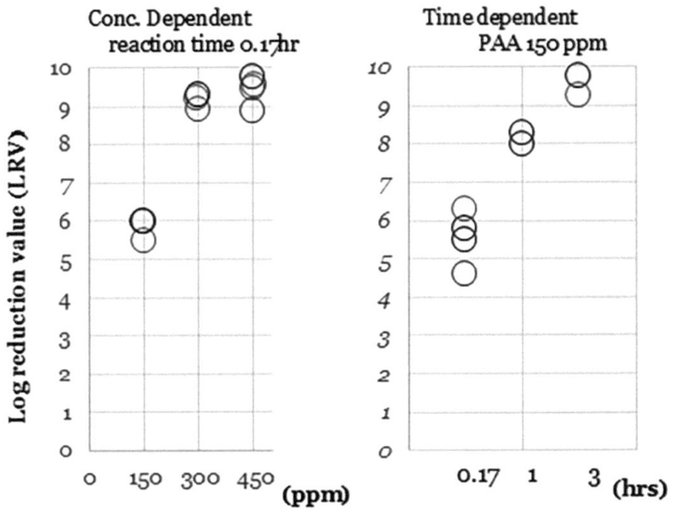

Figure 5.
Effects of different dilution rates of PAA and reaction time at high dilution rates on biofilms of M. radiotolerance. *Reprinted from Ref. [13]. Left: Dose-dependent. Dilution rate was at x100, x150, x300. Right: Time-dependent. Reaction time was extended for 1 to 3 hours at x300.*

alternatives for routine cleaning and disinfection following dialysis treatments, although strong oxidizing forces may damage components, causing leaks and equipment failure. Their ability to achieve significant biofilm reduction, coupled with their effectiveness at varying concentrations and reaction times, makes them valuable tools in dialysis system maintenance.

2.3 Hot water rinsing as a disinfection method

Hot water disinfection works by denaturing proteins and lipids through heat-induced structural changes and dehydration, which damage the outer membrane, cell membrane, and cytoplasm, ultimately resulting in bacterial death [14]. This method is widely used in pharmaceutical manufacturing processes, such as pasteurization, where water for injection is maintained at a temperature of 70°C or higher. Despite its efficacy, the high initial costs of heat-resistant equipment and heat sources limit its widespread adoption in dialysis facilities. Additionally, aquatic bacteria like *Methylobacterium radiotolerans*, which do not grow at 42°C [15], are generally susceptible to heat, but cooling during pipe transit or insufficient thermostatic maintenance can compromise the disinfection process.

For example [16], Hot water maintained at 80°C in a thermostatic bath was highly effective in disinfection, with the LRV against biofilm achieved 7 (6.69-8.85) in 10 minutes (**Figure 6**, upper panel, closed circles). On the other hand, when the 80°C water was left at room temperature, the LRV was only 2.68 (2.54-2.95) (**Figure 6**, upper panel, open circles). During this process, the actual water temperature in the bath ranged between 75 and 78°C, with an accumulated lethality value (Ao) of 120–280 seconds (80°C equivalent; **Figure 6**, middle panel) after 10 minutes. When left to cool at room temperature, the cumulative Ao value was only 15–34 seconds, as shown by continuous temperature measurements (**Figure 6**, lower panel).

Shorter reaction times (2–5 minutes) under constant temperature conditions were also tested (bold open circle in **Figure 6**, upper-right panel). The relationship

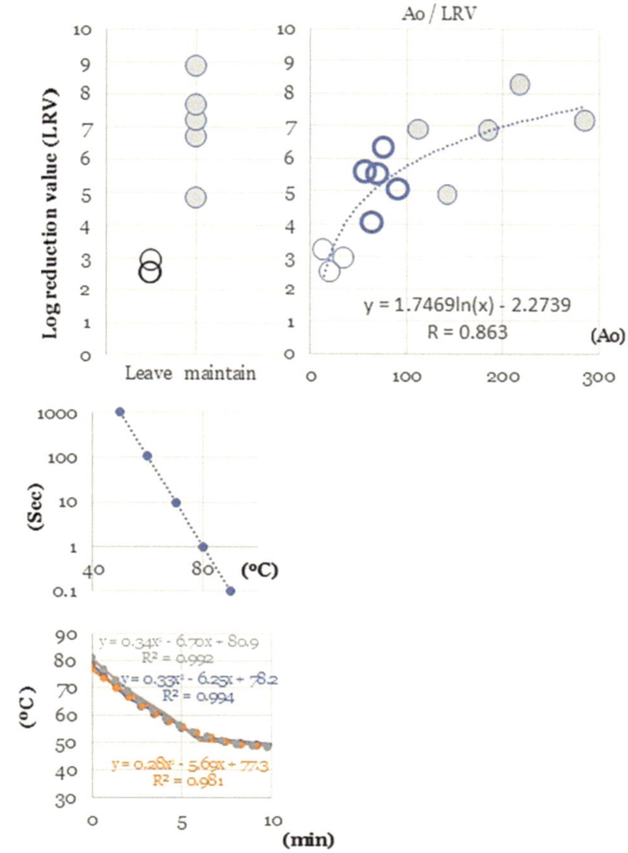

Figure 6.
Effect of hot water rinsing on M radiotolerance *biofilm. Reprinted from Ref. [16]. Upper-left: LRV by hot water. Open circle: left at room temperature, closed circle: maintain constant temperature. Upper-right: Relationship between Ao value and the bactericidal effect. Middle: Time length at each measured temperature that becomes Ao (80°C conversion 1 second). Vertical axis: second, Horizontal axis: Measured temperature. A change of 10°C results in a one-digit difference. Lower: Actual change when hot water was left at room temperature. Vertical axis: Measured temperature, horizontal axis: time after leaving.*

between Ao and LRV showed a strong correlation ($R = 0.863$, $p = 0.001$) in a semi-logarithmic plot. An Ao of 113 seconds was sufficient to reach an LRV of 6, but the sterilizing effect decayed rapidly below that.

Hot water disinfection has notable advantages, including leaving no harmful residues and supporting sustainable development goals (SDGs) by naturally reverting to water. However, it is not a comprehensive solution for biofilm removal or for use after dialysis sessions. Its limitations, such as inconsistent biofilm removal and potential deterioration of system components [17], highlight the need for it to be used as a supplementary method alongside chemical disinfection for optimal results.

2.4 Ozon and hydrogen peroxide

In facilities without effluent treatment systems, discharging disinfectants can damage sewage infrastructure, necessitating compliance with effluent standards (e.g., pH 5–9 and temperature < 50°C) [18]. Hydrogen peroxide (H_2O_2) is broken down by bacterial catalase releasing reactive oxygen species with disinfectant properties [12]. Even at low concentrations, H_2O_2 damages both bacterial cell wall and membranes [19]. However, residual H_2O_2 may interfere with biological assays, leading to overestimated disinfectant effects. In this study, a neutralizing agent (polysorbate, lecithin, and catalase) effectively halted reactions, ensuring no residual H_2O_2 remained 10 minutes after neutralization.

Ozone (O_3), itself a reactive oxygen species, considered for application in dialysis systems, was tested using Nikkiso's Handlex (Nikka Micron Co., Misato) for ozonized water production. At standard O_3 concentrations of 4 ppm and a maximum capacity of 10 ppm, the log reduction value (LRV) against planktonic bacteria was around 3 at 4 ppm but only 0.90 (0.61-1.26) against biofilms. At 10 ppm, the LRV for biofilms improved to 1.88 (1.85-1.93) (**Figure 7**, left panel) [16]. Ozone has the advantage of rapid degradation, making it a viable option for certain applications, such as during multi-use dialysis sessions.

For H_2O_2 (3.5% Kenei Pharma, Osaka), the LRV against planktonic bacteria was 2.45 (2.12-2.78) at 100x dilution, while it was only 0.37 (0.29-0.45) against biofilms (**Figure 7**, right panel). As the concentration increased, the LRV rose significantly. At a 10x dilution, the LRV reached 9 for planktonic bacteria and 2.72 (2.12-3.67) for biofilms, while the undiluted solution achieved an LRV of 7.49 (6.72-8.05). Undiluted H_2O_2, commonly used for cleaning and disinfecting skin wounds, showed strong efficacy against biofilms. However, its effectiveness decreased dramatically with dilution: the LRV dropped from 4 at a 10x dilution.

These results suggest that simple dilution is insufficient for complete removal, and thorough rinsing is required, as with other chemical disinfectants.

2.5 Antiseptics

Iodine, released from povidone-iodine (PI) in aqueous solutions, penetrates bacterial cell membranes and oxidizes water to form H_2OI^+, which denatures proteins by targeting SH groups, tyrosine, and histidine residues [20]. Chlorhexidine (CHX) disrupts bacterial cell membranes at low concentrations, causing irreversible leakage of cytoplasmic components and enzyme inhibition. At higher concentrations, CHX

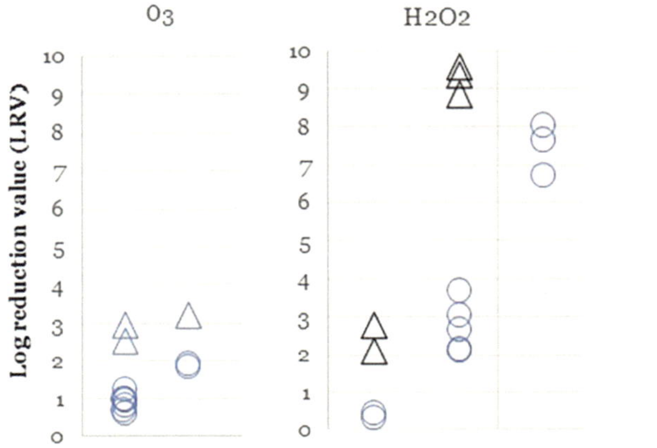

Figure 7.
Effect of ozone and hydrogen peroxide concentration on M radiotolerance *biofilm. Reprinted from Ref. [16].*
△: TMSM ○: CDC-BFR.

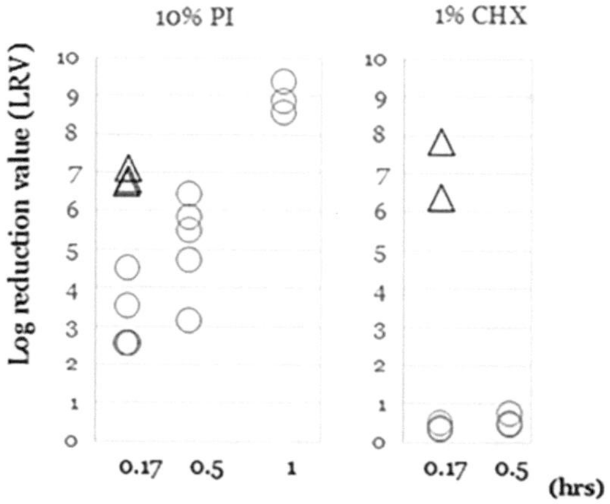

Figure 8.
Effect of reaction time of antiseptics on M radiotolerance *biofilm. Reprinted from Ref. [22].* △*: TMSM* ○*: CDC-BFR.*

precipitates intracellular proteins and nucleic acids [21]. Both PI (10%, Meiji Seika Pharma, Tokyo) and CHX (1% Yoshida Pharma, Osaka) are antiseptics that can also act as disinfectants for medical devices and environments where complete sterility is not feasible. These agents are typically used to disinfect dialysis fluid collection points prone to biofilm formation but are not applied directly to dialysis system piping.

PI showed significant efficacy against biofilms, achieving a log reduction value (LRV) of 3.10 (2.49–4.49) after 10 minutes of immersion, which increased to 5.09 (3.09–6.41) at 30 minutes and 8.92 (8.55–9.36) at 60 minutes, meeting the European sterilizer standard [22]. In contrast, against suspended bacteria, PI reached an LRV of 6.83 within just 10 minutes, demonstrating that biofilms present greater resistance (**Figure 8**, left panel). Similarly, CHX achieved an LRV of 7.06 against suspended bacteria after appropriate neutralization. However, its efficacy against biofilms was limited, with an LRV of 0.34 (0.28–0.44) after 10 minutes and only 0.51 (0.40–0.69) after 30 minutes, even with extended immersion time (**Figure 8**, right panel).

PI is highly effective against biofilms and has the potential to act as a chemical sterilant with sufficiently prolonged exposure times. Notable historical applications include sterilizing the Apollo 11 spacecraft after its return from the moon in 1969 [23] and maintaining sterility in permanent bio-implants, such as titanium connectors in peritoneal dialysis catheters. CHX, while less effective against biofilms, serves as an important biological disinfectant in hemodialysis, particularly for ensuring the cleanliness of vascular access sites. After thoroughly washing with soap, removing sebum, and decreasing the amount of bacteria, CHX effectively prevents bacterial growth during the 4 hours that the needle is inserted for hemodialysis [24].

3. Mechanisms of biofilm formation in dialysis system and challenges in evaluating disinfection

3.1 Evidence of biofilm formation in dialysis system contamination

Biofilms are often implicated in the recurring contamination long after disinfection observed in dialysis systems. For example [25], after periodic hot water

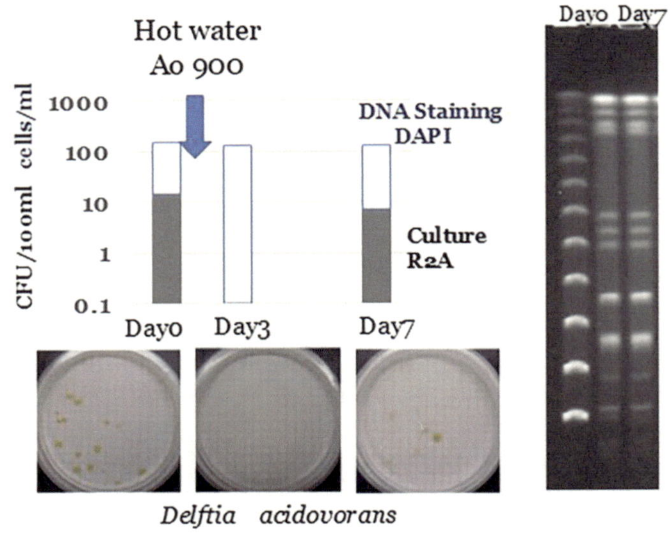

Figure 9.
Trend in bacteria isolated from dialysis fluid in dialysis equipment before and after hot water treatment. Reprinted from Ref. [25]. Provided by Dr. Okamatsu of Komagome Aoba Clinic. Left: Changes in bacterial counts assessed using R2A culturing and DNA fluorescence staining. Right: Genotypes of Delftia acidovorans *isolated before and 7 days after treatment, analyzed by Spe I digested pulsed-field gel electrophoresis (PFGE).*

disinfection under an aseptic procedure [2] that prevents hand-derived aquatic bacterial contamination [26], bacterial colonies are initially eradicated at 3 days post-disinfection (**Figure 9**). However, by the next disinfection cycle, the same bacterial strain, *Delftia acidovorans*, re-emerge, which is genomically identical, confirmed by pulsed-field gel electrophoresis (PFGE) analysis. This indicates that the bacteria entered a non-culturable state post-disinfection and later regained culturable as there was no fluctuation of cell count with DNA staining.

To further study when contamination was onset, large UF membranes were installed upstream of the brand-new dialysis equipment (Nipro, Osaka) [6]. Initial flushing under sterile procedure revealed high bacterial loads, which gradually decreased over time with daily cleaning and disinfection to a single dominant species, such as *Methylobacterium* spp. The genotypic analysis demonstrated that persistent colonization involved species from the initial contamination (**Figure 10**). These findings suggest that biofilms not only resist disinfection but also regenerate bacteria inside of biofilm altered by cleaning processes.

3.2 Location and species prone to biofilm formation in dialysis equipment

Dialysis equipment incorporates complex flow paths with branches, parallel routes, and dead-legs (**Figure 11**), made from materials such as polycarbonate (PC), stainless steel (SUS), and silicone (Sil) [9]. These structural features, particularly areas with uneven flow or turbulence, are prone to biofilm formation. Initial flushing of newly installed equipment revealed diverse microbial populations, predominantly from the class α-Proteobacteria. *Methylobacterium spp.* were present in all tested devices, with *Sphingomonas* spp. appearing in two-thirds (**Table 1**) [6]. When aqueous systems are cleaned and disinfected, colony colors are commonly converted (e.g., brown to yellow to red), often leaving *Methylobacterium spp.* as the dominant

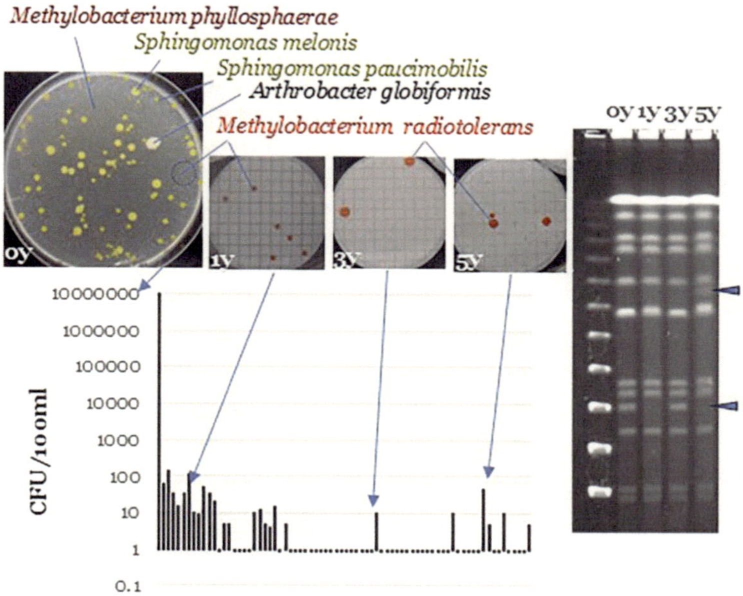

Figure 10.
Transition of bacteria isolated during the five-year clinical use of a newly installed dialysis device following initial cleaning. Reprinted from Ref. [25]. Dialysis fluid was cultured 1-2 times per week during initial cleaning and every 4 weeks after clinical use. If bacteria were detected, retested the following week. Left: Colony image and colony-forming units determined by the R2A culturing method. Right: Genotypes of Methylobacterium radiotolerans *analyzed by PFGE. Mutations up to three bands are considered to be the same strain.*

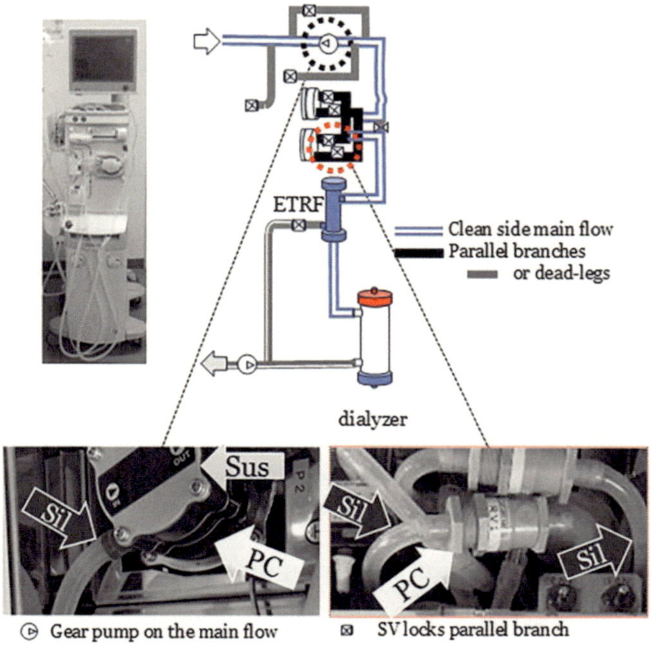

Figure 11.
Piping structure and main component materials of dialysis equipment. Reprinted from Ref. [8], partially modified. Upper: External appearance of the equipment & Piping diagram inside the equipment. Lower: gear pump and solenoid valves.

	Ratio (%)
Alfa-Proteobacteria	
Methylobacterium spp.	100
M. radiotolerance	100
M. phyllosphiae	50
M. aquaticum	42
Sphingomonas spp.	65
S. sanxanigenes	31
S. xenophagum	19
S. koreensis	15
S. paucimobilis	15
S. ginsenosidimutans	12
S. melonis	8
Brevundimonas nasdae	27
Bradyrhizobium spp.	23
B. elkanii	15
B japonicum	8
Afipia spp.	15
Beta Proteobacteria	
Aqubacterium spp.	38
Pelomonas saccharophila	15
Gamma Proteobacteria	
Aquincola tertiaricarbonis	8
Firmicutes	
Arthrobacter globiformis	8

Reprinted from Ref. [6], partially modified. Twenty-six instruments were included.

Table 1.
Microbial populations of newly installed equipment at the start of initial flushing identified by 16S ribosomal RNA gene sequence.

species (**Figure 10**). *Methylobacterium spp.* are notable for their resilience in extreme conditions and their ability to form biofilms with a robust extracellular matrix [15]. These bacteria frequently appear in water systems [27, 28], including clean and well-maintained piping [29]. Their survival and dominance in dialysis systems could be attributed to their metabolic versatility and biofilm-forming ability [6, 13].

3.3 Challenges in evaluating disinfectants for biofilm control

Accurate evaluation of disinfectants requires precise neutralization methods to prevent overestimating efficacy. For instance, high-concentration PAA and H_2O_2 can complicate testing. In this study, Gibson's formulation [30], a neutralizing agent containing catalase (Nacalai Tesque, Tokyo) effectively halted reactions (**Figure 12**,

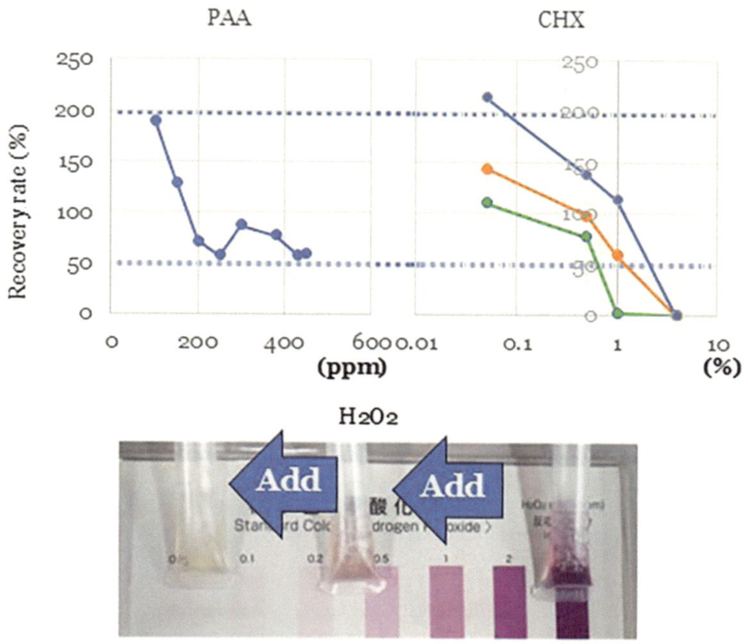

Figure 12.
Neutralization reactions. Reprinted from Ref. [22], partially modified. Upper: Recovery rate from prior neutralization of disinfectant by in the TMSM. Left: PAA products using the Gibson formula. Right: CHX using blue: Gibson formula; orange: DE formula; green: LP (lecithin + polysorbate). Lower: Residual hydrogen peroxide in PAA formulations after the addition of catalase, using Pack Test H_2O_2. Residuals were observed at the theoretical ratio of 0.3:1 and at double this amount.

upper-left panel). Neutralization efficacy was assessed using the TMSM, achieving recovery rates within 50–200% of the original bacterial count [3]. Catalase was added until no residual hydrogen peroxide was detected using a kit with a detection limit of 0.05 ppm (Pack Test H_2O_2, Kyoritsu Chemical, Yokohama, **Figure 12**, lower panel). For CHX, effective neutralization depended on concentration, with Gibson's formulation neutralizing 1% CHX but failing for 4% CHX (**Figure 12**, upper-right panel) [22].

3.4 Species-specific biofilm resistance and material interaction

To better understand biofilm resilience, species such as *Methylobacterium spp.* and *Sphingomonas spp.* were studied for their biofilm-forming abilities on dialysis materials (PC, Sil, and SUS) using a CDC-BFR [16]. *Methylobacterium radiotolerans* exhibited the highest biofilm viability across all materials, particularly on silicone, where surface roughness promotes adhesion (**Figure 13**). Stainless steel showed the least biofilm formation, though rust may enhance bacterial adhesion [31]. Disinfection tests revealed that *M. radiotolerans* showed notable resistance to NaOCl (**Figure 14**), explaining its persistence post-disinfection. While the BFR model provided insights closer to real-world conditions [32], its potential for overestimating resistance remains a concern. For instance, nutrient-deprived dialysis fluid may induce microbial starvation, increasing sterilization resistance compared to nutrient-rich conditions. Future investigations could explore advanced methods, such as the "Vickery" technique [33], to address these challenges.

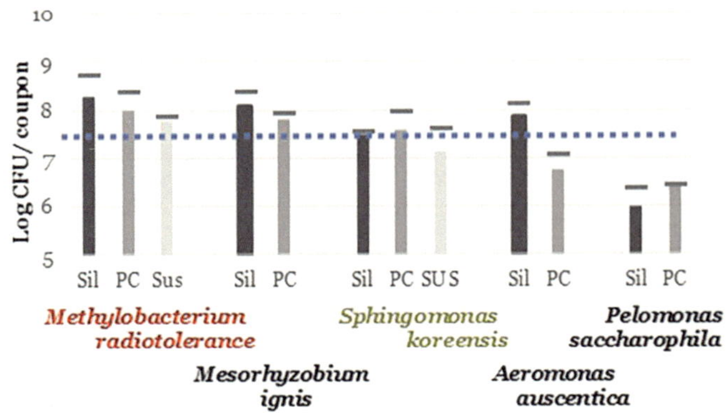

Figure 13.
Viable cell counts in biofilms formed on materials of internal components of dialysis equipment by bacteria isolated from dialysis fluid. Reprinted from Ref. [16]. Sil: Silicone; PC: Polycarbonate; Sus: Stainless Steel 304. All species were clinical isolated strains. M ignis *and* A auscentica *were separated multiple times before the introduction of the equipment shown in* **Table 1**. *The dashed line indicates the minimum viable cell count required to assess the disinfecting effect on biofilms, as defined by the EPA.*

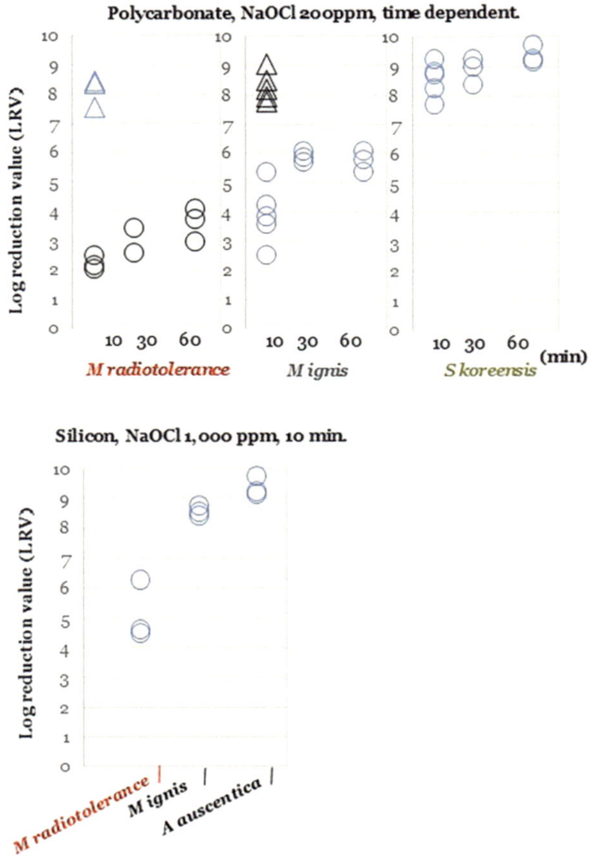

Figure 14.
Effect of NaOCl on different bacterial species. Reprinted from Ref. [16], partially modified. Bacteria species were selected that met the experimental conditions shown in **Figure 13** *for each material. Upper: Using polycarbonate coupons at 200 ppm, with exposure durations of 10, 30 and 60 minutes. Lower Using silicone coupons at 1000 ppm for 10 minutes.*

4. Conclusion

The investigation using the CDC-BFR demonstrated its utility as a method for evaluating the disinfection of dialysis equipment, particularly in its ability to compare disinfectants with different mechanisms of action on a unified scale. Disinfectants that penetrate cell membranes and act within the cytoplasm appear to be more effective against *M radiotolerance* biofilms. While commonly used products and methods currently available exhibit high efficacy, they appear to have limited applications for sustainable alternatives aligned with SDG principles, and replacing them will require further ingenuity.

Acknowledgements

The authors extend their heartfelt gratitude to Dr. Yoshihiko Norose, Dr. Toshio Akimoto, and the members of the Department of Microbiology and Immunology, Nippon Medical School, for their invaluable support, without which this work would not have been possible. This study aimed to provide a scientific background for the initiatives of the working group at the clinic in Koshigaya. The authors are also deeply indebted to Dr. Tetsuaki Tsuchido of Osaka Public University and Dr. Toshikazu Tomioka of Kansai University for their insightful guidance and logical frameworks, which greatly contributed to this work.

Additionally, this research was generously supported by funding from the Japanese Association of Dialysis Physicians (2016-8, 2018-11, 2021-14). The authors sincerely thank all individuals and organizations who made this work possible.

Author details

Eiichi Osono[1*] and Rimpei Morita[2]

1 Koshigaya Ohbukuro Clinic, Saitama, Japan

2 Department of Microbiology and Immunology, Nippon Medical School, Tokyo, Japan

*Address all correspondence to: e.osono@nms.ac.jp

References

[1] International Organization for Standardization. Strategies for microbiological control. In: ISO 23500-1, 2024, Preparation and Quality Management of Fluids for Hemodialysis and Related Therapies. Geneve: ISO; 2024. pp. 24-25

[2] Honda K, Inoue Y, Osono E, Ichimura K, Norose Y, Takahashi H, et al. Hand-hygiene is essential for avoiding bacterial contamination during hospital preparation of dialysis fluid. Journal of Japanese Society for Dialysis Therapy. 2010;**43**:361-366. DOI: 10.4009/jsdt.43.361

[3] Ministry of Health, Labor and Welfare, Japan. Disinfection and Decontamination Methods. The Japanese Pharmacopoeia. 18th ed. [Internet]. 2021. pp. 2698-2701. Available from: https://www.mhlw.go.jp/content/11120000/001372365.pdf [Accessed: February 14, 2025]

[4] U.S. Environmental Protection Agency. Efficacy Test Methods, Test Criteria, and Labeling Guidance for Antimicrobial Products with Claims against Biofilm on Hard, Non-Porous Surfaces. [Internet]. 2023. Available from: https://www.epa.gov/pesticide-analytical-methods/efficacy-test-methods-test-criteria-and-labeling-guidance [Accessed: January 21, 2025]

[5] ASTM International. Standard Practice for Preparing a *Pseudomonas aeruginosa* or *Staphylococcus aureus* Biofilm Using CDC Biofilm Reactor, E3161-21. West Conshohochen: ASTM International; 2021

[6] Osono E, Honda K, Inoue Y, Ichimura K, Kamano C, Kawamoto S, et al. Five-year trends in bacterial contamination of dialysis equipment. Journal of Microorganism control. 2023;**28**:68-75. DOI: 10.4265/jmc.28.3_69

[7] Fukusaki S. Mechanisms of actions of sodium hypochlorite in cleaning and disinfection processes. Biocontrol Science. 2006;**11**:147-157

[8] Osono E, Honda K, Inoue Y, Ichimura K, Kamano C, Akimoto T, et al. Sodium hypochlorite is effective against biofilms in dialysis equipment. Biocontrol Science. 2021;**26**:1-7. DOI: 10.4265/bio.26.1

[9] Osono E, Honda K, Inoue Y, Ichimura K, Negishi H, Kumagai T, et al. Evaluation of functional water for biofilm contamination of dialysis equipment. Bacterial Adherence & Biofilm. 2023;**37**:47-49

[10] Yoshida S, Fukusaki S, Urano H, Iwabuki J. Permeation and bactericidal action of hypochlorous acid through silicone rubber. Journal of Antibacterial and Antifungal Agents. 2020;**48**:247-253

[11] Sakamoto Z, Tsuchido T. Bacterial defense systems against oxidative stress and the mode of action of oxidative antimicrobial agents. Journal of the Japanese Society for Japan Food Microbiology. 2006;**23**:1-52. DOI: 10.5803/jsfm.23.41

[12] Alasri A, Roques C, Michel G. Bactericidal properties of peracetic acid and hydrogen peroxide, alone and in combination, and chlorine and formaldehyde against water strains. Canadian Journal of Microbiology. 1992;**38**:635-642. DOI: 10.1139/m92-104

[13] Osono E, Honda K, Inoue Y, Ichimura K, Negishi H, Kumagai T, et al.

Effect of peracetic acid cleaning agents on biofilms of *Methylobacterium* spp. derived from hemodialysis equipment. Journal of Microorganism Control. 2025;**30** [In review]

[14] Tsuchido T. Injury modes and physiological characteristics of injured microorganisms with a special reference to heat injury. Journal of Microorganism Control. 2023;**28**:187-200. DOI: 10.4265/jmc.28.4_187

[15] Kovaleva J, Degener JE, van der Mei HC. *Methylobacterium* and its role in health care-associated infection. Journal of Clinical Microbiology. 2014;**52**:1317-1321. DOI: 10.1128/JCM.03561-13

[16] Osono E, Honda K, Inoue Y, Ichimura K, Norose Y, Takaku S, et al. Science-based selection of cleaning and disinfection methods for hemodialysis systems–Verification of cleaning and disinfection efficacy against hard surfaces biofilms using the CDC biofilm reactor. Journal of Japanese Association of Dialysis Physicians. 2024;**39**:167-174

[17] Fukui R. Hot water disinfection and component replacement and deterioration. Journal of Antimicrobial Antifungal Agents. 2013;**41**:483-490

[18] Metropolitan Government of Tokyo. Dialysis drainage and sewage pipes. [Internet]. 2018. Available from: https://www.gesui.metro.tokyo.lg.jp/contractor/pdf/r4_touseki.pdf [Accessed: January 21, 2025]

[19] Koike K, Sakamoto J, Furuta M, Osono E, Tsuchido T. Biocontrol of aquatic bacteria after hemodialysis system disinfection–Heating and hydrogen peroxide treatment damaged bacteria on dialysis fluid. The Journal of Japanese Association of Dialysis Physicians. 2018;**33**:527-535

[20] Gottardi W. Iodine and iodine compounds. In: Block SS, editor. Disinfection, Sterilization, and Preservation. Philadelphia: Lippincott Williams & Wilkins; 2001. pp. 159-184

[21] Denton GW. Chlorhexidine. In: Block SS, editor. Disinfection, Sterilization, and Preservation. Philadelphia: Lippincott Williams & Wilkins; 2001. pp. 321-336

[22] Osono E, Honda K, Inoue Y, Ichimura K, Nakano M, Yoshida J, et al. Effect of anti-septics on aquatic biofilm. Bacterial Adherence & Biofilm. 2025;**39**. [In print]

[23] Uri J. 50 Years Ago: Hornet + 3 – The Recovery of Apollo 11. [Internet]. 2019. Available from: https://www.nasa.gov/history/50-years-ago-hornet-3-the-recovery-of-apollo-11/ [Accessed: February 14, 2025]

[24] Akahori Y, Sudoh T, Nakano M, Ichimura K, Osono E, Kurihara R, et al. Instant insertion wipe method of 10% povdone-iodne sites can disinfect the needle insertion sites of the skin on patients receiving chronic hemodialysis. Journal of Japanese Society for Dialysis Therapy. 2003;**36**:1539-1544. DOI: 10.4009/jsdt.36.1539

[25] Osono E, Ichimura K. Dialysis fluid. In: Editorial Board of the Publication Commemorating the 50th Anniversary of the Japanese Society for Antimicrobial Antifungal Agents Editor. The Encyclopedia of Antimicrobial and Antifungal Agents. Kouseisha Kouseikaku: Tokyo; 2025. in press

[26] Osono E, Honda K, Inoue Y, Norose Y, Takahashi M, Ichimura K, et al. Detection method for aquatic bacteria of the fingers, as a potential origin of the aqueous solution contamination.

Biocontrol Science. 2017;**22**:61-65. DOI: 10.4265/bio.22.61

[27] Feazel LM, Baumgartner LK, Peterson KL, Frank DN, Harris JK, Pace NR. Opportunistic pathogens enriched in showerhead biofilms. Proceedings of the National Academy of Sciences of the United States of America. 2009;**106**:16393-16399. DOI: 10.1073/pnas.0908446106

[28] Yano T, Kubota H, Hanai J, Hitomi J, Tokuda H. Stress tolerance of *Methylobacterium* biofilms in bathroom. Microbes and Environments. 2013;**28**:87-95. DOI: 10.1264/jsme2.me12146

[29] Hiraishi A, Furuhata K, Matsumoto A, Koike KA, Fukuyama M, Tabuchi K. Phenotypic and genetic diversity of chlorine resistant *Methylobacterium* strains isolated from various environment. Applied and Environmental Microbiology. 1995;**61**:2099-2107. DOI: 10.1128/aem.61.6.2099-2107.1995

[30] Gibson H, Taylor JH, Hall KE, Holah JT. Effectiveness of cleaning techniques used in the food industry in terms of the removal of bacterial biofilms. Journal of Applied Microbiology. 1999;**87**:41-48. DOI: 10.1046/j.1365-2672.1999.00790.x

[31] Nakamura M, Okayama M, Hagiwara S, Nawa T, Yokota S. Effects of metal corrosion in the pump of a dialysis machine on the sterility of the terminal dialysate by spike-and-recovery testing with bacteria. Renal Replacement Therapy. 2024;**10**:6. DOI: 10.1186/s41100-024-00522-6

[32] Buckingham-Meyer K, Goeres DM, Hamilton MA. Comparative evaluation of biofilm disinfectant efficacy tests. Journal of Microbiological Methods. 2007;**70**:36-244. DOI: 10.3390/antibiotics12071189

[33] Almatroudi A, Hu H, Deva A, Gosbell IB, Jacombs A, Jensen SO, et al. A new dry-surface biofilm model: An essential tool for efficacy testing of hospital surface decontamination procedures. Journal of Microbiological Methods. 2015;**117**:171-176. DOI: 10.1016/j.mimet.2015.08.003

Chapter 2

Effects of Bacterial Biofilm on Immunity in Chronic Tonsillitis

Fuat Bulut and Aylin Turksever Tetiker

Abstract

A great number of children suffer from recurrent tonsillitis attacks in which antimicrobials can only provide temporary relief. Underlying cause of this type of recurrent infections is largely biofilm formation, formed in tonsils. Biofilm development is a major virulent factor behind a vast number of chronic bacterial infections. Once a biofilm is formed, planktonic cells that grow around any tissue can enter a resting phase and begin to generate biofilm matrix. Biofilm is a primitive form of multicellular life and refers to biological systems formed by the functional groups of the bacteria with coordination ability. It is reported that biofilm is not necessarily pathologic on mucosal surfaces. A "healthy" and "pathologic" microbiome has to be present. Pathologic mucosal biofilm can be formed *via* microorganisms and viruses that are no good for mucosa. Recent studies have verified the connection of pathologic biofilm, on mucosal tissue in particular, with human diseases. In this review, effects of the biofilm in chronic tonsillitis on mucosal immunity, advantages and limitations of mucosal biofilm, chronic diseases emerging in biofilms, and latest treatment options focusing on biofilms have been explored collectively.

Keywords: palatine tonsil, immunity, mucosal, bacteria, tonsillitis, biofilms

1. Introduction

Palatine tonsils has strategic position in oropharynx, upper respiratory tract and gastrointestinal system and plays a major immunological role against the potential infections in these regions [1]. A series of cytokines regulate adhesive molecules in endothelium and epithelium cells; thereby increasing the migration of eosinophils to mucosa. In all these tissues, expression of Toll-like receptors indicates a substantial immunological function of upper airway mucosa [2]. Both humoral and cellular immunological phases are initiated in lymphoid follicles and extra follicles, which exist in crypt epithelium of lymphoids and dendritic cells [3].

2. Chronic tonsillitis and biofilm

It is safe to claim that in specific forms of tonsillitis, the cause of recurrence and chronicity is bacterial biofilm in the crypt inside infected tonsil. If pathologically, in follicular lymphoid hyperplasia and interfollicular region plasma cell infiltrate to fibrosis or non-fibrosis lymphoid, this phenomenon is named as chronic tonsillitis. Morphological classification of chronic tonsillitis is lymphoid hyperplasia, crypt dilation and parenchymal fibrosis. It is possible to detect heavily calcified structures in crypts. Clinical symptoms can be halitosis, tonsil stones and permanent lymphadenopathies. While the bacteria protect themselves from antibiotics and host defense, they simultaneously secrete endotoxins to the environment. As a result, local endotoxin inside tonsillar crypt leads to chronic inflammation. As is the case in various infections, in chronic tonsillitis too, polysaccharides also known as mucoid extracellular polymers secreted by the bacteria, proteins and teichoic acid are responsible for biofilm formation. Mucosal biofilm hampers the treatment and multiplies the likelihood of complications. Chronic tonsillitis is particularly of great importance because it requires frequent use of antibiotics, develops resistance to antibiotics, causes complications induced by chronic tonsillitis and calls for frequent need for surgical operation. Biofilms can be formed *via* a single type of microorganism or comprised of more than one type. Bacteria in the biofilm exist embedded into a matrix that acts like mud or slum containing a set of polysaccharide, nucleic acid and protein. They are named as non-cellular polymeric agents. Biofilm matrix may integrate non-cellular mineral crystals, corrosion particles and blood components [4]. Different biofilm architecture determines the exposure of bacteria to phages [5]. The polysaccharides that are synthesized by biofilm microorganisms form the main extracellular component of biofilm. As for the cellular structure of biofilm; 97% consists of water, 2–3% consists of microorganisms, 1% consists of polysaccharide, 1% consists of protein and 1% consists of the DNA and ions. Biofilm development takes place in five stages. Development stages of the biofilm are as shown in **Figure 1** [6].

1. Adhesion of microorganism: Organic and/or inorganic materials adhere to the surface. Next, microorganisms stick to the same surface. This adhesion stage is reversible. In these stages, biofilms are activated by the changes in environmental factors (food concentrations, pH, temperature, oxygen concentration, osmolality and iron)

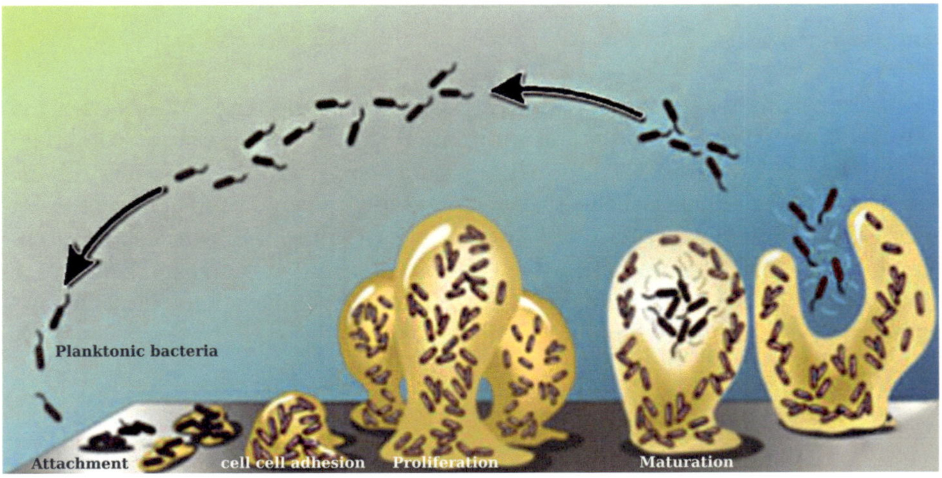

Figure 1.
Stages of biofilm development: attachment, proliferation and maturation. Graphics by Peg Dirckx, David Davies and Karin Sauer, courtesy of Dr. Gregory Schultz, WUWHS 2008, Toronto [6].

2. Irreversible adhesion: In this stage, microorganisms get connected and formed. Those microorganisms are dynamic. Biofilm layer quickly becomes thicker than 10 μm. As signal changes are activated, exopolysaccharide production occurs *via* genetic mechanisms and planktonic bacteria and food traps also contribute to this compound.

3. Colonization stage I: Bacteria on the surface form microcolonies

4. Colonization stage II: Once biofilm thickness exceeds 100 mm, the 4th stage of the colonization, also known as maturation II, occurs. Planktonic bacteria in the environment also attach on these colonies. A few days following this process, the 5th stage emerges.

5. Detachment: In this stage, cells break up. Certain bacteria that form planktonic phenotype disconnect from the biofilm. A range of bacteria types such as *Pseudomonas*, *Staphylococcus* and *Haemophilus* all have surface adhesion capacity.

Once the microorganism adheres to the surface, it then secretes complex polysaccharides that thus embed the bacteria. These micro-colonies gradually expand and named as "Quorum sensing" to refer to a large and wide form of settled bacteria. These are resistant toward treatment with various mechanisms implemented *via* planktonic bacteria [7]. Biofilm becomes infectious the moment it is formed. After the bacteria adhere to a surface and form the biofilm, they can no longer be detached from the surface *via* gentle rinsing [8].

Additionally, although microorganisms settled in biofilm are quite sensitive toward antimicrobials in culture plates under planktonic conditions, under high concentrations, they can survive even under the presence of bacteria killing antimicrobials [9]. Microbial biofilms are visible in more than 65–80% of all human bacterial infections [10]. The significance of biofilm among recurrent tonsillitis and peritonsillar abscess patients has been put forth [11]. Studies have reported the capacity to form biofilm in tonsil tissues of chronic tonsillitis patients [12]. Bacterial biofilm has been detected in saliva stones in mouth [13].

3. Effects of biofilm on mucosal immunity

A recent study has revealed the role of biofilms in immunity [14]. Bacterial biofilms in mouth suppress β6 integrin by weakening TGF-β1 signaling, which then leads to a developed pro-inflammatory response [15]. There is connection between bacterial infections and autoimmunity [16]. As a response to aggressive periodontitis treatment, the gravity of local IL-10 level has been demonstrated [17]. Mouth bacteria secrete pro-inflammatory cytokines, and through inflammation, it affects systemic diseases [18]. Inborn immunity plays role in the development of biofilm in pediatric respiratory infections [19]. Stress hormones have effects on microbial infections [20]. Pro-inflammatory cytokine IL-1β strongly increases biofilm formation [21]. *S. epidermidis* biofilms, immune-activating cytokines and TNFα elevate the expression of IL-6, IL-10, IL-1β and IFNγ [22, 23]. It has been acknowledged that biofilm plays direct role in pathogenesis. In chronic mucosal inflammation, self-antigens or allergens enable the formation of biofilm as a response. Local inflammation cytokines or excess mucus can also back up biofilm development [24]. It has been argued that some other factors also render the potential effect in mucosal biofilm pathogenesis. These include mucus compound and liquid flow, specific inborn epithelium defense mechanisms and epithelium's capacity to synthesize the antimicrobial molecules. In order to grasp mucosal role of the biofilm, it is vital to clearly manifest its host response against biofilm in chronic diseases.

In most of the chronic diseases, the role of biofilm is generally indirect. The context of regional lesions or tissue damage depends on the contribution of virulent factors specific to the disease inducting mucosal biofilm. In order to fully understand the pathogenesis of mucosal biofilms, it is quite important to conduct a local analysis of tissue virulence and the stage of biofilm. It has been reported that *P. aeruginosa*, *Staphylococcus aureus*, *Streptococcus pneumoniae*, *Haemophilus influenzae*, *Moraxella catarrhalis* and many other mucosal pathogens can form biofilm. The bacteria sticking to tonsillar epithelium particularly stay within tonsillary crypt and can become a mixed colony of the bacteria. While the bacteria protect themselves from the antibiotics and host defense, they simultaneously release their endotoxins to the environment. Biofilm's mixed microorganisms and virulence factors result in tissue damage. In human diseases, the role of mucosal biofilm can best be defined through the two pathogenesis models of host inflammatory response. Biofilm's mixed microorganisms and virulence factors result in tissue damage. In diseases, the role of mucosal biofilm can best be defined through the two pathogenesis models of host inflammatory response. In the first model, mucosal biofilms indirectly starts excessive pro-inflammatory response [25]. In the second model, on the other hand, biofilm components such as extracellular matrix can lower mucosal inflammatory response of the infection and develop phagocytic cell function disorder [26]. This phenomenon offers an advantage in the early development of biofilm organisms. Similar to mucosal tissue, host receptor microbial adhesion system also contributes to the feeding environment of biofilm organisms. In the biofilm that is formed *via Streptococcus pyogenes* in tissue and abiotic surfaces, there is approximately 50% variance in gene expression [27]. Extracellular matrix of the biofilm leads to antibiotic resistance upon secreting polymers that bind and deactivate the antimicrobials [28]. Compared to their planktonic counterparts, microorganisms in biofilms can be 500–1.000 times more tolerant toward antibacterial components [29]. In chronic mucosal inflammations self-antigens or allergens allow the formation of biofilm as a response. Locally inflammatory cytokines or excessive mucus can also contribute to biofilm formation [24]. In mucosal biofilm, there is biofilm formation associated with adaptive T and B cells in which innate immune response is due to tissue destruction by plenty of neutrophils and macrophages, matrix metallo proteinases and reactive oxygen species (ROS) and inflammatory cytokines (IL-1, PGE2, TNF-a, IL-1b) [30]. Host response contributes to the improvement of oral biofilm through collecting pro-inflammatory cells (neutrophils and macrophages), secretion of inflammatory mediator (interleukin-1 [IL-1] and prostaglandin E2) and matrix metallo proteinases (MMPs) [31] In inflammation, firstly, by releasing ROS to which neutrophils are hypersensitive in periodontal diseases, they contribute to disease progress which in turn damage proteinases, host gum and periodontal ligaments [32]. Neutrophils promote proinflammatory cytokines such as leukotriene B4, IL-6, tumor necrosis factor-a (TNF-a) and IL-1b [33]. Between biofilm and human immune system, a number of complex and multidimensional interactions, which alter host environment, condition biofilm phenotype and affect the functionality of host immune cells emerge [34]. Biofilms induce apoptotic process [35]. In a previous study we conducted, we exhibited the similarity between clinical picture of pediatric patients whose both mother and father have chronic tonsillitis and periodic fever, aphthous stomatitis, pharyngitis, adenitis (PFPA syndrome) [36]. On the other hand, it has been detected that bacterial biofilms substantiate the conditions that lead to oncogenic transformation of epithelium cells [37]. In otolaryngology, a review on biofilms and pathogenesis, diagnosis and treatment strategies has been conducted **Figure 2** [38].

Tonsil surface swab bacterial culture results are different from tonsil core in recurrent tonsillitis [39]. It demonstrates *ex vivo* the quantity and spatial distribution of gram-positive biofilms in multimodal optic mesoscopy tonsillary [40]. A number of studies focusing on increasing the biological significance of biofilm models have been reported [41]. Studies have been conducted to expedite the emergence productive biofilms in biology-based production stages [42]. Although in chronic tonsillitis we have clinically observed the effects of bacterial mucosal biofilms on immunological figures there is still need for biochemical, genetic and molecular studies in this field.

3.1 Beneficial biofilms

In animal models of biofilm, it has been demonstrated that in oral mucosa cancer treated with tretinoin, biofilm proves to be of use in the prevention or limitation of the tumor [43]. Biofilms are effective in the treatment of industrial wastes and removal of nitrogen and phosphorus [44]. They are, as studies show, effective in increasing bioelectric production [45]. Studies have documented the relationship between bacterial biofilms and immuno-modulation specific to anatomical site [46]. They are used in waste water treatment [47]. Biofilms can greatly diminish necrotizing enterocolitis incidence and its frequency [48]. Biofilms are a membrane system resistant to contamination [49]. Beneficial oral biofilms are used as smart bioactive interfaces [50]. Studies have reported specific biofilms that can be useful for tomato roots [51].

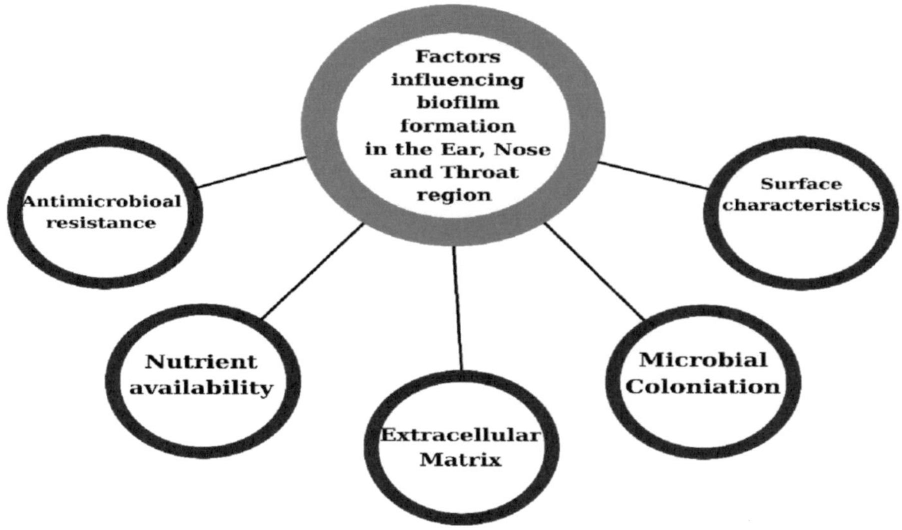

Figure 2.
Biofilms in ENT: understanding the pathogenesis, diagnosis and treatment. GhoshMoulic et al. [38].

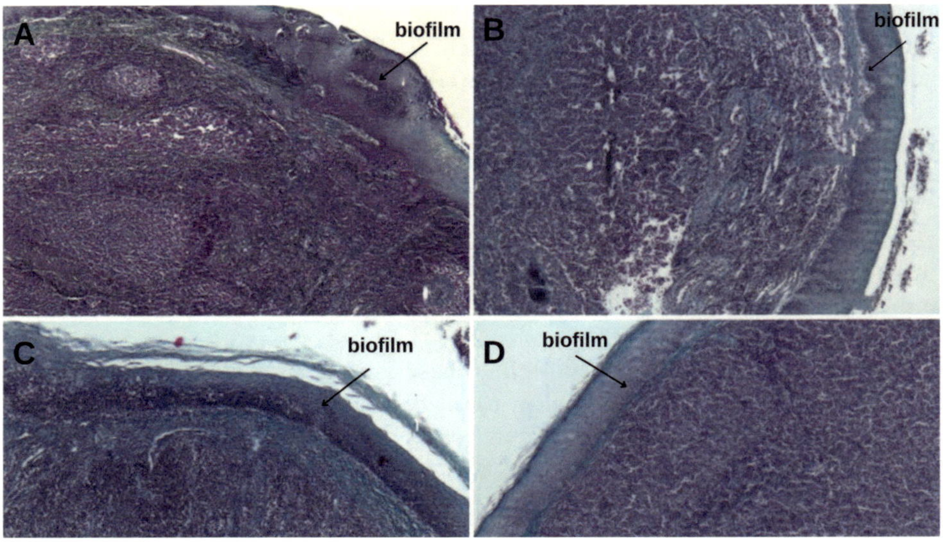

Figure 3.
Mucosal biofilm in tonsil tissue of children with a history of recurrent/chronic tonsillitis [52].

3.2 The near future of biofilm

In otorhinolarynologist infections, biofilm-induced infections have gained more popularity each new year. In a previous study we conducted, we have put forth the thickness and significance of bacterial biofilm in children with chronic tonsillitis whose mother and father both have chronic tonsillitis as shown in **Figure 3** [52].

Some studies have pointed at the relationship between cancer and bacterial biofilm [53]. As is the case in most of the chronic contagious diseases, biofilm-induced infections are also usually asymptomatic in early stages of chronic tonsillitis. When host defense is low, planktonic or free-living microorganisms can disintegrate from biofilm when host resistance is weak and can cause acute infection. Microbial biofilms significantly impact human health by rising morbidity, mortality and health care costs. The importance of anti-biofilm treatments in sleep disorders and recurrent chronic tonsillitis has been detected [54]. It has been reported that ROS impedes biofilm formation [55]. Biofilm morphology has been designed for high sensitivity of bioelectrochemical sensor [56]. Studies have exhibited the role of biofilm distribution-based nanoparticles in the prevention of re-infection [57]. Besides, it has been reported that local anesthetics create antimicrobial impact [58]. As an alternative treatment ultrasound can efficiently kill the bacteria *via* cavitation and peroxide production inside or onto bacteria cells and thus can increase the efficiency of antibiotic treatment [59]. Nanoparticles have been suggested for oral biofilm treatments [60]. It has been reported that mechanically induced saliva has impact on the oral biofilm formation [61]. Magnesium has been detected to exhibit antimicrobial effects [62]. Microrobots are suggested to have effects on oral biofilms [63].

4. Conclusion

In recent years, studies related to mucosal biofilms in otorhinolarynology have gained impetus. Emerging pathological mucosal biofilms are the main cause of resistance toward medical treatment and render negative effects on mucosal immunity. Mucosal biofilms are the primary reason of recurrent tonsillitis in both pediatric and adult patients. Upon the development of experimental models in biofilm-induced infections, therapeutic strategies that can be effective on biofilm can also be developed. By this way, potential complications likely to occur in many types of chronic infections can be diminished. Drug therapies in chronic infectious diseases can be modeled by prioritizing the biofilm. Hence, different drug combinations according to experimental models can be developed. In near future, more detailed and comprehensive studies will shed light on the effects of bacterial biofilms on mucosal immunity of patients with chronic tonsillitis.

Conflict of interest

No potential conflict of interest relevant to this article was reported.

Author details

Fuat Bulut[1]* and Aylin Turksever Tetiker[2]

1 Department of Otorhinolaryngology, University of Health Sciences, Bursa Faculty of Medicine, Bursa Yüksek Ihtisas Training and Research Hospital, Bursa, Turkey

2 Independent Researcher, Tekirdag, Turkey

*Address all correspondence to: bulutfuat40@yahoo.com

References

[1] Bernstein JM, Baekkevold ES, Brandtzaeg P. Immunobiology of the tonsils and adenoids. In: Mestecky J, Bienenstock J, Lamm ME, Mayer L, McGhee JR, Strober W, editors. Mucosal Immunology. 3rd ed. Amsterdam: Elsevier/Academic Press; 2005. pp. 1547-1572

[2] Claeys S, de Belder T, Holtappels G, Gevaert P, Verhasselt B, van Cauwenberge P, et al. Human beta-defensins and toll-like receptors in the upper airway. Allergy. 2003;**58**(8):748-753. DOI: 10.1034/j.1398-9995.2003.00180.x

[3] Nave H, Gebert A, Pabst R. Morphology and immunology of the human palatine tonsil. Anatomy and Embryology. 2001;**204**(5):367-373

[4] Fux CA, Costerton JW, Stewart PS, Stoodley P. Survival strategies of infectious biofilms. Trends in Microbiology. 2005;**13**:34-40

[5] Winans JB, Wucher BR, Nadell CD. Multi species biofilm architecture determines bacterial exposure to phages. PLoSBiology. 2022;**20**(12):e3001913. DOI: 10.1371/journal.pbio.3001913

[6] Dirckx P, Davies D, Sauer K. Stages of Biofilm Development Attachment, Proliferation Maturaion Graphics by Courtesy of Dr. Gregory Schultz. Toronto: WUWHS; 2008

[7] Stewart PS, Costerton JW. Antibiotic resistance of bacteria in biofilms. Lancet. 2001;**358**:135-138

[8] Stoodley P, Wilson S, HallStoodley L, Boyle JD, Lappin Scott HM, Costerton JW. Growth and detachment of cell clusters from mature mixed-species biofilms. Applied and Environmental Microbiology. 2001;**67**:5608-5613

[9] Anderl JN, Franklin MJ, Stewart PS. Role of antibiotic penetration limitation in *Klebsiella pneumoniae* biofilm resistance to ampicillin and ciprofloxacin. Antimicrobial Agents and Chemotherapy. 2000;**44**(7):1818-1824

[10] Costerton JW, Stewart PS, Greenberg EP. Bacterial biofilms: A common cause of persistent infections. Science. 1999;**284**(5418):1318-1322

[11] Klagisa R, Racenis K, Broks R, Balode AO, Kise L, Kroica J. Analysis of microorganism colonization, biofilm production, and antibacterial susceptibility in recurrent tonsillitis and peritonsillar abscess patients. International Journal of MolecularSciences. 2022;**23**(18):10273. DOI: 10.3390/ijms231810273

[12] Kostić M, Ivanov M, Babić SS, Tepavčević Z, Radanović O, Soković M, et al. Analysis of tonsil tissues from patients diagnosed with chronic tonsillitis-microbiological profile, biofilm-forming capacity and histology. Antibiotics (Basel). 2022;**11**(12):1747. DOI: 10.3390/antibiotics11121747

[13] Perez-Tanoira R, Aarnisalo A, Haapaniemi A, Saarinen R, Kuusela P, Kinnari TJ. Bacterial biofilm in salivary stones. European Archives of Oto-Rhino Laryngology. 2019;**276**(6):1815-1822. DOI: 10.1007/s00405-019-05445-1. Epub 2019 Apr 26

[14] Campoccia D, Mirzaei R, Montanaro L, Arciola CR. Hijacking of immune defences by biofilms: A multifront strategy. Biofouling. 2019;**35**(10):1055-1074.

DOI: 10.1080/08927014.2019.1689964. Epub 2019 Nov 25

[15] Bi J, Koivisto L, Dai J, Zhuang D, Jiang G, Larjava M, et al. Epidermal growth factor receptor signaling suppresses αvβ6 integrin and promotes periodontal inflammation and bone loss. Journal of Cell Science. 2019;**133**(5):jcs236588. DOI: 10.1242/jcs.236588

[16] Nicastro L, Tükel Ç. Bacterial amyloids: The link between bacterial infections and autoimmunity. Trends in Microbiology. 2019;**27**(11):954-963. DOI: 10.1016/j.tim.2019.07.002. Epub 2019 Aug 15

[17] Taiete T, Monteiro MF, Casati MZ, do Vale HF, GMB A, Nociti FH, et al. Local IL-10 level as a predictive factor in generalized aggressive periodontitis treatment response. Scandinavian Journal of Immunology. 2019;**90**(6):e12816. DOI: 10.1111/sji.12816. Epub 2019 Oct 3

[18] Chattopadhyay I, Lu W, Manikam R, Malarvili MB, Ambati RR, Gundamaraju R. Can metagenomics unravel the impact of oral bacteriome in human diseases? Biotechnology & Genetic Engineering Reviews. 2023;**39**(1):85-117. DOI: 10.1080/02648725.2022.2102877. Epub 2022 Jul 21

[19] Hamilos DL. Biofilm formations in pediatric respiratory tract infection: Part 1: Biofilm structure, role of innate immunity in protection against and response to biofilm, methods of biofilm detection, pediatric respiratory tract diseases associated with mucosal biofilm formation. Current Infectious Disease Reports. 2019;**21**(2):6. DOI: 10.1007/s11908-019-0658-9

[20] Sarkodie EK, Zhou S, Baidoo SA, Chu W. Influences of stress hormones on microbial infections. Microbial Pathogenesis. 2019;**131**:270-276. DOI: 10.1016/j.micpath.2019.04.013. Epub 2019 Apr 11

[21] Gutierrez Jauregui R, Fleige H, Bubke A, Rohde M, Weiss S, Förster R. IL-1β promotes *Staphylococcus aureus* biofilms on implants in vivo. Frontiers in Immunology. 2019;**10**:1082. DOI: 10.3389/fimmu.2019.01082

[22] Boelens JJ, Dankert J, Murk JL, Weening JJ, van der Poll T, Dingemans KP, et al. In pericateter macrophages relational permanence of Staphylococcus epidermidis with biomaterial. Journal of Infectious Diseases. 2000;**181**:1337-1349. DOI: 10.1086/315369

[23] Boelens JJ, van der Poll T, Zaat SA, Murk JL, Weening JJ, Dankert J. Compared to wild rats, lab rats with Interleukin-1 receptor type I gene deficiency are less sensitive to infections connected with Staphylococcus epidermidis biomaterial. Infection and Immunity. 2000;**68**:6924-6931

[24] McLaughlin RA, Hoogewerf AJ. Interleukin-1 beta–induced growth enhancement of Staphylococcus aureus occurs in biofilm but not planktonic cultures. Microbial Pathogenesis. 2006;**41**(2-3):67-79

[25] Lyczak JB, Cannon CL, Pier GB. Lung infections associated with cystic fibrosis. Clinical Microbiology Reviews. 2002;**15**(2):194-222

[26] Hong W, Mason K, Jurcisek J, Novotny L, Bakaletz LO, Swords WE. Phosphorylcholine decrease early inflammation and promotes the establishment of stable biofilm communities of non-typeable haemophilus influenza estrain 86-028 NP in a chinchilla model of otitis

media. Infection and Immunity. 2007;**75**(2):958-965

[27] Cho KH, Caparon MG. Patterns of virulence gene expression differ between biofilm and tissue communities of Streptococcos pyogenes. Molecular Microbiology. 2005;**57**(6):1545-1556

[28] Høiby N. Recent advances in the treatment of Pseudomonas aeruginosa infections in cystic fibrosis. BMC Medicine. 2011;**9**:32

[29] Sedlacek MJ, Walker C. Antibiotic resistance in an in-vitro subgingival biofilm model. Oral Microbiology and Immunology. 2007;**22**(5):333-339

[30] Mancl KA, Kirsner RS, Ajdic D. Wound biofilms: Lessons learned from oral biofilms. Wound Repair and Regeneration. 2013;**21**(3):352-362. DOI: 10.1111/wrr.12034

[31] Darby I. Non-surgical management of periodontal disease. Australian Dental Journal. 2009;**54**(Suppl. 1):86-S95

[32] Gemmell E, Yamazaki K, Seymour GJ. Destructive periodontitis lesions are determined by the nature of the lymphocytic response. Critical Reviews in Oral Biology and Medicine. 2002;**13**:17-34

[33] Page RC, Offenbacher S, Schroeder HE, Seymour GJ, Kornman KS. Advances in the pathogenesis of periodontitis: Summary of developments, clinical implications and future directions. Periodontology 2000. 1997;**14**:216-248

[34] Hall-Stoodley L, Costerton JW, Stoodley P. Bacterial biofilms: From the natural environment to infectious diseases. Nature Reviews. Microbiology. 2004;**2**(2):95-108. DOI: 10.1038/nrmicro821

[35] Cantero D, Cooksley C, Bassiouni A, et al. Staphylococcus aureus biofilms induce apoptosis and expression of interferon-g, interleukin-10, and interleukin 17A on humans inonasal explants. American Journal of Rhinology & Allergy. 2015;**29**:23-28

[36] Bulut F, Cumbul A, Ballica B. Clinical importance of family history in recurrent chronic tonsillitis pediatric patients: Review. Journal of Pediatrics and Pediatric Medicine. 2020;**4**(3):1-5

[37] Dejea CM, Wick EC, Hechenbleikner EM, et al. Microbiota organization is a distinct feature of proximal colorectal cancers. Proceedings of the National Academy of Sciences of the United States of America. 2014;**111**:18321-18326

[38] Ghosh Moulic A, Deshmukh P, Gaurkar SS, Cureus A. Biofilms in ENT understanding the pathogenesis. Diagnosis, and Treatment. 2024;**16**(4):e57634. DOI: 10.7759cureus.57634

[39] Dickinson A, Kankaanpää H, Silén S, Meri S, Haapaniemi A, Ylikoski J, et al. Tonsillar surface swab bacterial culture results differ from those of the tonsillar core in recurrent tonsillitis. The Laryngoscope. 2020;**130**(12):E791-E794. DOI: 10.1002/lary.28403. Epub 2019 Nov 20

[40] Clapperton M, Kunanandam T, Florea CD, Douglas CM, McConnell G. Multimodal optical mesoscopy reveals the quantity and spatial distribution of gram-positive biofilms in ex vivo tonsils. Journal of Microscopy. 2024;**295**(2):121-130. DOI: 10.1111/jmi.13266. Epub 2024 Jan 31

[41] Rumbaugh KP, Whiteley M. Towards improved biofilm models. Nature Reviews. Microbiology. 2025;**23**(1):57-66.

DOI: 10.1038/s41579-024-01086-2. Epub 2024 Aug 7

[42] Edel M, Horn H, Gescher J. Biofilm systems as tools in biotechnological production. Applied Microbiology and Biotechnology. 2019;**103**(13):5095-5103. DOI: 10.1007/s00253-019-09869-x. Epub 2019 May 11

[43] Wang Z, Polavaram R, Fuentes CF, Shapshay SM. Topical chemo prevention of oral cancer with tretinoin "biofilm". Archives of Otolaryngology – Head & Neck Surgery. 2003;**129**:869-873

[44] Altinbas U, Ozturk I. Comparison of intermittently aerated continuous and batch biofilm reactor in nutrient removal. Water Science and Technology. 2003;**48**(11-12):371-376

[45] Lin Z, Long M, Liu W, Liu T, Li F, Wu Y. Distinct biofilm formation regulated by different culture media: Implications to electricity generation. Bioelectro Chemistry. 2021;**140**:107826. DOI: 10.1016/j.bioelechem.2021.107826. Epub 2021 Apr 27

[46] Morra CN, Orihuela CJ. Anatomical site-specific immuno modulation by bacterial biofilms. Current Opinion in Infectious Diseases. 2020;**33**(3):238-243. DOI: 10.1097/QCO.0000000000000643

[47] Gustavsson DJI, Suarez C, Wilén BM, Hermansson M, Persson F. Long-term stability of partial nitritation anammox for treatment of municipal waste water in a moving bed biofilm reactor pilot system. Science of the Total Environment. 2020;**714**:136342. DOI: 10.1016/j.scitotenv.2019.136342. Epub 2020 Jan 7

[48] Olson JK, Rager TM, Navarro JB, Mashburn-Warren L, Goodman SD, Besner GE. Harvesting the benefits of biofilms: A novel probiotic delivery system for the prevention of necrotizing enterocolitis. Journal of Pediatric Surgery. 2016;**51**(6):936-941. DOI: 10.1016/j.jpedsurg.2016.02.062. Epub 2016 Mar 2

[49] Wood TL, Guha R, Tang L, Geitner M, Kumar M, Wood TK. Living biofouling-resistant membranes as a model for the beneficial use of engineered biofilms. Proceedings of the National Academy of Sciences of the United States of America. 2016;**113**(20):E2802-E2811. DOI: 10.1073/pnas.1521731113. Epub 2016 May 2

[50] Gutt B, Ren Q, Hauser-Gerspach I, Kardas P, Stübinger S, AstasovFrauenhoffer M, et al. Beneficial oral biofilms as smart bioactive interfaces. Frontiers in Microbiology. 2018;**9**:107. DOI: 10.3389/fmicb.2018.00107

[51] Sato Y, Miwa T, Inaba T, Akachi T, Tanaka E, Hori T, et al. Microbially produced fertilizer provides rhizo bacteria to hydroponic tomato roots by forming beneficial biofilms. Applied Microbiology and Biotechnology. 2023;**107**(23):7365-7374. DOI: 10.1007/s00253-023-12794-9. Epub 2023 Sep 29

[52] Bulut F, Cumbul A, Safak AS. An analysis of the histomorphometric and clinical significance of mucosal biofilm in tonsil tissue of the children with a history of recurrent/chronic tonsillitis in both the mother and father. European Archives of Oto-Rhino-Laryngology. 2020;**277**(12):3381-3389. DOI: 10.1007/s00405-020-06111-7. Epub 2020 Jun 23

[53] Wang ZH, Liu JM, Li CY, Wang D, Lv H, Lv SW, et al. Bacterial biofilm bioinspired persistent luminescence nanoparticles with gut-oriented drug delivery for colorectal cancer imaging and chemotherapy. ACS

Applied Materials & Interfaces. 2019;**11**(40):36409-36419. DOI: 10.1021/acsami.9b12853. Epub 2019 Sep 26

[54] Mateus T, Seppanen EJ, de Gier C, Clark S, Coates H, Vijayasekaran S, et al. Sleep disordered breathing and recurrent tonsillitis are associated with polymicrobial bacterial biofilm infections suggesting a role for anti-biofilm therapies. Frontiers in Cellular and Infection Microbiology. 2022;**12**:831887. DOI: 10.3389/fcimb.2022.831887

[55] Guo L, Zhang C, Chen G, Wu M, Liu W, Ding C, et al. Reactive oxygen species inhibit biofilm formation of listeria monocytogenes. Microbial Pathogenesis. 2019;**127**:183-189. DOI: 10.1016/j.micpath.2018.11.023. Epub 2018 Nov 17

[56] Qi X, Liu P, Liang P, Hao W, Li M, Li Q, et al. Biofilm's morphology design for high sensitivity of bioelectrochemical sensor: An experimental and modeling study. Science of the Total Environment. 2020;**729**:138908. DOI: 10.1016/j.scitotenv.2020.138908. Epub 2020 Apr 23

[57] Li X, Lin S, Wang Y, Chen Y, Zhang W, Shu G, et al. Application of biofilm dispersion-based nanoparticles in cutting of reinfection. Applied Microbiology and Biotechnology. 2024;**108**(1):386. DOI: 10.1007/s00253-024-13120-7

[58] Razavi BM, FazlyBazzaz BS. A review and new insights to antimicrobial action of local anesthetics. European Journal of Clinical Microbiology & Infectious Diseases. 2019;**38**(6):991-1002. DOI: 10.1007/s10096-018-03460-4. Epub 2019 Jan 24

[59] Feizabadi N, Sarrafzadeh J, Fathali M, Vasaghi-Gharamaleki B, Dadgoo M, Kardan-Yamchi J, et al. The pulsed ultrasound strategy effectively decreases the *S. Aureus* population of chronic rhino sinusitis patients. NBMC Research Notes. 2019;**12**(1):576. DOI: 10.1186/p13104-019-4579-3

[60] Benoit DSW, Sims KR Jr, Fraser D. Nanoparticles for oral biofilm treatments. ACS Nano. 2019;**13**(5):4869-4875. DOI: 10.1021/acsnano.9b02816. Epub 2019 Apr 29

[61] Inui T, Palmer RJ Jr, Shah N, Li W, Cisar JO, Wu CD. Effect of mechanically stimulated saliva on initial human dental biofilm formation. Scientific Reports. 2019;**9**(1):11805. DOI: 10.1038/p41598-019-48211-3

[62] Demishtein K, Reifen R, Shemesh M. Antimicrobial properties of magnesium open opportunities to develop healthier food. Nutrients. 2019;**11**(10):2363. DOI: 10.3390/nu11102363

[63] Babeer A, Oh MJ, Ren Z, Liu Y, Marques F, Poly A, et al. Microrobotics for precision biofilm diagnostics and treatment. Journal of Dental Research. 2022;**101**(9):1009-1014. DOI: 10.1177/00220345221087149. Epub 2022 Apr 21

Chapter 3

Understanding the Role of Bacterial Biofilm in Antibiotic Resistance: Defensive Strategies and Clinical Challenges

Syed Hamza Abbas, Hafiza Sehrish Kiani, Faryal Gohar, Shama Zahra, Alisha Javed, Shahzar Khan and Dilawaiz Khan

Abstract

Bacterial biofilms significantly cause persistent exacerbation of infections in the clinical setting. These groups of microorganisms are highly resistant to host immune responses and conventional antibiotic therapies, whereas they are embedded in an extracellular matrix. This chapter provides more detailed information on the mechanism of biofilm formation involving key stages of adherence, maturation, and spread, including the composition and structure of a biofilm matrix. This chapter further explores how biofilms contribute to antibiotic resistance, including physical barriers to drug penetration, quorum sensing mechanisms, and adaptive resistance strategies such as genetic adaptation, stress responses, and the formation of persister cells. The role of horizontal gene transfer in the spread of antibiotic resistance within biofilm communities is also discussed. The chapter discusses the clinical challenges posed by biofilm-associated infections, focusing on the challenges of diagnosing and treating chronic and recurrent infections, the role of host factors in biofilm persistence, and the limitations of current therapeutic options. Finally, we address emerging countermeasures to counter resistance mediated by biofilms, such as enzymatic therapies, nanomedicine technologies, natural product-based inhibitors, quorum sensing inhibitory agents, photodynamic and sonodynamic antimicrobial therapy, and combinatorial therapies.

Keywords: bacterial biofilm, antibiotic resistance, clinical challenges, quorum-sensing, defensive strategies

1. Introduction

For over a century, various implications have been made by scientists and microbiologists regarding uniform bacterial cultures in portraying a faulty image of microbial life in terms of genetics and physiology. Initially, it was thought bacteria existed in the natural environment as free-floating (plankton) structures. Still, many studies later showed the presence of multicellular bacterial cells or communities that can live in biofilms that consist of extracellular substances and are fixed in extracellular polymers where one cell communicates with another and forms biofilm [1]. With the aid of a basic microscope, a Dutch researcher named Antoni van Leeuwenhoek made the basic observation of an "animalcule" on tooth surfaces in 1683–1708, which was called the discovery of the microbial biofilm for the first time. Over the past decade, the concept of biofilm has been very well-known and sufficiently studied. Further investigation proved that almost 99.8% of bacterial cells show the process of biofilm formation at least in some stage of their life. But the question arises: Why do bacterial cells need to accumulate and result in biofilm formation? This concept has many better reasons, such as to survive many harsh and unbearable environments and a variety of phenotypical variations to survive and resist the antibiotic's wide range [2].

Several types of bacterial communities interact and communicate with each other to live in the form of colonies. However, multispecies biofilms, having various species of bacteria, are better adapted to the environment, such as nutritional deficiency and instability, than single-species biofilms. We can say that a monofilm is defined as a biofilm made by a single species of bacteria. On the other hand, multifilms are those constructed by more than one species of bacteria [3]. Many medical illnesses, such as native valve endocarditis, lung infections in cystic fibrosis patients, infections linked to medical devices, infections from ocular implants, middle ear infections, carditis, and osteomyelitis, have been difficult to deal with because of the development of biofilm in all such illnesses. It is still very difficult to remove from the human body, as it can easily tolerate the required concentrations of antimicrobial treatment (10–1000 times) compared to the actual strength of the simple bacterial cells [4]. Moreover, a mature biofilm is unaffected by phagocytosis (cell eating). That is why, even after treating certain diseases due to biofilm, the disease can return after weeks or months. For this, the painful process of surgically removing affected tissues is more emphasized [5].

Microorganisms coexist with humans and play a vital role in influencing the host's overall health and physiology. Some bacteria, which live in harmony with the host, form biofilms that can be formed on various surfaces, such as the skin, vagina, intestines, and mucosa of the mouth [6]. Pathogenic bacteria that colonize hosts and form detrimental biofilms can lead to persistent infections and recurrence. Biofilms can evade the host's immune system and demonstrate the remarkable capacity to endure antibiotic treatment attributed to tolerance and resistance mechanisms. Resistance often occurs due to acquired mutations, which involve mechanisms such as modifications to antibiotic targets, efflux pumps, or enzymes that degrade antibiotics [7]. These changes enable bacteria to resist antibiotics outside biofilms by eliminating their molecular targets. However, within biofilms, antibiotic-resistant cells can survive exposure to high concentrations of antibiotics. Since Fleming discovered penicillin in 1928, numerous antibiotics have been developed to treat bacterial infections, saving countless lives. Unfortunately, the misuse and overuse of antibiotics have led to bacterial resistance, resulting in multi-drug resistance, marking the onset of a "post-antibiotic era." Biofilm infections are responsible for numerous diseases, posing a significant and persistent threat to public health and the economy due to their novel resistance mechanisms and high mortality rates. It has been observed that bacteria within biofilms often exhibit increased resistance due to the reduced effectiveness of antibiotics against biofilm-associated infections [8].

2. Biofilm formation

The biofilm usually includes grouping single bacterial cells together to make the community, which is further covered by the outer extracellular material that protects the biofilm and is attached to the solid surface for further development. The maximum dry mass, i.e., 90–91%, is constituted by the semi-liquid matrix; the remaining microorganisms occupy 9–10%. However, cell-cell contact, firm growth of microbial species on a surface, and intimate cell contact and communication are done by different physiological processes inside the cell [9]. Eventually, five basic stages of biofilm formation and development are highlighted. In the first step of biofilm formation, the adhesion mechanism helps the planktonic (single cell) attach to the surface material. In the second step of biofilm formation, the cell adjusts itself to adhere and multiply further. In the third step, the complexity starts as the biofilm formation is constructed by cell-to-cell communication with the help of certain molecules that play a major role in signaling. Later on, the architecture of a very mature biofilm is formed that also produces the outer extracellular polymeric substance [10]. Lastly, in the final step, the single small cells from the mature biofilm are released into their surrounding environment. It has been found that both environmental and genetic factors contribute their role in the formation and maturation of biofilm, as shown in **Figure 1**. Extracellular Polymeric substance, an important constituent of biofilm, comprises various components such as lipids, nucleic acids, and proteins. The biofilm's attachment to the surface and its architectural stability are usually contributed to by certain molecules such as lipopolysaccharides, glycopeptides, and lipids [11].

2.1 Steps in biofilm formation

2.1.1 Adherence

The first step involves the attachment of the planktonic cell to its substrate by the adhesion process. The free-flowing microorganisms in the isolated form get assembled into the proper community structures [12]. During this stage, microorganisms

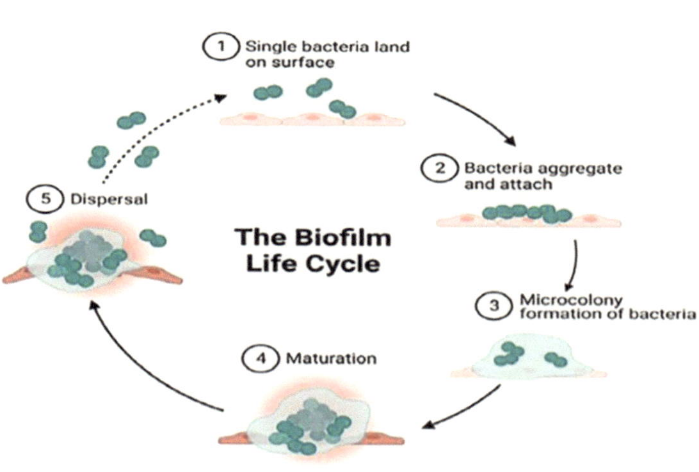

Figure 1.
Steps of biofilm formation [1].

can go back to their planktonic state as they are loosely connected to the surfaces and are reversible. The bacteria then change their orientation, and they begin synthesizing the adhesion molecules called extracellular polymeric substance (EPS), which enables the attachment of bacterial cells to their surface form, facilitating irreversible attachment. This irreversible attachment also makes them resistant to various environmental factors that hinder the formation of biofilms [13, 14]. The studies indicated that bis-(3′–5′)-cyclic dimeric guanosine monophosphate (c-di-GMP), which is an intracellular signaling molecule, plays a crucial role in the early stages of biofilm formation as it promotes the formation of a biofilm matrix and inhibits flagella-mediated swimming motility. Microorganisms have the Pil-Chp system, a surface-sensing mechanism; as bacteria attach or detach from surfaces, the concentration of c-di-GMP, a signaling molecule, increases. This increase in c-di-GMP levels triggers the transformation of planktonic bacteria into surface-sensing bacteria, leading to irreversible attachment and the initiation of biofilm formation [14].

2.1.2 Expansion or creation of microcolonies

Bacteria attach to the biological tissue or physical surface, and this binding eventually becomes stable, creating microcolonies. Chemical signals released by bacterial cells signaled the beginning of bacterial multiplication. These signals serve as a communication channel between the bacterial cells, creating the biofilm. When the signal strength crosses a particular level, the genetic mechanism for exopolysaccharide synthesis is started [15]. Therefore, the bacterial cell divisions occur within the implanted exopolysaccharide matrix in response to the chemical signal and in the presence of a high concentration of c-di-GMP, ultimately creating a microcolony. It is also believed that flagella and type IV pili-mediated motilities are essential for interacting microbes with surfaces and forming microcolonies by cell-cell aggregations [16].

2.1.3 Maturation

Some biofilm-related genes can be expressed after the microcolony stage of biofilm development. These genetic products are required for the EPS, the primary structural component of the biofilm. It has been studied that bacterial adhesion alone can cause the extracellular matrix to develop. Water-filled tubes are formed after matrix development to carry nutrients within the biofilm [17]. According to research, these water channels act as a kind of circulatory system, supplying various nutrients and eliminating waste by the groups in the microcolonies of biofilm. Extracellular polymeric substances (EPS) not only help the microorganisms to adhere to surfaces but also stabilize biofilm three-dimensional structure, cluster cells, protect the biofilm from a variety of stresses, including the host immune system response, antimicrobials, oxidative damage, and metallic cations, and encapsulate signaling molecules required for quorum sensing, metabolic products, and enzymes [18]. These factors make EPS crucial for biofilm maturation. Biofilm in a maturation phase consists of three layers: an inner layer that controls the biofilm, an outer layer that harbors microorganisms that are ready to be again in their planktonic/isolated condition, and a middle layer known as the microbial basement layer [19].

2.1.4 Spread

After maturation, bacterial cells regularly depart from biofilms either passively due to physical factors like liquid flow-dependent dispersion or actively (due to motility and EPS degradation-dependent dispersion). Bacteria can occasionally become isolated from the colony and enter the environment due to stress. In more instances, some bacteria stop the production of EPS and release it into the environment. Cells express genes for motility during dissociation of motile bacterial cells, including transcription of ribosomal protein and pilus, and are almost visible in planktonic cells [20]. Biofilms disperse because of various factors, such as lack of nutrients, intense competition, and outgrown population, which encourage the production of dispersion-related genes, for example, upregulation of genes involved in EPS degradation and cell motility and a downregulation of genes essential for polysaccharide and fimbriae synthesis.

3. Biofilm-associated antibiotic resistance

Biofilm is a bacteria colony wrapped in a self-produced polymeric matrix. The protective layer includes polysaccharides, proteins, and DNA, collectively called extracellular polymeric substances (EPS). Biofilms are important in the sense that they cause chronic and persistent infections. This is achieved by their incredible ability to reduce the effectiveness of antibiotics. In the biofilm state, the efficiency of antibiotics is reduced by 1000 times more than in the planktonic state. Biofilm-mediated antibiotic resistance is a relatively new clinical issue. Studying biofilms and resulting chronic infections is important because biofilms are not easily treatable with antibiotics, immune systems, or surfactants.

3.1 Physical barrier: EPS - Reducing the penetration of antibiotics

External nucleic acids (eDNA, eRNA), proteins, and polysaccharides are known to form a matrix. This matrix is called an extracellular polymeric substance (EPS). It is common in biofilms because it offers mechanical stability to biofilms. EPS is the physical barrier that is believed to be the first control against the use of antibiotics. EPS is a diverse matrix in terms of its structure and its roles in the process of amplification of antibiotic resistance. This matrix prevents the diffusion of antibiotics within the desired community and can also prevent the penetration of wanted antibiotics by rendering them useless. For example, the EPS layer reduces the ability of β-lactams to penetrate, affecting cell wall synthesis. This makes it possible for the bacteria to survive in biofilm [21]. Likewise, aminoglycosides that pass through porin channels and diffuse across the cell membrane are substantially less effective because of low mobility within the matrix against bacteria that develop biofilm [22]. The EPS layer is not necessarily uniform in composition, charge, and size for different types of bacteria and for the same type of bacteria. This is explicable in light of recent developments in imaging and microscopic technology due to the heterogeneous nature of biofilms, where some parts are less, and others are more resistant to treatment [23]. However, some are connected to biofilms as factors such as β-lactamases that break down the β-lactam antibiotics, increasing antibiotic resistance [24].

3.2 Quorum sensing

Bacteria have a method to communicate within an environment. This method is known as quorum sensing (QS). Communication is possible through the release of tiny molecules. This communication mechanism depends on the expression, regulation, and increase of antibiotic resistance. Both Gram-negative and positive bacteria have specialized molecules that enable them to communicate. Gram-negative QS systems depend on AHLs, and Gram-positive have peptide-based signals. These enable bacteria to form biofilms for regulating genes involved in pathogenicity, EPS synthesis, stress response, and synchronization. QS alters the rigidity of bacterial structures and controls its behavior, enhancing antibiotic resistance. Antibiotic resistance of *Pseudomonas aeruginosa* is higher toward Ciprofloxacin because QS systems enable it to activate the virulence factors and biofilm formation by using Las and Rhl systems for signaling [25]. QS also regulates the formation of efflux pumps besides matrix formation. These pump the antibiotics out of the cell, therefore increasing antibiotic resistance. It is important to alter quorum sensing to make commercially available antibiotics effective against bacteria and to limit antibiotic resistance [26].

3.3 Strategies of adaptive resistance

Through adaptive mechanisms, bacteria can overcome antibiotic stress, especially in biofilm. The distinct environment of biofilm facilitates the adaptive mechanism. These strategies that enable bacteria to go in such harsh environments include changes in the physiological environment, genetic changes as well as phenotypic changes.

3.3.1 Genetic mechanisms

Some of the genetic processes by which biofilm bacteria acquire adaptive resistance are now known from experimental investigations. One such strategy is the Horizontal Gene Transfer (HGT), or genetic modifications of overexpression of resistance genes, to give microbes a new set of functions. We can also notice that bacteria in a biofilm can be genetically different. Genetic mutants within certain subpopulations can contain antibiotic-resistance genes. These mutations can occur in antibiotic-degrading enzyme genes or antibiotic target genes of DNA gyrase or penicillin-binding protein [27]. Furthermore, the biofilms favor the exchange of genetic material among bacteria and thus the rate of emergence of resistance. In this mechanism, horizontal gene transfer, particularly conjugation, plays a significant role. Biofilm matrices enhance the transfer of the resistance plasmid and other genes because cells are in close contact. For example, plasmids with ESBL genes in *Escherichia coli* can be dispersed using biofilms, causing multi-drug resistance [28].

3.3.2 Physiological modifications

Besides, bacteria residing in biofilms display certain metabolic changes that will help them become antibiotic-resistant. Downregulation of metabolic activity, slow division, and nutrient restriction in the biofilm mode of growth are often cited causes for reduced antibiotic susceptibility [29]. It turns out that fluoroquinolones and β-lactams primarily target only actively dividing bacteria. These are less effective in biofilms because many cells are in a slow-growing phase or quiescent, aiding the biofilm population. Susceptibility is frequently the result of low metabolic activity, decreased cell division, and nutrition limitations in the biofilm environment [29]. The fluoroquinolones and β-lactams target the actively growing bacteria. As many cells are slowly growing and dormant, these drugs are less effective in biofilms. This helps the biofilm population to thrive even in the presence of antibiotics.

3.3.3 Mechanisms of stress response

Biofilm bacteria that form in difficult operating environments, including an environment containing antibiotics, activate stress response signal transduction pathways. Such processes may include lowered growth, metabolic variations, or the switching on of protective enzymes. The SOS response is one of the pathways, a deeply conservative bacterial response to DNA damage that leads to a higher probability of obtaining antibiotic resistance genes and a higher mutation rate [30].

3.3.4 Persister cells: Leading figure in biofilm resistance

It is important to understand that bacterial cells entering a dormant stage, a metabolically inactive state, are called persister cells. They are one of the toughest to handle from the aspect of being treatable with drugs. Such cells can be found most often in biofilms; they can also be found in the planktonic cultures. Antibiotics that act on bacteria that require an active metabolic state or bacterial cell division present a problem because persisters are not replicating or metabolizing. Stress response pathways, which include toxin-antitoxin systems that control cell growth and survival in unfavorable conditions, are involved in controlling the synthesis of persister cells [31]. Accumulation of toxins produced by certain bacterial species may enhance the formation of persister cells in biofilms. For instance, *Pseudomonas aeruginosa forms a subpopulation of persisters more resistant to antimicrobial agents,* hence the persistent biofilm-associated infections. These cells are very stubborn; thus, biofilms can regrow once the antibiotics are stopped, hence recurrent infections. In conclusion, recent research has shown that if the process of persister cell formation is controlled, this could lead to a fresh combating strategy to avoid infections connected to biofilms [32].

3.4 Horizontal gene transfer (HGT)

Recent studies have shown a connection between horizontal gene transfer and biofilm formation. During biofilm, conjugation is enhanced. Through this, the bacteria in biofilm are more resistant to antibiotics, and horizontal gene transfer helps the bacteria gain antibiotic-resistant genes from the surroundings. Three main transfer mechanisms, namely transduction, transformation, and conjugation, are involved [33]. During biofilm, the main process of transfer is via conjugation. The features of overlapping and the compact arrangement of bacterial cells in biofilms foster genetic exchange efficiently [34]. The mobile genetic elements that facilitate the exchange of antibiotic-resistance genes in biofilms include plasmids, transposons, and integrons, which may harbor multiple resistance genes [35]. Likewise, bacteria residing in biofilms are likely to develop resistance against many classes of antibiotics by horizontal gene transfer between species or strains [36]. Biofilm environments also contribute to the selection of antibiotic-resistant strains because, in microbial communities containing both susceptible and resistant strains, resistance is rapidly selected by the powerful adherence forces exerted by biofilms.

4. Chronic infections and the role of biofilms

Biofilms are also involved in acquiring chronic and recurrent infections [37]. These microbial communities are protected and maintained in a suitable environment and favorable circumstances, surrounded by an EPS matrix produced by the microbes. Pathogens often colonize host tissues or medical devices, leading to persistent infections [38]. This biofilm allows microorganisms to remain protected from immune responses and antimicrobial intervention. This persistence is due to the EPS matrix shielding immune recognition and antibiotic penetration [39]. Furthermore, when bacteria develop biofilms, they become dormant or slow-growing, and this also plays a role in their resistance to antimicrobial agents, which target actively proliferative cells. For instance, in pulmonary infections due to cystic fibrosis, biofilms allow a chronic infection with *Pseudomonas aeruginosa* to adhere to the surfactant layer of the lung. The situation worsens because these biofilms secrete toxins and inflammatory mediators, leading to lung disease [40].

4.1 Recurrent infections

Biofilms are difficult to eradicate since they contain persister cells, dormant forms of bacteria that exist after antibiotic use. They reside inside the biofilm structure, and on the withdrawal of antibiotics or any weakening of the immune system, they can wake up and grow back to give a relapse [41]. A good example of biofilm-mediated infection is recurrent urinary tract infections (UTIs). Uropathogenic *Escherichia coli* (UPEC) attaches to the bladder epithelium, forming biofilms that create reservoirs protected from antibiotics and host defenses [42]. However, these reservoirs can reinfect new cycles after removing stresses like antibiotics and host immune responses, particularly in patients with underlying diseases such as diabetes or anatomic deviations.

Recurrent infection with biofilms is also commonly related to chronic sinusitis. The bacteria *Haemophilus influenzae* and *Staphylococcus aureus* cause biofilm formation in the nasal mucosa, thus causing chronic inflammation and recurrent symptoms despite the treatment. The ability of biofilm to exist for long periods is attributed to its ability to withstand mucociliary clearance and antimicrobial agents [43]. CF is a disease resulting from a cystic fibrosis transmembrane conductance regulator (CFTR) gene mutation, leading to thick mucus in the respiratory and digestive systems. Due to biofilm formation in the thick mucus in the lungs, chronic and relapsing infections occur. Biofilm-forming bacteria are highly susceptible to colonization of the respiratory tract in CF patients [44]. The thick mucus provides the microbes with nutrients they can attach to and multiply. Bacteria that adhere to the mucus grow in biofilms, a shield from the host's immune system and other antimicrobial substances. Biofilms release extracellular polymeric substances (EPS) that create a physical barrier against the entry of antibiotics and shield bacteria from immune cells [45]. This invariably leads to worsening, poorer lung functioning, and enhanced mortality rates. *P. aeruginosa* biofilms are relatively hard to eliminate and are linked to the deterioration of lung function over time [46]. Moreover, CF patients also have biofilms of other pathogens, such as *S. aureus* and *H. influenzae*, which makes the problem worse and results in chronic infections.

Bacterial colonization is also a common characteristic of chronic wounds such as diabetic foot ulcers [47], venous leg ulcers [48], and pressure ulcers [49] due to the presence of biofilm. Biofilms are significant in the context of the inhibition of wound healing [48]. Biofilm formation especially prevails in chronic wounds since the microenvironment where biofilms are produced is highly suitable [50]. Moreover, bacterial colonization and formation of biofilms are further enhanced by factors such as moist conditions, necrotic tissue, and decreased blood circulation. As biofilms develop, they change the local inflammatory pattern, interfere with the healing of the tissues, and create conditions favorable for repeated infections. Bacteria can also form biofilm, and it can adhere to tissue base, dead tissue, and wound secretion to form a vast and long-lasting microbial conglomerate [50].

4.2 Role of host factors in chronicity and recurrence of biofilm infections

The duration and frequency of biofilm-associated infections have also been established to be host factors. Exopolysaccharide matrix hinders phagocytosis and cytokine signaling so microbial communities can survive in a secure niche; immune evasion is essential [51]. While inflammation is intended to eradicate infection, it can also destroy tissue and lead to biofilm persistence with external conditions. Host-related risks such as immune suppression, diabetes, or using indwelling medical devices also increase the risk of chronic and recurrent infections [52]. For instance, the biofilm on the catheter surface is the site of infection that leads to repeated bacterial colonization in the case of CAUTIs.

4.3 Challenges

Bacterial localization in a biofilm makes it hard to diagnose because of its structural and functional properties and the current diagnostic tools. Biofilm infections are challenging to diagnose because they cannot be detected by the immune system or standard microbiological assays [53]. The protective matrix produced by EPS also shields the bacteria and makes them less available for diagnostic procedures [54]. When in biofilm, bacteria have a different behavior; they are dormant, while the planktonic bacteria are free-floating and metabolically active. Traditional diagnostic methods like culture-based depend on the growth of microorganisms for identification [55] and cannot identify these metabolically dormant bacteria. Furthermore, biofilms are considered to have high-density structures. A bacterium in polymicrobial biofilms can be in various physiological statuses or in contact with other microorganisms, including fungi, in the same biofilm [58]. The diversity of the biofilm poses a challenge to the identification process since such diagnostic methods may not be able to identify the whole spectrum of microbial activity or even the microbial population density of the biofilm [56].

Biofilm-related infections are challenging to manage because biofilm bacteria are highly resistant to antibiotics than planktonic (free-living) bacteria. Due to biofilms' structural, metabolic, and genetic characteristics, this resistance is a multifactorial phenomenon. The EPS matrix, which is the outer layer of the biofilm, acts as a physical barrier that does not allow the antibiotics to penetrate the deeper layers of the biofilm. The matrix is gel-like and dense, hindering the diffusion of antibiotics, particularly big molecules [57]. For instance, aminoglycosides and beta-lactams are often entrapped or delivered slowly into the matrix, reducing their access to bacteria in deeper layers [58]. Furthermore, the EPS matrix can also adsorb with antibiotics, making them ineffective before interacting with the target cells. For instance, the negatively charged parts of the EPS, eDNA, or specific polysaccharides bind positively charged antibiotics, such as aminoglycosides [59]. This binding effect leads to a concentration gradient in which sublethal concentrations in the deeper zones can help bacteria survive.

Another characteristic is the metabolic heterogeneity of bacterial cells within the biofilm. Cells at the surface of the biofilm are in contact with nutrients and oxygen and are metabolically active. In contrast, the deeper cells are starved of nutrients [60] and become nonmetabolically active or even enter a dormant state. The metabolic stratification has profound significance for antibiotic resistance. Most antibiotics, including beta-lactams and fluoroquinolones, work on some cellular functions such as cell wall synthesis, protein synthesis, or DNA replication. These antibiotics' implementation methods are constrained because these cells are less metabolically active and thus less vulnerable to these antibiotics in biofilms where they are stationary or slow dividing within the matrix. Steady-state hypoxia is often observed in biofilms developed on mucosal tissues or the surface of medical implants [61]. When exposed to hypoxic conditions, the bacteria change their metabolic activity to glycolysis fermentation or nitrate reduction [62]. This metabolic switch changes bacterial phenotype and is a factor that contributes to resistance. The developing alterations under anaerobic growth led to the decreased absorption of some antibiotics requiring an electron transport chain, such as the aminoglycoside antibiotics.

4.4 Limited treatment options

Biofilm-related infections are challenging in clinical medicine because they are recurrent and resistant to traditional antimicrobial agents. The existing antibiotic therapies cannot remove biofilms completely, leading to chronic and recurring infections, which are dangerous to patients and a significant cost to the healthcare system. Due to the properties of biofilm bacteria, such as limited penetration and metabolic activity, antibiotics cannot reach bactericidal concentrations across the biofilm [63]. Not only can bacteria survive this sublethal exposure, but this exposure will also favor the emergence of antibiotic-resistant mutants. Antibiotics target fundamental bacterial functions, including synthesizing proteins and cell walls or replicating DNA [64]. Nonetheless, these antibiotics are ineffective in biofilms because bacteria within them are embedded in a layer of extracellular polymeric substances and metabolically distinct. In addition, quorum sensing systems control the formation and establishment of biofilms. However, current antibiotics cannot act on quorum-sensing pathways important for biofilm stability and synchronization, as shown in **Figure 2** [65].

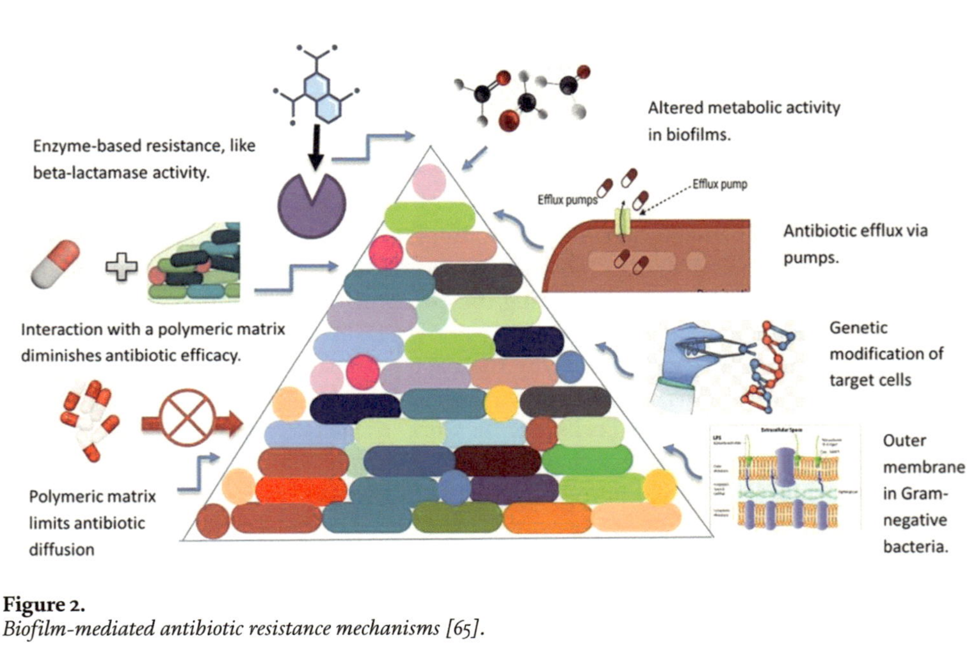

Figure 2.
Biofilm-mediated antibiotic resistance mechanisms [65].

5. Defensive strategies against biofilm-associated resistance

5.1 Novel approaches to preventing and treating biofilm infections

Recently, many advanced and novel methods are being analyzed to fight and remove the biofilms affecting different natural vicinities. These methods that are being focused on and effective for biofilm studies include the disruption of quorum sensing, certain natural substances, antimicrobial sonodynamic or photodynamic therapies, nanotechnology-based techniques, and enzymatic degradation. These approaches have shown promising results by targeting the physiological structure and functioning of biofilm and disturbing the single-cell bacterial populations in biofilm, proving the older method of antibiotic treatment to be efficient and still effective.

5.2 Enzymatic breakdown of biofilms

In enzymatic treatments, the mature biofilms normally divide into smaller fragments by the action of specific enzymes, which help their easy degradation. This treatment is not only safe to handle. Still, it is also applicable to different conditions and is nontoxic in nature, so it can be effectively implemented for various medical illnesses at hospitals [1]. Enzymatic biodegradation is an effective tool for biofilm removal that cannot be easily removed by using conventional cleaning methods. The areas that are difficult to deal with in medical cases, such as biomedical devices and medical implants, are useful for breaking the biofilm in **Table 1** [66]. The biofilm's cellular components, such as proteins, lipids, and carbohydrates, which provide the potential to the biofilm structure, are acted upon by various enzymes, such as lipases, amylases, and proteases, during the enzyme degradation strategy. Using the standard cleaning technique by cells, the waste is usually removed from the cells after enzymatic action. For instance, the lysozyme enzyme is responsible for unwinding

Aspect	Description	Clinical implications
Biofilm structure	Biofilms consist of a bacterial community encased in a self-produced matrix of EPS containing polysaccharides, proteins, and eDNA.	• Biofilms reduce the efficacy of antibiotics and immune responses, leading to persistent infections.
Resistance enhancement	Tight biofilm-dense structure limits antibiotic penetration and increases bacterial survival.	• Increases resistance up to 1000 times compared to planktonic (free-floating) bacteria. • Biofilms are difficult to treat with conventional antibiotics.
Role of Quorum Sensing (QS)	Bacteria in biofilms communicate through QS, which regulates gene expression for biofilm formation, stress response, and resistance.	• Increases biofilm stability, virulence factor production, and antibiotic resistance. • Targeting QS could enhance antibiotic effectiveness.
Adaptation mechanisms	Biofilms allow bacteria to adapt through genetic, physiological, and stress responses.	• Genetic mutations, metabolic changes, and stress response pathways enable bacteria to survive harsh conditions like antibiotics.

Table 1.
Biofilm formation and its role in chronic infections [66].

the components of bacterial cell walls, thus releasing the biofilm layer. By breaking the peptidoglycan layer of the bacterial cell wall, the bacterial cells become much more at risk of being targeted by the respective immune system and antibiotics [67]. Moreover, one of the enzymes, Dispersion B, known for its biodegradable nature, targets the cell by making the Extrapolysaccharides soluble and easier to eradicate. The various factors on which the action of enzymes depends are the biofilm's composition and nature, the prevailing surrounding environment, and the biofilm and enzymatic types utilized [68]. Furthermore, one more important enzyme responsible for degrading is DNAse, which degrades the bacterial DNA in biofilm and helps efficiently remove DNA components [69].

5.3 Advanced strategies utilizing nanotechnology

Nanotechnology-based strategies offer substantially promising avenues in addressing biofilm-based infections. In this approach, biofilms are usually degraded using components such as specified nanoparticles that can have a powerful impact on biofilm eradication. This emerging strategy works by focusing on the nanoparticle's actions to treat and stop the biofilm formation [70]. Nanomaterials have also been studied to detect biofilm formation at the initial stage and diagnose and identify various biofilm-related infections and illnesses. For example, a more rapid and easy diagnosis is made by binding bacterial cells with real-time signals with nanomaterial-based biosensors. Different factors such as infection dissemination, bacterial cell attachments with the surface, and biofilm formation and maturation can be stopped by coating nanomaterials with certain medical devices to make them functional properly against bacterial cells. A thin layer of nano-sized particles is being applied on various coatings to make it more antimicrobial and protective against the biofilm consisting of mature cells. These nanoparticles form a strong barrier that stops the bacterial cell from penetrating the medical devices by highlighting their power to remove and degrade the biofilm components [71]. They are also preferred to be used in the drug delivery process to treat and stop the infections related to biofilm to combat the other side effects of older methods of antibiotics, such as allergic reactions, organ toxicity, and gastrointestinal or stomach-related issues in the body [72]. Several metals are associated with their action in biofilm destabilization and degradation. Certain key mechanisms are related to these nanoparticle methods for their anti-biofilm effects, such as disturbance of outer polysaccharides having various components, attachment of biofilm, penetration of cell wall and membrane, and disruption of quorum sensing. By studying these aspects, the nanoparticles have potential anti-biofilm progress against a wide range of pathogenic and disease-causing bacterial species. For instance, the catheters coated with the Ag particles help stop the Gram-positive bacteria antibiotic-resistant settlement, such as Staphylococcus. aureus and S. epidermis. But, it is more effective against gram-negative bacteria such as *E. coli* and *Pseudomonas aeruginosa*. Similarly, Cu metal has also been found to effectively target the fungal cells while grouping by impacting and blocking the quorum sensing [73].

5.4 Natural compounds

Natural compounds, including plant extracts, essential oils, and substances derived from marine sources, have demonstrated considerable potential in preventing biofilm formation. Due to their lower likelihood of side effects and natural origin than synthetic drugs, these compounds are emerging as promising anti-biofilm agents [74].

Plant-based compounds such as eucalyptus (*Eucalyptus globulus*), garlic (*Allium sativum*), oregano (*Oreganum vulgare*), and grape (*Vitis vinifera*) possess antimicrobial activity against a variety of pathogens, including drug-resistant strains. Their antibacterial effects result from mechanisms such as interfering with metabolic processes, disrupting bacterial membranes and walls, and inhibiting protein synthesis. These natural compounds also present a more environmentally friendly, cost-effective, and sustainable alternative to synthetic antimicrobials. Additionally, their ability to selectively target specific bacteria enhances the precision of anti-biofilm treatments, making them effective against a broad spectrum of bacterial strains [75]. Thymol, a natural compound derived from *Thymus vulgaris*, has proven effective against antibiotic-resistant bacteria such as *Escherichia coli* and *Staphylococcus aureus*. It achieves this by inhibiting survival and growth by disrupting bacterial cell walls and preventing biofilm formation. Plant-derived terpenoids, known for their antibacterial properties, are potential sources for developing new antibiotics. These compounds exhibit strong antioxidant effects that damage bacterial cell walls, interfere with quorum sensing and biofilm formation, and inhibit bacterial replication, thereby curbing infection spread. Similarly, polyphenols from *Vitis vinifera* are effective against infections caused by antibiotic-resistant bacteria. They exhibit potential anti-biofilm activity and possess anti-inflammatory and antioxidant properties that may be beneficial for treating various health conditions [76]. Quercetin, a flavonoid with antibacterial activity, is effective against Gram-negative and Gram-positive bacteria, including resistant strains. It functions as an antioxidant, disrupts bacterial membranes, and inhibits bacterial growth and reproduction while preventing the formation of biofilms that protect bacteria under harsh conditions. Curcumin, a polyphenolic compound obtained from the rhizome of *Curcuma longa*, exhibits broad-spectrum antimicrobial activity. Its anti-inflammatory properties help reduce infection risks, especially in individuals with chronic inflammation. Additionally, curcumin exhibits biofilm formation, making it a promising candidate for combating infections caused by antibiotic-resistant bacteria [77].

5.5 Quorum-sensing inhibition

The inhibition of quorum sensing is a new strategy adopted to curtail the formation of biofilms. This method interferes with bacterial communication, which hinders the formation of biofilms. Quorum-sensing molecules are chemical signals released by the biofilm-forming organisms that are essential for coordinating behavior within bacterial communities. These chemicals signal the start of biofilm development when a specific bacterial threshold is achieved. Quorum-sensing inhibitors serve by averting the synthesis of auto-inducer molecules, which is vital for bacterial communication. Bacteria cannot form biofilms when the synthesis of these molecules is inhibited, hence stopping the spread of diseases. Additionally, by reducing bacterial contamination in the environment, these inhibitors can aid in preventing infections. Quorum-sensing inhibitors are, therefore, significant tools for controlling and treating bacterial diseases. Moreover, quorum-sensing inhibitors have demonstrated efficacy in reducing antibiotic resistance in bacterial strains, providing a viable strategy to fight infections caused by multidrug-resistant bacteria. Notably, quorum-sensing inhibition is nontoxic and environmentally safe, making it a desirable substitute for traditional therapeutic approaches. Various quorum-sensing inhibitors have been created, including phages and small compounds to fight bacterial infections. For example, the small chemical acyldepsipeptide (ADEP) has demonstrated potential as a strong inhibitor for bacterial infections by recently being found to be effective in blocking quorum-sensing in multidrug-resistant *Acinetobacter baumannii* as shown in **Figure 3** [78]. ADEP inhibits the virulence factors that cause infection by interfering with bacterial communication. Incredibly, ADEP is harmless to mammalian cells, making it a promising option for new treatments for biofilm infections. Numerous other small peptide molecules, such as furanone, AHL, 2-heptyl-4-hydroxyquinoline sulfonamide (HQSA), and N-(3-(4-fluorophenyl)-2-propynyl)-4-quinolone, are being studied as possible anti-biofilm agents as they exhibit the ability to inhibit the production of quorum-sensing molecules in a variety of bacterial species [79]. A subclass of bacteriophages known as quorum-sensing inhibitor phages works by interfering with the quorum-sensing systems of bacteria. These phages impede the synthesis of quorum-sensing signals, which are essential for bacterial communication and the formation of biofilm. Notably, this approach is more persistent than previous anti-biofilm therapies since phages are less likely to acquire resistance.

5.6 Antimicrobial photodynamic/sonodynamic therapy

Antimicrobial photodynamic therapy (aPDT) and antimicrobial sonodynamic therapy (aSDT) are innovative approaches for combating biofilms, utilizing sound waves and light to eliminate bacteria and inhibit biofilm formation. In aPDT, light-sensitive compounds known as photosensitizers are activated by specific wavelengths of light, generating reactive oxygen species (ROS) that destroy bacterial cells. Conversely, aSDT uses ultrasound waves to create vibrations in bacterial cell walls, ultimately causing cell death. These therapies are considered safe and have diverse applications in medical settings, particularly in managing biofilm-associated infections. aPDT is a non-invasive method well-suited for treating infections in hard-to-reach areas, while aSDT, being minimally invasive, is effective for addressing infections located in deeper tissues [80]. Both treatments demonstrate effectiveness against antibiotic-resistant

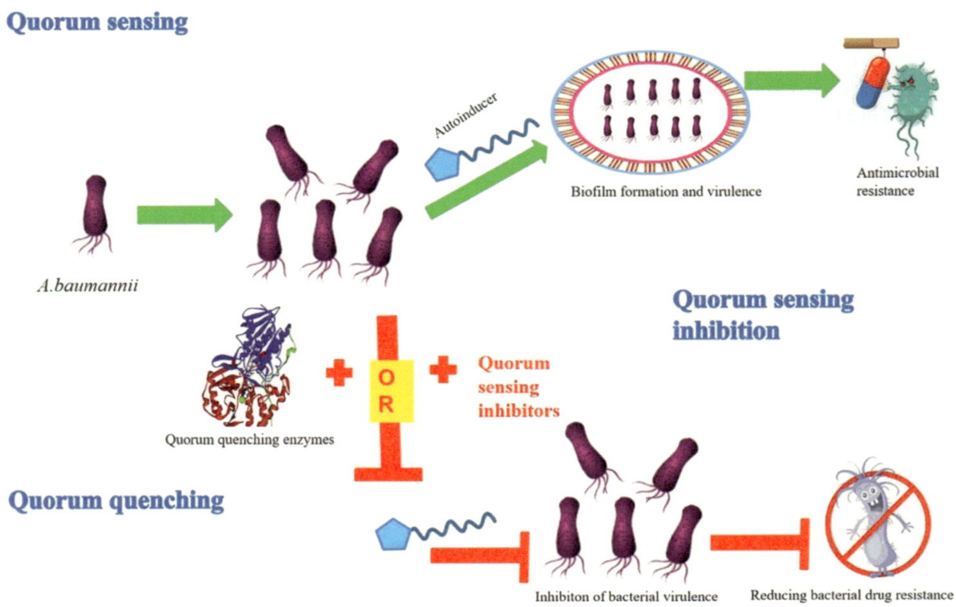

Figure 3.
Quorum-sensing inhibition [78].

bacteria due to their unique mechanism of action. The reactive oxygen species (ROS) generated by aPDT are toxic to biofilm-forming bacteria. However, prolonged exposure to light may lead to bacterial resistance, necessitating regular monitoring and periodic treatments every few months to maintain its effectiveness. Combating aPDT with lipid-coated nanoparticles containing peptide nucleic acid (PNA) has emerged as a promising approach for managing biofilm-associated infections. This method effectively combats biofilm-related infections by utilizing gene-specific PNAs to target pathogens. The purine and pyrimidine components in PNAs enable them to bind with DNA and RNA, expanding their applications in biological research. Antimicrobial sonodynamic therapy (aSDT) is a valuable complement to biofilm treatments. Ultrasound waves can disrupt the structural integrity of biofilms, enhancing the efficacy of antimicrobial photodynamic therapy (aPDT) by activating photosensitizers. Additionally, ultrasound can be paired with antibiotics to improve their penetration into biofilm matrices, increasing their effectiveness. The mechanism by which ultrasound disrupts biofilms involves breaking hydrogen bonds between biofilm cells, thereby boosting the efficiency of other anti-biofilm methods and promoting bacterial cell destruction [81]. Combating aPDT and aSDT leverages the strengths of both therapies to provide a more comprehensive treatment strategy. While aPDT is particularly effective at eradicating bacteria, aSDT excels at reducing the size and density of biofilms. The synergistic use of these therapies maximizes their potential, offering a more effective solution for managing biofilm-associated infections [82].

5.7 Combination anti-biofilm therapies

Combination therapies, an integration of multiple treatments against the diseases, help researchers to attack multiple pathways simultaneously, enabling a more thorough approach to treating different infectious diseases [83]. These treatments have more significance than individual treatments, as they are frequently less harmful and more cost-effective, making them a desirable choice for infection prevention. Combination therapies can be used to reduce the alarming issue of antibiotic resistance by customizing their levels. It has been observed that combining antibiotics with other agents, such as probiotics and surfactants, reduced biofilm production levels. Antibiotics work by limiting the growth of bacteria, while surfactants and probiotics aid in disrupting the biofilms. Due to their ability to target multiple aspects of biofilms, they are effective in treating different chronic infections. Some examples of effective combination therapies are demonstrated in **Table 2** [84].

Sr. No.	Combination therapies	Effect	References
1	Combining ambroxol with vancomycin	Enhanced effectiveness of vancomycin against *Staphylococcus epidermidis* biofilms	[84]
2	Quorum-sensing inhibitors with bacteriocins	Lull the bacteria and disrupt their communication simultaneously	[85]
3	Combining RNAIII inhibiting peptide (RIP) FSio with the antibiotic tigecycline	Effective in treating *Staphylococcus aureus* wound infections in mice	[86]
4	Combining antimicrobial peptide, GioKHc, antibiotic tobramycin	Effective against *Pseudomonas aeruginosa*	[87]

Table 2.
Effective combination anti-biofilm therapies.

6. Conclusion

Advanced nanomaterial-based solutions offer a promising and innovative approach to tackling biofilms and other persistent substances. The unique properties of nanomaterials have revolutionized numerous fields, including medicine. These materials can be engineered to mimic the size and structure of bacterial internal components and proteins. In chronic wound infections, effectively eliminating biofilms and managing infections are crucial steps for promoting improved wound healing. To achieve improved therapeutic outcomes, focusing on targeting specific stages of the biofilm life cycle is essential. For persistent wound infections associated with biofilms, one strategy involves disrupting the initial attachment of microorganisms to the wound site. This can be achieved by inhibiting their interaction with the wound surface, such as cell surface-associated adhesions and polymeric extracellular substances (EPS), including proteins and appendages. The early stages of biofilm production can be prevented by targeting cell and EPS production. Established biofilms can be disrupted through various strategies such as breaking down the EPS, interfering with microbial interactions, physically removing the biofilms, eradicating dominant cells, or altering the pathogenic environment (e.g., addressing hypoxia or reducing pH). Bacteriophages, viruses specifically engineered to target bacteria by recognizing bacterial cell surface receptors, are emerging as a promising alternative in the fight against antimicrobial resistance.

Acknowledgements

All authors have equal contributions in this publication.

Conflicts of interest

No conflicts of interest are associated with this publication.

Author details

Syed Hamza Abbas[1*], Hafiza Sehrish Kiani[1], Faryal Gohar[1], Shama Zahra[1], Alisha Javed[1], Shahzar Khan[1] and Dilawaiz Khan[2]

1 Department of Microbiology, Quaid-i-Azam University, Islamabad, Pakistan

2 Department of Animal Sciences, Quaid-i-Azam University, Islamabad, Pakistan

*Address all correspondence to: habbas@bs.qau.edu.pk

References

[1] Sharma S, Mohler J, Mahajan SD, Schwartz SA, Bruggemann L, Aalinkeel R. Microbial biofilm: A review on formation, infection, antibiotic resistance, control measures, and innovative treatment. Microorganisms. 2023;**11**(6):1614

[2] Kanematsu H, Barry DM. Formation and Control of Biofilm in Various Environments. Singapore: Springer Nature, Singapore Pte Ltd; 2020

[3] Rather MA, Gupta K, Mandal M. Microbial biofilm: Formation, architecture, antibiotic resistance, and control strategies. Brazilian Journal of Microbiology. 2021;**52**(4):1701-1718. Springer Science and Business Media Deutschland Gmb H. DOI: 10.1007/s42770-021-00624-x

[4] Costerton JW, Cheng KJ, Geesey GG, Ladd TI, Nickel JC, Dasgupta M, et al. Bacterial Biofilms in Nature and Disease. Annual Review of Microbiology. 1987;**41**:435-464. DOI: 10.1146/annurev.mi.41.100187.002251

[5] Anju VT, Busi S, Imchen M, Kumavath R, Mohan MS, Salim SA, et al. Polymicrobial infections and biofilms: Clinical significance and eradication strategies. Antibiotics. MDPI; 2022;**11**(12):1731. DOI: 10.3390/antibiotics11121731

[6] Bowler P, Murphy C, Wolcott R. Biofilm exacerbates antibiotic resistance: Is this a current oversight in antimicrobial stewardship? Antimicrobial Resistance and Infection Control. BioMed Central Ltd. 2020;**9**(1):162. DOI: 10.1186/s13756-020-00830-6

[7] Liu S, Lu H, Zhang S, Shi Y, Chen Q. Phages against pathogenic bacterial biofilms and biofilm-based infections: A review. Pharmaceutics. MDPI; 2022;**14**(2):427. DOI: 10.3390/pharmaceutics14020427

[8] Asma ST, Imre K, Morar A, Imre M, Acaroz U, Shah SRA, et al. Natural strategies as potential weapons against bacterial biofilms. Life. MDPI; 2022;**12**(10):1618. DOI: 10.3390/life12101618

[9] Gilmore BF, McDougald D, Beloin C. Editorial: Insights in biofilms: 2021. Frontiers in Cellular and Infection Microbiology. 2022;**12**:1093692. Frontiers Media S.A. DOI: 10.3389/fcimb.2022.1093692

[10] Schilcher K, Horswill AR. Staphylococcal Biofilm Development: Structure, Regulation, and Treatment Strategies. 2020. Available from: https://journals.asm.org/journal/mmbr

[11] Vani S, Vadakkan K, Mani B. A narrative review on bacterial biofilm: Its formation, clinical aspects and inhibition strategies. Future Journal of Pharmaceutical Sciences. 2023;**9**(1):50. DOI: 10.1186/s43094-023-00499-9

[12] Grooters KE, Ku JC, Richter DM, Krinock MJ, Minor A, Li P, et al. Strategies for combating antibiotic resistance in bacterial biofilms. Frontiers in Cellular and Infection Microbiology. 2024;**14**:1352273. Frontiers Media SA. DOI: 10.3389/fcimb.2024.1352273

[13] Fu B, Yan Q. Exopolysaccharide is required for motility, stress tolerance, and plant colonization by the endophytic bacterium Paraburkholderia phytofirmans PsJN. Frontiers in Microbiology. 2023;**14**:1218653. DOI: 10.3389/fmicb.2023.1218653

[14] Park S, Sauer K. Controlling biofilm development through cyclic di-GMP signaling. In: Advances in Experimental Medicine and Biology. Vol. 1386. Switzerland, AG: Springer; 2022. pp. 69-94. DOI: 10.1007/978-3-031-08491-1_3

[15] Abbott C, Grout E, Morris T, Brown HL. Cutibacterium acnes biofilm forming clinical isolates modify the formation and structure of Staphylococcus aureus biofilms, increasing their susceptibility to antibiotics. Anaerobe. 2022;**76**:102580. DOI: 10.1016/j.anaerobe.2022.102580

[16] Banerjee P, Singh M, Sharma V. All rights reserved. International Journal of Pharma Research and Health Sciences. 2015;**3**(2):556-560. Available from: www.pharmahealthsciences.net

[17] McDougald D, Rice SA, Barraud N, Steinberg PD, Kjelleberg S. Should we stay or should we go: Mechanisms and ecological consequences for biofilm dispersal. Nature Reviews. Microbiology. 2011;**10**:39-50

[18] Pechaud Y, Derlon N, Queinnec I, Bessiere Y, Paul E. Modelling biofilm development: The importance of considering the link between EPS distribution, detachment mechanisms and physical properties. Water Research. 2024;**250**:120985. DOI: 10.1016/J.WATRES.2023.120985

[19] Islayem M, Agha A, Al Bataineh MT, Bataineh MS, Alazzam A. Modification of surface topographies to inhibit candida biofilm formation. PLoS One. 2024;**19**(10):e0308705. DOI: 10.1371/journal.pone.0308705

[20] Guzmán-Soto I, McTiernan C, Gonzalez-Gomez M, Ross A, Gupta K, Suuronen EJ, et al. Mimicking biofilm formation and development: Recent progress in in vitro and in vivo biofilm models. IScience. 2021;**24**(5):102443. DOI: 10.1016/J.ISCI.2021.102443

[21] Yang L et al. Biofilm formation and its association with antibiotic resistance in Staphylococcus epidermidis. Journal of Antimicrobial Chemotherapy. 2019;**74**(7):1813-1822

[22] Patel S et al. Antibiotic resistance in biofilms: Mechanisms and emerging strategies for overcoming resistance. Infectious Disease Reports. 2020;**12**(1):14-27

[23] Duarte S et al. The biofilm matrix: A dynamic interplay of components and their role in antibiotic resistance. Pathogens. 2020;**9**(3):195

[24] Nguyen et al. Biofilm-associated antibiotic resistance in clinical pathogens. Journal of Clinical Microbiology. 2018;**56**(4):e01579-e01517

[25] Sandoz KM et al. Quorum sensing in Pseudomonas aeruginosa: Implications for biofilm formation and antibiotic resistance. Microbiology Insights. 2020;**13**:1-12

[26] Gonzalez M et al. Quorum sensing and antibiotic resistance in biofilms. Microbial Drug Resistance. 2019;**25**(7):1024-1034

[27] Lo CK et al. Genetic diversity and antibiotic resistance of Staphylococcus aureus biofilms. Microbial Ecology. 2018;**76**(3):764-773

[28] Gomi R et al. Horizontal gene transfer in Escherichia coli biofilms: Implications for the spread of antibiotic resistance. Antimicrobial Agents and Chemotherapy. 2020;**64**(5):e00412-e00420

[29] Jin W et al. Biofilm formation, antimicrobial resistance, and

treatment strategies: The emerging role of metabolism. Critical Reviews in Microbiology. 2019;**45**(1):1-14

[30] Foster PL. Stress-induced mutagenesis in bacteria. Critical Reviews in Biochemistry and Molecular Biology. 2007;**42**(4):261-285

[31] Chowdhury N et al. Toxin-antitoxin systems and bacterial persistence: Implications for antimicrobial therapy. Journal of Antimicrobial Chemotherapy. 2020;**75**(2):369-376

[32] Li B et al. Persister cells in bacterial biofilms: Mechanisms and strategies for combating antibiotic resistance. Frontiers in Microbiology. 2019;**10**:1253

[33] Liao H, Friman VP, Geisen S, Zhao Q, Cui P, Lu X, et al. Horizontal gene transfer and shifts in linked bacterial community composition are associated with maintenance of antibiotic resistance genes during food waste composting. Science of the Total Environment. 2019;**660**:841-850

[34] Hall CW, Mah TF. Molecular mechanisms of biofilm-based antibiotic resistance and tolerance in pathogenic bacteria. FEMS Microbiology Reviews. 2017;**41**(3):276-301

[35] McCarthy AJ, Loeffler A, Witney AA, Gould KA, Lloyd DH, Lindsay JA. Extensive horizontal gene transfer during Staphylococcus aureus co-colonization in vivo. Genome Biology and Evolution. 2014;**6**(10):2697-2708

[36] Peters G et al. Biofilm formation and its impact on antibiotic resistance. Clinical Microbiology and Infection. 2019;**25**(6):707-714

[37] Nag M, Lahiri D, Mukherjee D, Garai S, Banerjee R, Ray RR. Biofilms and acute and chronic infections. In: Biofilm-Mediated Diseases: Causes and Controls. Springer nature, Singapore Pte Ltd; 2021. pp. 73-100

[38] Caldara M, Belgiovine C, Secchi E, Rusconi R. Environmental, microbiological, and immunological features of bacterial biofilms associated with implanted medical devices. Clinical Microbiology Reviews. 2022;**35**(2):e00221-e00220

[39] Shree P, Singh CK, Sodhi KK, Surya JN, Singh DK. Biofilms: Understanding the structure and contribution towards bacterial resistance in antibiotics. Medicine in Microecology. 2023;**16**:100084

[40] Moser C, Jensen PØ, Thomsen K, Kolpen M, Rybtke M, Lauland AS, et al. Immune responses to Pseudomonas aeruginosa biofilm infections. Frontiers in Immunology. 2021;**12**:625597

[41] Roy S. A new strategy for persister control (Doctoral Dissertation). New York: Syracuse University; 2023. Available from: https://surface.syr.edu/etd/1692

[42] Zhou Y, Zhou Z, Zheng L, Gong Z, Li Y, Jin Y, et al. Urinary tract infections caused by uropathogenic Escherichia coli: Mechanisms of infection and treatment options. International Journal of Molecular Sciences. 2023;**24**(13):10537

[43] Rouillard KR, Esther CP, Kissner WJ, Plott LM, Bowman DW, Markovetz MR, et al. Combination treatment to improve mucociliary transport of Pseudomonas aeruginosa biofilms. PLoS One. 2024;**19**(2):e0294120

[44] Kodori M, Nikmanesh B, Hakimi H, Ghalavand Z. Antibiotic susceptibility and biofilm formation of bacterial isolates derived from pediatric patients

with cystic fibrosis from Tehran, Iran. Archives of Razi Institute. 2021;**76**(2):397

[45] Guillaume O, Butnarasu C, Visentin S, Reimhult E. Interplay between biofilm microenvironment and pathogenicity of Pseudomonas aeruginosa in cystic fibrosis lung chronic infection. Biofilms. 2022;**4**:100089

[46] Elborn JS, Flume PA, Van Devanter DR, Procaccianti C. Management of chronic Pseudomonas aeruginosa infection with inhaled levofloxacin in people with cystic fibrosis. Future Microbiology. 2021;**16**(14):1087-1104

[47] Afonso AC, Oliveira D, Saavedra MJ, Borges A, Simões M. Biofilms in diabetic foot ulcers: Impact, risk factors and control strategies. International Journal of Molecular Sciences. 2021;**22**(15):8278

[48] Versey Z, da Cruz Nizer WS, Russell E, Zigic S, DeZeeuw KG, Marek JE, et al. Biofilm-innate immune interface: Contribution to chronic wound formation. Frontiers in Immunology. 2021;**12**:648554

[49] Levine JM. Pressure injury and chronic wounds. In: Geriatric Medicine: A Person Centered Evidence Based Approach. Cham: Springer International Publishing; 2024. pp. 1185-1212

[50] Drago F, Gariazzo L, Cioni M, Trave I, Parodi A. The microbiome and its relevance in complex wounds. European Journal of Dermatology. 2019;**29**:6-13

[51] Campoccia D, Montanaro L, Arciola CR. Extracellular DNA (eDNA). A major ubiquitous element of the bacterial biofilm architecture. International Journal of Molecular Sciences. 2021;**22**(16):9100. DOI: 10.3390/ijms22169100

[52] Rodríguez-Rodríguez N, Martínez-Jiménez I, García-Ojalvo A, Mendoza-Mari Y, Guillén-Nieto G, Armstrong DG, et al. Wound chronicity, impaired immunity and infection in diabetic patients. MEDICC Review. 2022;**24**:44-58

[53] Magana M, Sereti C, Ioannidis A, Mitchell CA, Ball AR, Magiorkinis E, et al. Options and limitations in clinical investigation of bacterial biofilms. Clinical Microbiology Reviews. 2018;**31**(3):10-1128

[54] Albalawi T. Strategies for detecting bacterial biofilms: Unveiling the hidden world of microbial aggregates. Egyptian Journal of Soil Science. 2024;**64**(3):1069-1096. DOI: 10.21608/ejss.2024.285393.1756

[55] Franco-Duarte R, Černáková L, Kadam S, Kaushik S, Salehi B, Bevilacqua A, et al. Advances in chemical and biological methods to identify microorganisms—From past to present. Microorganisms. 2019;7(5):130

[56] Lof M, Janus MM, Krom BP. Metabolic interactions between bacteria and fungi in commensal oral biofilms. Journal of Fungi. 2017;**3**(3):40

[57] Banerjee A, Chowdhury P, Bauri K, Saha B, De P. Inhibition and eradication of bacterial biofilm using polymeric materials. Biomaterials Science. 2023;**11**(1):11-36

[58] Singh A, Amod A, Pandey P, Bose P, Pingali MS, Shivalkar S, et al. Bacterial biofilm infections, their resistance to antibiotics therapy and current treatment strategies. Biomedical Materials. 2022;**17**(2):022003

[59] Panlilio H, Rice CV. The role of extracellular DNA in the formation, architecture, stability, and treatment of bacterial biofilms. Biotechnology and Bioengineering. 2021;**118**(6):2129-2141

[60] Salgar-Chaparro SJ, Lepkova K, Pojtanabuntoeng T, Darwin A, Machuca LL. Nutrient level determines biofilm characteristics and subsequent impact on microbial corrosion and biocide effectiveness. Applied and Environmental Microbiology. 2020;**86**(7):e02885-e02819

[61] Wu Y, Klapper I, Stewart PS. Hypoxia arising from concerted oxygen consumption by neutrophils and microorganisms in biofilms. Pathogens and Disease. 2018;**76**(4):fty043

[62] Ciemniecki JA, Newman DK. The potential for redox-active metabolites to enhance or unlock anaerobic survival metabolisms in aerobes. Journal of Bacteriology. 2020;**202**(11):10-1128

[63] Uruén C, Chopo-Escuin G, Tommassen J, Mainar-Jaime RC, Arenas J. Biofilms as promoters of bacterial antibiotic resistance and tolerance. Antibiotics. 2020;**10**(1):3

[64] Baquero F, Levin BR. Proximate and ultimate causes of the bactericidal action of antibiotics. Nature Reviews Microbiology. 2021;**19**(2):123-132

[65] Abdelhamid AG, Yousef AE. Combating bacterial biofilms: Current and emerging antibiofilm strategies for treating persistent infections. Antibiotics. 2023;**12**(6):1005

[66] Su Y, Yrastorza JT, Matis M, Cusick J, Zhao S, Wang G, et al. Biofilms: Formation, research models, potential targets, and methods for prevention and treatment. Advanced Science. John Wiley and Sons Inc; 2022;**9**(29):e2203291. DOI: 10.1002/advs.202203291

[67] Opdensteinen P, Dietz SJ, Gengenbach BB, Buyel JF. Expression of biofilm-degrading enzymes in plants and automated high-throughput activity screening using experimental Bacillus subtilis biofilms. Frontiers in Bioengineering and Biotechnology. 2021;**9**:708150. DOI: 10.3389/fbioe.2021.708150

[68] Wang S, Zhao Y, Breslawec AP, Liang T, Deng Z, Kuperman LL, et al. Strategy to combat biofilms: A focus on biofilm dispersal enzymes. npj Biofilms and Microbiomes. 2023;**9**(1):63. Nature Research. DOI: 10.1038/s41522-023-00427-y

[69] Shineh G, Mobaraki M, Perves Bappy MJ, Mills DK. Biofilm formation, and related impacts on healthcare, food processing and packaging, industrial manufacturing, marine industries, and sanitation–a review. Applied Microbiology. Multidisciplinary Digital Publishing Institute (MDPI); 2023;**3**(3):629-665. DOI: 10.3390/applmicrobiol3030044

[70] Sahli C, Moya SE, Lomas JS, Gravier-Pelletier C, Briandet R, Hémadi M. Recent advances in nanotechnology for eradicating bacterial biofilm. Theranostics. 2022;**12**(5):2383-2405. Ivyspring International Publisher. DOI: 10.7150/thno.67296

[71] Kumar L, Bisen M, Harjai K, Chhibber S, Azizov S, Lalhlenmawia H, et al. Advances in nanotechnology for biofilm inhibition. ACS Omega. 2023;**8**(24):21391-21409. American Chemical Society. DOI: 10.1021/acsomega.3c02239

[72] Blanco-Cabra N, Alcàcer-Almansa J, Admella J, Arévalo-Jaimes BV, Torrents E. Nanomedicine against biofilm infections: A roadmap of challenges and limitations. Wiley Interdisciplinary Reviews: Nanomedicine and Nanobiotechnology. John Wiley and Sons Inc; 2024;**16**(1):e1944. DOI: 10.1002/wnan.1944

[73] Mukherjee A, Bose S, Shaoo A, Das SK. Nanotechnology based therapeutic approaches: An advanced strategy to target the biofilm of ESKAPE pathogens. Materials Advances. 2023;**4**(12):2544-2572. Royal Society of Chemistry. DOI: 10.1039/d2ma00846g

[74] Kashi M, Noei M, Chegini Z, Shariati A. Natural compounds in the fight against Staphylococcus aureus biofilms: A review of antibiofilm strategies. Frontiers in Pharmacology. 2024;**15**:1491363. DOI: 10.3389/fphar.2024.1491363

[75] Qi W, Qi W, Xiong D, Long M. Quercetin: Its antioxidant mechanism, antibacterial properties and potential application in prevention and control of toxipathy. Molecules. MDPI; 2022;**27**(19):6545. DOI: 10.3390/molecules27196545

[76] Masyita A, Mustika Sari R, Dwi Astuti A, Yasir B, Rahma Rumata N, Emran TB, et al. Terpenes and terpenoids as main bioactive compounds of essential oils, their roles in human health and potential application as natural food preservatives. Food Chemistry: X. 2022;**13**:100217. DOI: 10.1016/j.fochx.2022.100217

[77] Nguyen TLA, Bhattacharya D. Antimicrobial activity of Quercetin: An approach to its mechanistic principle. Molecules. 2022;**27**(8):2494. DOI: 10.3390/molecules27082494

[78] Brackman G, Coenye T. Quorum sensing inhibitors as anti-biofilm agents. Current Pharmaceutical Design. 2015;**21**(1):5-11. DOI: 10.2174/1381612820666140905114627

[79] Hetta HF, Ramadan YN, Rashed ZI, Alharbi AA, Alsharef S, Alkindy TT, et al. Quorum sensing inhibitors: An alternative strategy to win the Battle against multidrug-resistant (MDR) bacteria. Molecules. Multidisciplinary Digital Publishing Institute (MDPI); 2024;**29**(15):3466. DOI: 10.3390/molecules29153466

[80] Pang X, Li D, Zhu J, Cheng J, Liu G. Beyond antibiotics: Photo/Sonodynamic approaches for bacterial theranostics. Nano-Micro Letters. Springer; 2020;**12**(1):144. DOI: 10.1007/s40820-020-00485-3

[81] Li Y, Sun G, Xie J, Xiao S, Lin C. Antimicrobial photodynamic therapy against oral biofilm: Influencing factors, mechanisms, and combined actions with other strategies. Frontiers in Microbiology. Frontiers Media S.A; 2023;**14**:1192955. DOI: 10.3389/fmicb.2023.1192955

[82] Pourhajibagher M, Bahrami R, Bahador A. Application of antimicrobial sonodynamic therapy as a potential treatment modality in dentistry: A literature review. Journal of Dental Sciences. 2024;**19**(2):787-794. Association for Dental Sciences of the Republic of China. DOI: 10.1016/j.jds.2023.11.006

[83] Tits J, Cammue BPA, Thevissen K. Combination therapy to treat fungal biofilm-based infections. International Journal of Molecular Sciences. 2020;**21**(22):1-19. MDPI AG. DOI: 10.3390/ijms21228873

[84] Zhang Y, Fu Y, Yu J, Ai Q, Li J, Peng N, et al. Synergy of ambroxol with vancomycin in elimination of catheter-related Staphylococcus epidermidis biofilm in vitro and in vivo. Journal of Infection and Chemotherapy. 2015;**11**:808-815

[85] Doostmohammadi A, Jooya H, Ghorbanian K, Gohari S, Dadashpour M. Potentials and future perspectives of

multi-target drugs in cancer treatment: The next generation anti-cancer agents. Cell Communication and Signaling. BioMed Central Ltd; 2024;**22**(1):228. DOI: 10.1186/s12964-024-01607-9

[86] Simonetti O, Cirioni O, Ghiselli R, Goteri G, Scalise A, Orlando F, et al. RNAIII-inhibiting peptide enhances healing of wounds infected with methicillin-resistant Staphylococcus aureus. Antimicrobial Agents and Chemotherapy. 2008;**52**(6):2205-2211. DOI: 10.1128/AAC.01340-07

[87] Eckert R, Brady KM, Greenberg EP, Qi F, Yarbrough DK, He J, et al. Enhancement of antimicrobial activity against Pseudomonas aeruginosa by coadministration of G10KHc and tobramycin. Antimicrobial Agents and Chemotherapy. 2006;**50**(11):3833-3838. DOI: 10.1128/AAC.00509-06

Chapter 4

pH Homeostasis during Dual-Species Biofilm Formation by *Bacillus subtilis* and *Escherichia coli* Strains

Ivo Ganchev

Abstract

In a large part of ecological niches, bacterial species are united in communities and develop together in the form of heterogeneous structures called biofilms, which are formed on different surfaces by the participation of one or more species as a result of their interaction. The main objective of the present work is to study the effects of pH-value in the culture medium on the biofilm development and architecture of biofilms of the bacterium (*B. subtilis*) during their interactions with *Escherichia coli* K-121655 strain. Effects of pH-value in the culture medium on bacterial biofilm formation and the mechanisms were analyzed by the crystal violet staining method combined with cultivated microbial analysis, and confocal laser scanning microscopy. In the presence of phosphate at pH-value of pH 6,0, the bacterial growth rates of single-species biofilms of *Bacillus subtilis* strains and biofilms as result of their interaction with *Escherichia coli* strains were similar and determines the mutualism between two strains in the structure of biofilms, formed by the participation of *B. subtilis* 170 and *E. coli* K-121655, *B. subtilis* 168 and *E. coli* K-121655 strains. Considering that static growth in a biofilm is a highly relevant growing state for many soil bacteria, more research on phosphate acquisition and pH homeostasis by model soil bacteria in static cultures is required to draw a more comprehensive picture of the role of biofilm production in phosphate use efficiency and pH homeostasis.

Keywords: pH homeostasis, confocal laser scanning microscopy, *Bacillus subtilis*, multispecies biofilm, microbial relationships

1. Introduction

In a large part of ecological niches, bacterial species are united in communities and develop together in the form of heterogeneous structures called biofilms, which are formed on surfaces of different nature and nature with the participation and as a result of the interaction of two or more bacterial species [1, 2]. At the basis of their formation and their resistance to the various effects of the external environment are the relationships between microorganisms, which include competition for nutrients from the composition of the medium for cultivating biofilms, antagonism, and symbiosis. The structure of biofilms and the composition of the microbial community in them are determined by the fluctuation in the values of environmental factors [3]. Changes in the values of environmental factors affect the physiological state of the cells in the structure of the forming biofilm. In the process of development, conditions are created for contacts between bacterial cells and contacts of cells with the surface on surfaces that are different in nature and morphology. Changes in environmental conditions have an impact on the properties of the bacterial cell, expressed in a change in the level of gene regulation for the implementation of the process of biofilm formation or in the charge of the cell surface, as well as on the physicochemical characteristics of the substrate [4].

The growth and development of microbial biofilms is accompanied by the biosynthesis of exocellular polysaccharides, which ensure intercellular contacts in them and their attachment to the surface of the substrate, protecting microbial cells from the influence of adverse environmental factors—the formation and secretion of surfactants produced by other microbial species, which stimulate the transition from attached state to plankton, toxic compounds, and oxidative and acid stress [5]. The formation of biofilms and the composition of the matrix forming them depend on the characteristics of the growth medium and the bacterial surface; its course is affected by the pH-value and temperature of the environment [6].

The pH-value of the environment affects the surface charge of the cells of the microbial species and the substrate, and the interaction between them in the process of biofilm formation is reversible and is based on the formation of hydrogen bonds and vander-Waals interactions. At pH 7.0, the bacterial cell and the surface layer of the substrate are distinguished by a different charge, which creates prerequisites for the adhesion of microbial cells on the surface and the formation of biofilms [3]. Maximum cell adhesion of *E. coli* O157:H7 strains to biotic surfaces was observed at a pH-value of the medium of pH 7.0, which was reduced when the pH decreased to pH 5.5 [7]. The expression of the ycfR gene in the biofilm, encoding the formation of the YcfR protein from the composition of the outer side of the cell wall, occurs when the pH-value of the culture medium is changed from pH 8.0 to pH 5.5 [8]. It includes in its structure the low molecular weight subunits YcfR, YahO, YbiJ, YbiM, YdgH, YhcN, YjfN, YjfO, and YjfY [8], and its formation inhibits the process of development of E. coli strains to biofilms as a result of the inhibition of intercellular contacts and the contact of cells with the surface layer of the substrate [9], the increase in the level of secreted indole in the intercellular space [5], and the reduction of cell hydrophobicity through the expression of other cell surface proteins such as lipoprotein OsmB [10]. Deletion in the ycfR gene in *E. coli* strains is accompanied by the expression of 30 genes that encode the biosynthesis of proteins from the structure of the periplasmic space and the outer layer of the cell wall, which leads to a change in the character of the bacterial cell surface [11] and the increase in the level of cell aggregation and the biomass of the formed biofilms [9]. The course of these regulatory processes during the formation of biofilms is also a result of the increase in the intracellular level of acetyl-phosphate from the change in pH, as a result of which conditions are created for the formation of type 1 pili and fringes, ensuring the adhesion of cells on the surface layer of the substrate and their development to the formation of biofilms [12].

The regulation of acid stress in *B. subtilis* strains in the process of their development into biofilms is carried out by extracytoplasmic σ-factors, the increase in whose activity creates conditions for increasing the resistance of their cells to the effects of antibiotic agents of a protein nature and other agents inhibiting cell wall biosynthesis [13].

DOI: http://dx.doi.org/10.5772/intechopen.1009887

Their structure contains the subunits SigO and RsoA [14], the formation of which is initiated by the decrease in the acidity value of the medium [15], while the increase in pH to pH 7.0 leads to the activation of *rsiO* gene responsible for the synthesis of the anti-sigma factor RsiO [3]. RsiO binds to the N-terminal region of SigO and thus inhibits the transcription of genes encoding the biosynthesis of alkaline stress proteins [14]. Its activation is the result of the formation of the RSiO-SigO-RsoA complex, which occurs under conditions of high acidity (pH 5.4) [13]. The formation of the σ-factors σ^X and σ^W during the development of *B. subtilis* strains on the surface layer of substrates of different nature and structure, which is stimulated by the decreasing pH value of the culture medium, leads to the activation of *abh* gene responsible for the formation of the Abh regulatory protein, which positively regulates the expression of *eps* and *yqxM* operons by reducing the level of repression initiated by the regulator AbrB, carrying the information about the biosynthesis of exocellular polysaccharides and TasA protein from the matrix structure of biofilms. At the basis of this mechanism lie the processes of expression of *slrR* gene, encoding the positive regulator for the transcription of *yqxM* operon, and activation of the eps operon in the way of increasing the expression of *slrR* gene for the transcriptional regulator SlrR, positively controlled by Abh [16].

The biosynthesis of cytoplasmic σ-factors under conditions of high acidity is accompanied by the production of antibiotic compounds of a protein nature by strains of *B. subtilis* [17], and the regulation of its synthesis takes place with the participation of the regulatory proteins AbrB, Abh, and Rok [18]. Acid stress leads to an increase in the intracellular level of the phosphorylated form of the regulator Spo0A, which specifically binds to the promoter region of *abrB* gene [19], encoding the master regulator AbrB, which represses the formation of the antibacterial peptide toxins SdpC and factors of cannibalism Skf [20]. Negative regulation on the activity of the promoter regions of *skfA* and *sdpA* genes is also carried out by the regulator Abh [21], which positively affects the synthesis of suplancin [22]. The operon for its formation during the development of *B. subtilis* strains to biofilms is part of the SPβ prophage genome, including sunA, sunT, bdbA, yolJ, and bdbB genes [23, 24]. Suplancin, secreted by *B. subtilis* strains in the process of biofilm formation, is characterized by an oligopeptide nature and includes in its structure β-methyllanthoid and disulfide bonds [25], thanks to which it is distinguished by its antagonistic activity against gram-positive bacterial species such as *Bacillus cereus*, *Staphylococcus aureus*, and *Streptococcus pyogenes* [26]. The structural *sunA* gene encodes the biosynthesis of the starting peptide containing 56 amino acid residues [24]. The transcription of the adjacent *sunT* gene determines the activity of an ABC-type transport system, including a domain with proteolytic activity, which catalyzes the hydrolysis of the peptide structure of suplancin in the process of its transfer across the cytoplasmic membrane [25]. The BdbB and BdbA domains possess a region with thiol oxidoreductase activity, thanks to which they take part in the posttranslational regulation of coplancin synthesis by *B. subtilis* strains during their development into biofilms [26].

The expression of extracytoplasmic factors creates conditions when the pH of the medium decreases to increase the activity of the regulatory protein Abh, which positively affects the formation of suplancin by *B. subtilis* strains during their development into biofilms [27]. The transcription of *abh* gene increases upon the activation of σ^X or σ^M, which leads to an increase in the amount of the synthesized antibiotic compound [28] and ensures the competitive advantage of *B. subtilis* strains in the spatial structures formed on the surface layer of the substrate at their association with other gram-positive and gram-negative bacterial species [28]. The basis of their antagonistic effect, determined by the synthesis of suplancin, is the increase in the activity of *sunA* operon, which limits the repressive influence of the negative regulator AbrB on the operon for the σ^W factor [29]. The increase in its intracytoplasmic level ensures the resistance of the antibiotics of *B. subtilis* strains in the process of biofilm formation against the effect of their secreted suplancin [30], which inhibits the spread of cells of *S. epidermidis* strains [28], *E. coli* [26], and *S. aureus* in the structure of biofilms [28]. The induction of extracytoplasmic factors in *B.subtilis* strains during the formation of biofilms, their role in the synthesis of the compound with antimicrobial effect in their association with other microbial species is carried out by different pathways and appears to be a mechanism by which they adapt to the unfavorable factors of environment. Their clarification necessitates the need to look for a relationship between the oxygen content and the formation of biofilms with the participation of two or more bacterial species. This circumstance is complemented by the peculiarities of the synthesis of the YcfR protein in *E. coli* strains, which is induced by lowering the pH-value of the medium, increasing the temperature of cultivation of vegetative cells and biofilms, the formation of H_2O_2 as a result of the course of intracellular oxidative processes or in the presence of heavy metal ions [30]. Most natural biofilms are polymicrobial in composition, but the mechanism remains unclear about how pH regulates polymicrobial biofilm development and the biofilm matrix component and spores in their structures.

The main objective of the present work is to study the effects of pH-value in the culture medium on the biofilm development and architecture of biofilms of the bacterium (*B. subtilis*) during their interactions with *Escherichia coli* K-121655 strain. Effects of pH-value in the culture medium on bacterial biofilm formation and the mechanisms were analyzed by the crystal violet staining method combined with cultivated microbial analysis, and confocal laser scanning microscopy. Taken together, the results of this study demonstrate a close link between biofilm formation and phosphates acquisition in *B. subtilis* and *E. coli* strains, allowing a better comprehension of how bacteria can cope with unfavorable pH-value under environmental conditions.

2. Material and methods

2.1 Experimental design

In the first part of this research, a dual-species model biofilm consisting of *Bacillus subtilis* and *Escherichia coli* was developed. In order to obtain a strongly adherent and mature model biofilm, different (incubation) conditions were altered, that is, growth medium. The adherence of the biofilm at each of the different (incubation) conditions was quantified by means of crystal violet staining and subsequent optical density (OD) measurements. To determine the cell density/maturity of the biofilm, viable plate counts were used. General and selective media were applied to determine the total biofilm cell density and the contribution of each individual species to this total cell density.

2.2 Bacterial strains and culture media

In this research, *Bacillus subtilis* and *Escherichia coli*, both acquired from the BCCM/LMG bacteria collection of NBIMCC, NCIPD and the “Stephan Angeloff ”Institute of Microbiology in Sofia, were used. Stock-cultures were stored

DOI: http://dx.doi.org/10.5772/intechopen.1009887

at −80°C in Luria Bertani Broth (LB, NCIPD, Sofia), which were both supplemented with 20 (v/v) % glycerol (NCIPD, Sofia). For every experiment, a purity plate was prepared by spreading a loopful of stock-culture onto a LB agar plate [Plate Count Agar (NCIPD, Sofia). The purity plates for *Bacillus subtilis* and *Escherichia coli* were incubated for 24 h at 37°C.

Starting from the purity plates, pre-cultures were prepared by transferring one colony into an Erlenmeyer flask containing 20 mL of LB medium (LB, NCIPD, Sofia). *Bacillus subtilis* and *Escherichia coli* pre-cultures were incubated for 24 h at 37°C. Following this incubation period, stationary phase cultures with a cell density of ~109 CFU/mL were obtained.

2.3 Biofilm development conditions

The stationary phase pre-cultures were used to develop a 100-fold diluted inoculum with a cell density of ~107 CFU/mL. The investigated pre-culture ratios (*Bacillus subtilis* and *Escherichia coli*) were 1:1, and the growth media was Luria Bertani Broth (NCIPD, Sofia), which proved to be the optimal media for single-species and multi-species biofilm development by *Bacillus subtilis* and *Escherichia coli*, respectively.

To develop the biofilms, 1.2 mL of the inoculum was transferred to a small Petri dish made out of polystyrene (50 mm diameter, 9 mm height, Simport, Canada). After inoculation, Petri dishes were closed and gently shaken to make sure the inoculum covered the entire surface. Dependent on the applied (incubation) conditions, Petri dishes were incubated for 24 h at 20°C, which were the optimal temperatures for *Bacillus subtilis* and *Escherichia coli* single-species and multispecies biofilm formation, respectively.

2.4 Crystal violet assay

Bacterial biofilms were developed into 96-well microtiter plates (Greiner Bio-One, Kremsmünster, Austria) with 100 μL of bacteria in post-exponential growth phase in VNSS per well. In parallel, 100 μL of cell-free culture supernatant of another strain were collected in VNSS at the beginning of the stationary growth phase and were added on the bacterial biofilms (the addition of VNSS alone was used as a control). The final OD600 nm was 0.4 into each well. After 24 h of growth in static conditions and a temperature of 20°C, samples were washed thrice with NaCl (36 $g.l^{-1}$) and dried during 30 min at room temperature. Biofilms were stained during 15 min with 200 μL of Crystal Violet at 0.01% (w/v) and rinsed thrice with NaCl (36 $g.l^{-1}$) and dried for 10 min. The quantification of biofilm was evaluated by releasing the stain from the biofilm with absolute ethanol for 10 min at 20°C, at 120 rpm and measuring the absorbance of the Crystal Violet solution at 595 nm. The final OD595 nm of each sample was divided by the blank (i.e., VNSS medium only treated with Cristal Violet).

2.5 Quantification of colonies

Each specimen was individually placed in a centrifuge tube containing 4.5 mL of sterile physiological solution, and these tubes were vortexed for 1 min to detach the biofilms from the acrylic samples. After this, aliquots of 25 μL of serial dilutions (10^{-1}, 10^{-2}, 10^{-3}, and 10^{-4}) were seeded in duplicate on Plate Count Agar (NCIPD, Sofia) and MacCocey Agar (NCIPD, Sofia) for the identification of *Bacillus subtilis* and *Escherichia coli*, respectively. Red and pink colonies grown on MacCocey Agar (NCIPD, Sofia) were presumptively identified as *Escherichia coli*. After incubation at 37°C for 24 h, the colony-forming unit per milliliter (CFU/ml) was determined and log-transformed (log10).

2.6 Multispecies biofilm formation

For the dual-species biofilm, bacteria in post-exponential growth phase were suspended in ASW and inoculated in 24 well plates (Corning Incorporated Costar®, New York, NY, United States) to a final OD600 nm of 0.3 (0.15 per strain). For the biofilms involving two bacterial strains, the final OD600 nm was 0.3 or 0.4 (0.1 per strain). Controls included single species biofilms formed in the same concentrations and conditions than the multispecies biofilm. To study the influence of the pH value of the medium on biofilm growth, nutrient media were prepared with different ratios of KH_2PO_4 and K_2HPO_4 so that the pH values were 5.0, 6.0, 7.0, and 8.0. For the purposes of the task, 18-hour cultures of *B. subtilis* 170, *B. subtilis* 168, and *E. coli* k-121,655 strains were prepared in advance in a medium broth (BulBio Laboratory - Sofia). 50 μl of the liquid cultures was inoculated into 5 cm3 liquid medium M63 (0.02 M KH_2PO_4, 0.04 M K_2HPO_4, 0.02 M $(NH_4)_2SO_4$, 0.1 mM $MgSO_4$, and 0.04 M glucose) (pH 7.0) and M63 at different ratio of KH_2PO_4 and K_2HPO_4 so that the pH of the medium is pH 5.0, pH 6.0, and pH 8.0. For each factor, the experiment was carried out in five test tubes, in the first one only 50 μl of the liquid culture of *B.subtilis* 170 strain was seeded, in the second - *B.subtilis* 168, in the third - *E.coli* K-12 1655, in the fourth tube inoculate 50 μl of the liquid culture of *B.subtilis* 170 strain and 50 μl of the liquid culture of *E.coli* K-12 1655 strain, in the fifth place inoculate 50 μl of the liquid culture of *B.subtilis* 168 strain and 50 μl of the liquid culture culture of *E.coli* K-12 1655 strain. Fresh cultures are distributed in 96-well plates. Each fresh culture was dispensed into 12 wells, placing 150 μl of the liquid fresh culture in each well. 150 μl of distilled water is dripped into the final unseeded wells. The first plate is placed at a temperature of 20°C. The cultivation of the biofilms on the plates was carried out for a duration of 24 h. After that, the plankton was separated from each well and washed three times with saline (0.85% NaCl); 150 μl of saline was placed in half of the wells, and the biofilm was peeled off using a knife previously burned and cooled in sterile saline of them, and for each variant of the experiment, the suspension is collected from 6 wells in one Eppendorf.

2.7 Matrix components staining

For matrix staining, a static biofilm of 48 h was performed. Each biofilm was stained with DAPI at 5 μg/mL (Sigma-Aldrich, Darmstadt, Germany) and one of the following matrix dyes. Exopolysaccharides were stained with the Wheat Germ Agglutinin (WGA) associated with the Alexa FluorTM 555 conjugate (Thermo Fisher Scientific, Waltham, MA, United States) at 100 μg/mL to label N-acetyl-glucosamine. After 30 min of incubation of each probe, each coverslip was washed 3 times in PBS 1×. Finally, the coverslips were mounted with a drop of ProlongTM Diamond Antifade before observation with confocal laser scanning microscopy **Leica TCS SPE** at wavelength of 540 nm.

2.8 Data extraction from images and statistics

At least three replicates and five pictures per replicate were performed and used for data extraction. The pictures have been acquired by epifluorescence microscopy or by CLSM. The percentages of recovery of epifluorescence microscopy were determined using an algorithmic method with RStudio 0.98.1025 (RStudio, Boston, MA, United States), where the brightness pixel was determined by threshold's definition of small area of picture around the pixel and against the background. Each picture has been divided in 36 pieces, which permitted empirically to render the distortion of objective negligible, and the threshold was defined as two multiplied by percentile 5th of pixel values on a small area in which the pixel was measured (Supplementary Figure S2). The biovolume, the average thickness, and the evaluation of the maximum coverage in the CLSM pictures were determined with the COMSTAT software developed in MATLAB R2015a (MathWorks, Natick, MA, United States) as previously performed [31].

To test for statistically significant differences ($P < 0.05$) between two conditions, a t-test was performed, and between different time points, a two-way analysis of variance including the Bonferroni post-test was performed using SPSS 13.0 (IBM, Armonk, NY, United States).

3. Results and discussion

The increase in the pH value of the medium between pH 5.0 and pH 6.0 in the conducted study did not create the conditions for a statically significant increase in the optical density at 540 nm ($p > 0.05$) in the co-cultivation of *B. subtilis* and *E. coli* strains. Increasing its value to pH 8.0 leads to a statistically significant decrease in the biomass of mixed biofilms ($p < 0.05$). A maximum optical density value of 0.236 ± 0.11 for the co-culture of *B. subtilis* 170 and *E. coli* K-121655 strains and 0.155 ± 0.63 for the co-cultivation of *B. subtilis* 168 and *E. coli* K-121655 strains was reached at pH value of the medium pH 6,0, which significantly ($p < 0.05$) exceeds their indicators in monospecies biofilms of *B. subtilis* and *E. coli* strains (**Figure 1**).

A number of extra cytoplasmic σ-factors take part in the regulation mechanism of the formation of biofilms by *B. subtilis* strains under conditions of changing pH-value of the medium, which affect the activity of a number of gene regions encoding resistance to the effects of antibiotic substances [24, 26], the low acidity of the environment [8], and regulation of the biosynthesis of the extracellular polymers that make up the matrix [16]. The increase in the activity of the σm-factor in *B. subtilis* 168 strain is activated at low acidity of the medium [19, 21]. Its activation plays an important role in the development of strains to form biofilms [24]. Deletion in the σ^m-factor gene in *B. subtilis* 168 strain led to a decrease in biofilm biomass in the study by Nagorska et al. [32]. These results confirm the role of the σ-factor in the process of biofilm formation at low acidity [24, 26], which can explain the exponential decrease in the optical density value at 540 after crystal violet staining of the biofilms of *B. subtilis* 170 and *B. subtilis* 168 strains and in the process of their association with *E .coli* K-121655 strain when changing the pH-value of the culture medium in the range from pH 6.0 to pH 8.0. The higher value of optical density of biofilms of *B. subtilis* 168 strain and in its association with *E. coli* K-121655 strain compared to *B. subtilis* 170 strain was associated with the different expression level of genes for σ- and anti-σ factor in the process of their cultivation at pH 5.0–6.0.

The low pH value of the biofilm culture medium of pH 4.0–5.0 inhibits the process of indole formation [6]; increasing its value to pH 9.0 induces the expression of *tnaA* gene responsible for the biosynthesis of indole [6, 8], which reduced the biomass of biofilms of *E. coli* BW25113 strains [24]. The optical density at 540 nm after staining the biofilms of *E. coli* K-121655 strain was distinguished by a value of 0.215 ± 0.09,

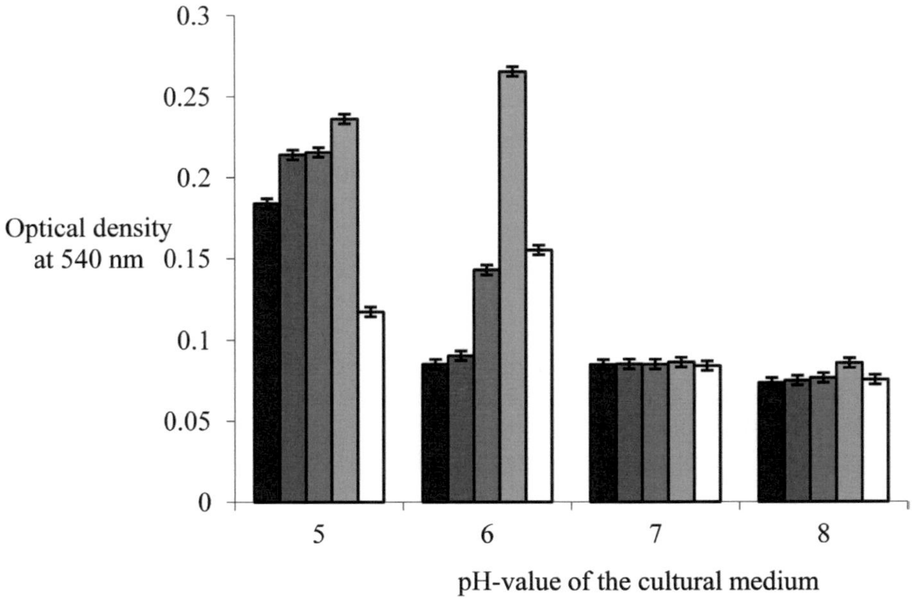

Figure 1.
The Influence of pH-value in the culture medium on the biofilm growth: ■ B. subtilis *170;* ■ B. subtilis *168;* ■ E. coli *1655;* ■ B. subtilis *170+* E. coli *1655;* □ B. subtilis *168+* E. coli *1655. The growth of biofilms was carried out in 96-well plates for a time of 24 h at temperature of 20°C in a medium M63 with different pH-value. The optical density was measured at 540 nm after staining of biofilms with 0,1% crystal violet solution.* $y = 0{,}0219.x^2 - 0{,}1428.x + 0{,}2994$, $r^2 = 0{,}9253$, $p < 0{,}05$ - B. subtilis *170.* $y = 0{,}0284.x^2 - 0{,}1842.x + 0{,}3686$, $r^2 = 0{,}9408$, $p < 0{,}05$ - B. subtilis *168.* $y = 0{,}016.x^2 - 0{,}1278.x + 0{,}329$, $r^2 = 0{,}9951$, $p < 0{,}05$ - E. coli *K-121655.* $y = -0{,}1041.x^2 + 0{,}3413.x - 0{,}001$, $r^2 = 1$, $p < 0{,}05$ - B. subtilis *170*-E. coli *K-121655.* $y = -0{,}0544.x^2 + 0{,}2009.x - 0{,}0292$, $r^2 = 1$, $p < 0{,}05$ - B. subtilis *168*-E. coli *K-121655.*

which significantly decreased to a level of 0.085, when the pH of the culture medium was changed from pH 5.0 to pH 8.0 in the present study and confirms the results of a study of Leo et al. [24]. The formation of indole by *E. coli* strains was initiated by the presence of antibiotics in the medium [5], which in the present study appeared to be the result of the development of *B. subtilis* strains. In other studies, the accumulation of indole creates the conditions for inhibiting the process of biofilm formation by inhibiting cell motility [24] and inhibiting chemotaxic movement [24–26].

The pH-value of the culture medium affected the nature of the relationships between *B. subtilis* 170 and *E. coli* K-121655 and *B. subtilis* 168 and *E. coli* K-121655 strains in the process of their co-development into biofilms in the study conducted. At pH 5.0, the microbial population of the mixed biofilm structure was dominated by *B. subtilis* 170 strains with a number reached of $9.55 \pm 0.13.10^6$ cfu/cm^3, while for *B. subtilis* 168 strain, the value was $6.38 \pm 0.\ 29.10^6$ cfu/cm^3 and statistically does not differ from their value in monospecies biofilms ($p > 0.05$). A similar regularity between the number of colonies in the structure of monospecies and mixed biofilms was found in *E. coli* K-121655 strain, whose population number was lower compared to *B. subtilis* strains. The pH-value of the medium in the range of pH 5.0 to pH 6.0 ensures the presence of cells of *E. coli* K-121655 strains in the population structure of biofilms in their association with *B. subtilis* 170 and *B. subtilis* 168 strains, as their numbers decreased from $3.16 \pm 0.12.10^6$ cfu/cm^3 to $0.40 \pm 0.05.10^6$ cfu/cm^3 in the structure of mixed biofilms when co-cultivated with *B. subtilis* 170 strain, as well as from $5.21 \pm 0.22.10^6$ cfu/cm^3 to $0.63 \pm 0.04.10^6$ cfu/cm^3 in their interaction with *B. subtilis*

168 strain. Their values are higher than their numbers in the structure of monospecies biofilms of *E. coli* K-121655 strain (**Tables 1** and **2**).

The biosynthesis of surfactin by *B. subtilis* BS5 strain is favored by an increase in the pH value of the culture medium in the range of pH 5.0 to pH 6.8 according to the study of Abdel-Mawgoud et al. [33], which corresponds to the significant increase in the number of colonies of *B. subtilis* 170 and *B. subtilis* 168 strains in their monospecies culture and in their interaction with *E. coli* K-121655 strain during the formation of biofilms in the present study. *B. subtilis* strains are distinguished by their antagonistic activity in their association with other microbial species in the rhizosphere layer of different crops thanks to their ability to synthesize surface-active agents of a lipoprotein nature that specifically inhibit cell motility and colonization of the cells of the companion species on the surface of the substrate [19, 26, 27]. The ability to secrete surfactants with anti-adhesion actions underlies the antagonistic activity of *B. subtilis* strains against *Pseudomonas syringae* strains in the rhizosphere layer of tomato plants [19].

At higher pH values of the culture medium above pH 6.0, conditions are created for the occurrence of antagonistic relationships, as a result of which biofilms are formed only with the participation of cells of *B. subtilis* strains. However, a significant decrease in population numbers of *B. subtilis* 170 and *B. subtilis* 168 strains was reported, which was found to values of 1.48 ± 0.07.10^6 cfu/cm^3 and 6.18 ± 0.20.10^6 cfu/cm^3 at reaching the pH-value of the environment of pH 8.0, which exceeds their value in monospecies biofilms, where a similar regularity is established

№	pH	Colony forming units in biofilms of *B. subtilis* 170 cfu/cm^3	Colony forming units in biofilms of *E. coli* K-121655, cfu/cm^3	Colony forming units in dual-species biofilms, cfu/cm^3	
				B. subtilis 170	*E. coli* 1655
1.	5,0	9,05 ± 0,18.10^6	1,62 ± 0,12.10^6	9,55 ± 0,13.10^6	3,16 ± 0,12.10^6
2.	6,0	8,11 ± 0,07.10^6	0,26 ± 0,03.10^6	35,91 ± 0,05.10^6	0,40 ± 0,05.10^6
3.	7,0	0,56 ± 0,07.10^6	0	10,95 ± 0,13.10^6	0
4.	8,0	0,23 ± 0,03.10^6	0	6,18 ± 0,20.10^6	0

Table 1.
The impact of pH-value of the cultural medium on colony forming units of B. subtilis *170 and* E. coli *1655 strains in the structures of single-species and dual-species biofilms.*

№	pH	Colony forming units in biofilms of *B. subtilis* 168, cfu/cm^3	Colony forming units in biofilms of *E. coli* K-121655, cfu/cm^3	Colony forming units in dual-species biofilms, cfu/cm^3	
				B. subtilis 168	*E. coli* K-121655
1.	5,0	8,08 ± 0,20.10^6	1,62 ± 0,12.10^6	6,38 ± 0,29.10^6	5,21 ± 0,22.10^6
2.	6,0	7,66 ± 0,07.10^6	0,26 ± 0,03.10^6	39,01 ± 0,16.10^6	0,63 ± 0,04.10^6
3.	7,0	0,36 ± 0.05.10^6	0	9,05 ± 0,05.10^6	0
4.	8,0	0,27 ± 0,06.10^6	0	1,48 ± 0,07.10^6	0

Table 2.
The impact of pH-value of the cultural medium on colony forming units of B. subtilis *168 and* E. coli *1655 strains in the structures of single-species and dual-species biofilms.*

in the investigated pH-interval. Media pH above 7.0 inhibits the formation and secretion of surfactin in *B. subtilis* strain [33], which appears to be a signaling molecule during its development in a surface-attached state [26] and contributes to the maturation of the formed structures [2]. Inhibition of surfactin synthesis at pH in the range of pH 7.0 to pH 8.0 explains the decrease in population numbers of *B. subtilis* 170 and *B. subtilis* 168 strains in the structure of mixed biofilms in their interaction with *E. coli* K-121655 strain in the present study.

Indole, formed by *E. coli* strains in its association with other bacterial species, represses the formation of biofilms [24], which is determined by its binding to SdiA, which is distinguished by the property of forming complexes with homoserine lactones [8, 24]. The same lactone exerts a stimulating effect on the formation of biofilms by *Pseudomonas* strains, which are characterized by oxygenase activity, allowing the reduction of its concentration in the process of biofilm formation [24]. An increase in the activity of SdiA is accompanied by a decrease in the transcription level of *ftsQ2p* gene, responsible for the acid resistance of *E. coli* strains [24, 25], which explains the lower number of their population in the structure of biofilms compared to *E. coli* K-121655 strains, when changing the pH in the range of pH 5.0 to pH 6.0.

In acidic media (pH 5.0), *B. subtilis* and *E. coli* strains formed biofilms with a rough surface with an average thickness of 8.14 ± 0.48 μm to 8.46 ± 0.37 μm at a roughness factor of 0, 04 ± 0.03 to 0.03 ± 0.01, which increased to a value of 10.35 ± 0.41 μm upon reaching the pH-value of the medium of pH 6.0 in the co-cultivation of the pair of *B. subtilis* 170 and *E. coli* K-121655 strains, and the inequality coefficient kept a relatively constant value ($p < 0.05$) (**Figures 2** and **3**). The average thickness of the structures formed as a result of the development of the pair of *B. subtilis* 170 and *E. coli* K-121655 strains is characterized by a value of 10.78 ± 0.37 μm under the same cultivation conditions. In neutral and alkaline media, the relative proportion of biofilm dispersion zones increases, which correlates with a decrease in the diameter o the structures in the narrow range of 3.02 ± 0.23 μm and 3.01 ± 0.05 μm in the pair of *B. subtilis* 170 and *E. coli* K-121655 strains, while in *B. subtilis* 168 and *E. coli* K-121655 strains, single structures with the same size of the average thickness were found at the pH of the medium in the range of pH 7.0 to pH 8 .0 in the conducted survey. These results positively correlate with optical density values at 570 nm after crystal violet staining and with the change in population numbers of *B. subtilis* strains in the structure of mixed biofilms, which changes inversely with the magnitude of the ratio of the area of the structures formed to their volume during the conducted survey. It reached a minimum value of 0.09 ± 0.006 $\mu m^2.\mu m^{-3}$ for the pair of *B. subtilis* 170 and *E. coli* K-121655 strains and 0.09 ± 0.009 $\mu m^2.\mu m^{-3}$ for *B. subtilis* 168 and *E. coli* K-121655 strains at a pH of 6.0 of the biofilm culture medium, immediately after which an increase in its size was observed as a result of the change in the pH value to pH 7.0, which remained at the same level at pH 8,0 (**Table 3**).

An important feature in the formation of biofilms, involving cells of *B. subtilis* strains, is the biosynthesis of the exocellular matrix [34], the formation of which is encoded by *epsA-O* and *tapA-sipW-tasA* operons [7, 35]. Their transcription is determined by the activity of the regulatory proteins AbrB and Abh, whose activity is determined by the intracellular expression level of σ-factors [8], which increases under conditions of alkaline stress [24]. The Abh regulatory protein positively affects the biosynthesis of the biofilm matrix, and the activation of the transcription of the abh gene encoding occurs as a result of the interaction of the σ-factor with the RNA polymerase to activate the transcription of *abh* gene [25]. The transcription of the

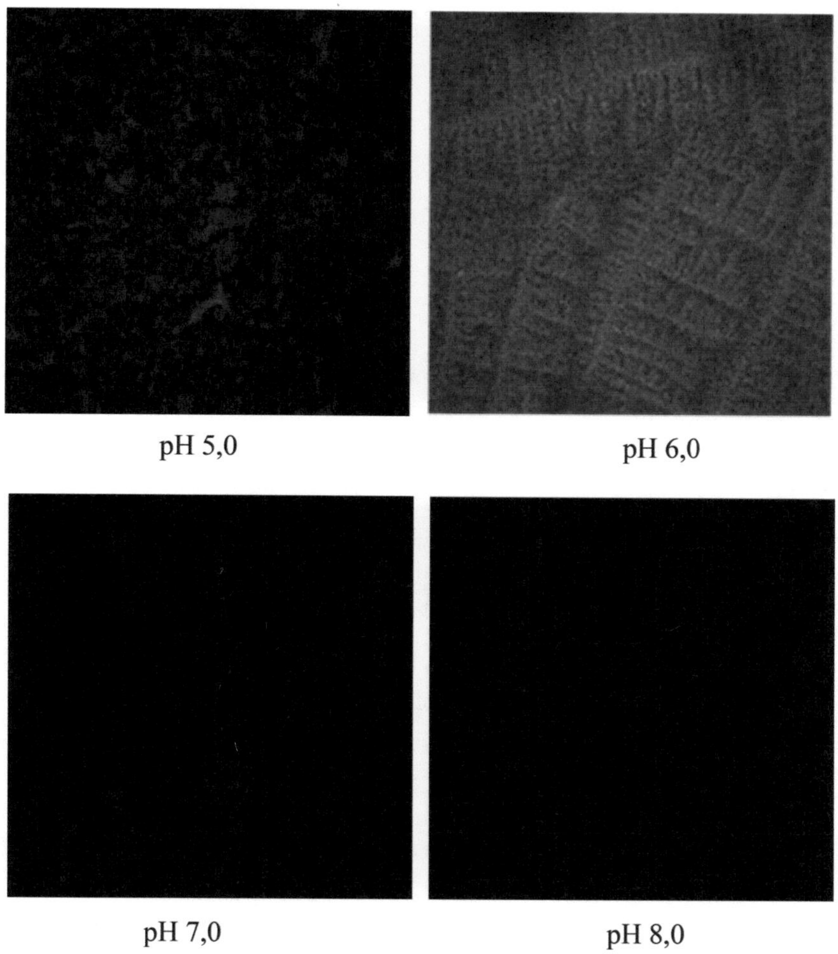

Figure 2.
Microscope study of biofilms of Bacillus subtilis *170 and* Escherichia coli *K-121655 strains at different pH-values of the cultural medium. Biofilm growth was carried out on the cover glasses for a time of 24 h at temperature of 20°C. The staining was carried out by using of complex fluorescence dye Live Bacterial Gram Stain Kit (Biotum), but the observations were carried out by using of confocal laser scanning microscopy Leica TCS SPE at wavelength of 540 nm.*

operons is not carried out directly by the regulatory protein, but with the help of the intermediary molecule RsiW, which by its nature is a protease and performs the role of an anti-sigma factor [27], as a similar regulatory mechanism is also observed in *E. coli* strains under the conditions of alkaline stress with the participation of the anti-sigma factor RseP [19]. The occurrence of this genetically complex regulatory mechanism explains the decrease in the average thickness and relative volume of the structures formed as a result of the co-development of *B. subtilis* 170 and *E. coli* K-121655, *B. subtilis* 168 and *E. coli* K- 121655 strains when changing the pH value of the culture medium in the range of pH 6.0 to pH 8.0 in the present study. The reduction of the relative volume per unit area of the formed structures is the result of the inhibition of the synthesis of the exocellar matrix, which determines the hydrophobic nature of the biofilms and ensures their adhesion to the surface of the substrate. The established regularity is in agreement with the results of the study by Helman et al. [27], according to which mutations in *yoaW* and *sipW* genes, responsible for

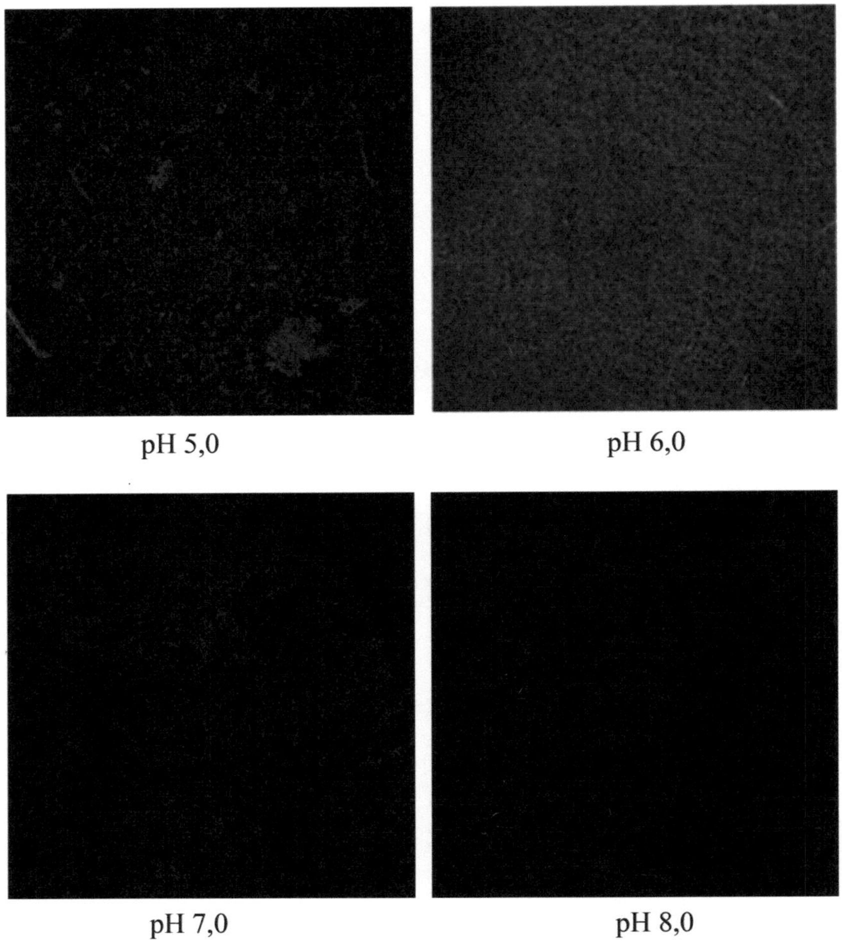

Figure 3.
Microscope study of biofilms of Bacillus subtilis *168 and* Escherichia coli *K-121655 strains at different pH-values of the cultural medium. Biofilm growth was carried out on the cover glasses for a time of 24 h at temperature of 20°C. The staining was carried out by using of complex fluorescence dye Live Bacterial Gram Stain Kit (Biotum), but the observations were carried out by using of confocal laser scanning microscopy Leica TCS SPE at a wavelength of 540 nm.*

the biosynthesis of the exocellular proteins of the biofilm matrix composition and negatively regulated by the regulator AbrB, do not lead to a change in the adhesion properties of cells of *B. subtilis* 170 strain in comparison with the starting strain. These strains form biofilms with a thickness of 8.0 ± 0.5 μm, while in the original strain, this value is of the order of 14 ± 0.7 μm [27]. A similar mechanism of reduction of the thickness of the formed structures was observed in the development of the *wcaF* mutant *E. coli* strain in the attached state [Danese et al., 2000]. Between *B. subtilis* and *E. coli* strains, there is a similarity in terms of inhibition of the process of biofilm formation, expressed in suppression of the biosynthesis of exocellular polysaccharides when the pH-value of the medium is increased [27].

The relative spreading area of the mixed biofilms formed by the co-cultivation of the pair of *B. subtilis* 170 and *E. coli* K-121655, *B. subtilis* 168 and *E. coli* K-121655 strains increases with a change in the pH value of the medium for cultivation from pH 5.0 to pH 6.0, immediately after which a strong decrease occurs when pH 7.0 is

pH	Mean thickness, µm*	Coefficient of unevenness	Relative area, μm^{2}**	Relationship area/volume, $\mu m^{2}.\mu m^{-3}$***
Dual-species biofilms of *B. subtilis* 170 and *E. coli* K-121655 strains				
5,0	8,14 ± 0,48	0,04 ± 0,03	0,65 ± 0,01	0,12 ± 0,007
6,0	10,35 ± 0,41	0,02 ± 0,06	0,99 ± 0,12	0,09 ± 0,006
7,0	3,02 ± 0,23	0,05 ± 0,02	0,23 ± 0,01	0,33 ± 0,002
8,0	3,01 ± 0,05	0,06 ± 0,04	0,15 ± 0,02	0,34 ± 0,001
Dual-species biofilms of *B. subtilis* 168 and *E. coli* K-121655 strains				
5,0	8,46 ± 0,37	0,03 ± 0,01	0,70 ± 0,01	0,11 ± 0,004
6,0	10,78 ± 0,37	0,03 ± 0,01	0,99 ± 0,00	0,09 ± 0,009
7,0	3,39 ± 0,48	0,06 ± 0,07	0,23 ± 0,01	0,30 ± 0,004
8,0	3,39 ± 0,48	0,06 ± 0,07	0,23 ± 0,01	0,30 ± 0,004

* *y = −4,77.x2 + 16,52.x-3,61,r2 = 1,p < 0,05 – B. subtilis 170-E. coli K-121655; y = −4,85.x2 + 16,85.x-3,57,r2 = 1, p < 0,05 – B. subtilis 168-E. coli K-121655.*
** *y = −0,55.x2 + 1,99.x-0,79,r2 = 1,p < 0,05 – B. subtilis 170-E. coli K-121655; y = −0,525.x2 + 1,86.x-0,64,r2 = 1, p < 0,05 – B. subtilis 168-E. coli K-121655.*
*** *y = 0,135.x2–0,435.x + 0,42,r2 = 1,p < 0,05 – B. subtilis 170-E. coli K-121655;y = 0,115.x2–0,36.x + 3,57,r2 = 1, p < 0,05 – B. subtilis 168-E. coli K-121655.*

Table 3.
Morphometric features of dual-species biofilms of B. subtilis *170 and* E. coli *K-121655 and* B. subtilis *168 and* E. coli *K-121655 strains, depending on pH-value of the cultural medium.*

reached ($p < 0.05$). Its value at pH 6.0 is 0.99 ± 0.12 μm^2 for the biofilms of the pair of *B. subtilis* 170 and *E. coli* K-121655 strains and 0.99 ± 0.00 μm^2 for the pair of *B. subtilis* 168 and *E. coli* K-121655 strains and was approximately fourfold higher as the pH of the medium increased to pH 7.0. Reaching its value to pH 8.0 is accompanied by a statistically insignificant decrease in the size of the relative area of spread of the formed structures of 0.15 ± 0.02 µm2 in the dual-species biofilms of the co-culture of *B. subtilis* 170 and *E. coli* K-121655 strains, while in *B. subtilis* 168 and *E. coli* K-121655 strains, it keeps a constant value.

The main function of the regulatory protein AbrB is reduced to the inhibition of *sipW* gene, responsible for the biosynthesis of the signal peptidase SipW, whose role in the process of biofilm formation is reduced to the secretion of proteins to the cell surface, which contributes to the adhesion and spreading of cells on the surface layer of the substrate [27] and can explain the decrease in the value of the relative spreading area of the formed biofilms as a result of the co-cultivation of the co-culture of *B. subtilis* 170 and *E. coli* K-121655, *B. subtilis* 168 and *E. coli* K-121655 strains, which was linear as the pH of the medium changed from pH 6.0 to pH 8.0 in the study. According to other studies, peptidase SipW plays an important role in the formation of adhesion of peptide nature, which ensures intercellular contacts and the biosynthesis of structures for cell motility in B. subtilis strains [19]. The inhibition of its biosynthesis explains the correlation found in the present study between the change in optical density at 540 nm after crystal violet staining of the formed mixed biofilms in the co-cultivation of the pair of *B. subtilis* 170 and *E. coli* K-121655 and *B. subtilis* 168 and *E. coli* K-121655 strains, their average thickness, and relative volume per unit area. According to other studies, regulatory proteins take part in the process of cell differentiation until the development of competence associated with the acceptance of exogenous DNA from the lysis of part of the cell population and their germination into spores [27].

The obtained results for the morphological characteristics of biofilms when the pH-value of the culture medium is changed do not correlate with the number of spores in their structure. The number of spores with the structure of multispecies biofilms of *B.subtilis* and *E.coli* strains remains relatively constant when the pH changes in the range from pH 5.0 to pH 6.0, while under the same cultivation conditions a statically insignificant increase in numbers is observed them from $0.2.10^3$ cfu/cm^3 to $0.7.10^3$ cfu/cm^3 in the co-culture of *B. subtilis* and *E. coli* strains. The increase in its value is accompanied by a significant increase in the number of spores in the structure of the mixed biofilms during the course of the study ($p < 0.05$), which at the pH of the medium of pH 8.0 reaches a value of $2.0.10^3$ cfu/cm^3 in the biofilms of *B. subtilis* 170 and *E. coli* K-121655 strains and $2.5.10^3$ cfu/cm^3 in the co-culture of *B. subtilis* 168 and *E. coli* K-121655 strains. The number of spores changed inversely proportional to the biomass of the structures formed in the conducted study, and statistically significant differences were found in the number of spores in the structure of monospecies and mixed biofilms in the present study ($p < 0.05$).

The results of the dependence of the number of spores in the structure of biofilms in the present study, formed with the participation of *B. subtilis* strains, depending on the pH value of the culture medium confirm the studies of Illades-Aguiar and Setlow [36], in which low pH ensured vegetative growth of the studied strains and inhibited sporulation. The indole formed by *E. coli* K-121655 strain in the process of its co-cultivation with *B. subtilis* 170 and *B. subtilis*168 strains at pH—the value of the medium in the range from pH 7.0 to pH 8.0—has an inducing effect on the formation of spores in the structure of biofilms [24]. The regulatory protein AbrB negatively affects the expression of genes for the formation of the biofilm matrix, and the gene encoding is activated by a high intracellular level of the core regulatory protein SpoOA, which is formed when the pH of the culture medium increases. The course of this regulatory mechanism leads to the activation of *abrB* gene, which is accompanied by an increase in the activity of *spoIIE*, *spoIIE*, and *spoIIG* genes encoding the processes occurring during the second stage of ferrospore formation in *B. subtilis* strains [22, 23]. Mutations in the genes encoding the σ-factors of the mother cell and for ferrospore formation did not significantly affect the biofilm-forming ability compared to the original or wild-type strains, suggesting that spore formation is not an obligatory mechanism for biofilm formation when the factors are changed of the environment [22], which explains the lack of correlation between the optical density at 540 nm of monospecies

№	pH	Spore forming units in biofilms of *B. subtilis* 170, cfu/cm^3	Spore forming units in biofilms of *B. subtilis* 168, cfu/cm^3	Spore forming units in dual-species biofilms, cfu/cm^3	
				B. subtilis 170 + *E. coli* 1655	*B. subtilis* 168 + *E. coli* 1655
1.	5,0	$(6{,}66 \pm 0{,}5).10^3$	$(10 \pm 0.1).10^3$	$(2{,}54 \pm 0{,}47).10^3$	$(2{,}66 \pm 0{,}5).10^3$
2.	6,0	$(0{,}2 \pm 0{,}05).10^2$	$(0{,}4 \pm 0.02).10^2$	$(0{,}12 \pm 0{,}44).10^2$	$(0{,}3 \pm 0.30).10^2$
3.	7,0	$(5{,}66 \pm 0{,}21).10^2$	$(5{,}74 \pm 0.12).10^2$	$(0{,}56 \pm 0{,}57).10^2$	$(1{,}3 \pm 0{,}46).10^2$
4.	8,0	$(6{,}01 \pm 0{,}29).10^2$	$(6{,}12 \pm 0.17).10^2$	$(2{,}96 \pm 026).10^2$	$(4{,}0 \pm 0{,}07).10^2$

Table 4.
The impact of pH-value of the cultural medium on spore forming units of B. subtilis *170,* B. subtilis *168, and* E. coli *1655 strains in the structures of single-species and dual-species biofilms.*

and mixed biofilms and the number of spores in them when the pH value of the culture medium is changed in the range of pH 5. 0 to pH 8.0 in the present study (**Table 4**).

4. Conclusion

In the presence of phosphate at pH-value of pH 6.0, the bacterial growth rates of single-species biofilms of *Bacillus subtilis* strains and biofilms as result of their interaction with *Escherichia coli* strains were similar and determines the mutualism between two strains in the structure of biofilms, but pH-value above and over of pH 6.0 lead to the impeded growth and affect adversely the process of biofilm formation by the participation of *B.subtilis* 170 and *E.coli* K-12 1655, *B.subtilis* 168 and *E.coli* K-12 1655 strains, as a result of which a decrease in the value of the optical density, average thickness, and relative spreading area and an inversely proportional increase in the ratio of the spreading area of the structures to their volume, but inhibits spore formation. Many studies on pH homeostasis by soil-drawing bacteria of *B. subtilis* strains have been performed in shaken cultures.

The importance of the interplay between extracellular matrix production and efficient phosphate acquisition and pH homeostasis might have been overlooked. Considering that static growth in a biofilm is a highly relevant growing state for many soil bacteria, more research on phosphate acquisition and pH homeostasis by model soil bacteria in static cultures is required to draw a more comprehensive picture of the role of biofilm production in phosphate use efficiency and pH homeostasis.

Acknowledgements

This research is supported by Bulgarian Ministry of Education and Science under National Science Found, Contract № KP-06-PM67/6 - SUNY BG-175467353-2022-2103-0019.

Conflict of interest

The authors declare no conflict of interest.

Author details

Ivo Ganchev
Trakia University of Stara Zagora, Stara Zagora, Bulgaria

*Address all correspondence to: ivotg@abv.bg

References

[1] Domka J, Lee J, Wood T. YliH (BssR) and YceP (BssS) regulate Escherichia coli K-12 biofilm formation by influencing cell signaling. Applied and Environmental Microbiology. 2006;**72**(4):2449-2459

[2] Rendueles O, Ghigo J. Multi-species biofilms: How to avoid unfriendly neighbors. FEMS Microbiology Reviews. 2012;**36**:972-989

[3] Moons P, Van Houdt R, Aertsen A, Vanoirbeek K, Engelborghs Y, Michiels CW. Role of quorum sensing and antimicrobial component production by *Serratia plymuthica* in formation of biofilms, including mixed biofilms with *Escherichia coli*. Applied and Environmental Microbiology. 2006;**72**:7294-7300

[4] Garcia-Gutierrez L, Zeriouh H, Romero D, Cubero J, de Vicente A, Perez-Garcia A. The antagonistic strain *Bacillus subtilis* UMAF6639 also confers protection to melon plants against cucurbit powdery mildew by activation of jasmonate- and salicylic acid-dependent defence responses. Microbiotechnology. 2013;**6**:264-274

[5] Kingston AW, Liao X, Helmann JD. Contributions of the sigma (W), sigma (M) and sigma (X) regulons to the lantibiotic resistome of *Bacillus subtilis*. Molecular Microbiology. 2013;**90**:502-518

[6] Hamon MA, Lazazzera BA. The sporulation transcription factor Spo0A is required for biofilm development in *Bacillus subtilis*. Molecular Microbiology. 2001;**42**(5):1199-1209

[7] Chagnot C, Agus A, Renier S, Peyrin F, Talon R, Astruc T, et al. *In vitro* colonization of the muscle extracellular matrix components by *Escherichia coli* O157:H7: The influence of growth medium, temperature and pH on initial adhesion and induction of biofilm formation by collagens I and III. PLoS One. 2013;**8**:e59386

[8] Yang K, Meng J, Huang YC. The role of the QseC quorum-sensing sensor kinase in epinephrine-enhanced motility and biofilm formation by *Escherichia coli*. Cell Biochemistry and Biophysics. 2014;**70**:391-398

[9] Dudin O, Geiselmann J, Ogasawara H, Ishihama A, Lacoura S. Repression of Flagellar genes in exponential phase by CsgD and CpxR, two crucial modulators of *Escherichia coli* biofilm formation. Journal of Bacteriology. 2013;**196**(3):707-715

[10] Hobley L, Ostrowski A, Rao FV, Bromley KM, Porter M, Prescott AR, et al. BslA is a self-assembling bacterial hydrophobin that coats the *Bacillus subtilis* biofilm. Proceedings of the National Academy of Sciences of the United States of America. 2013;**110**:13600-13605

[11] Stancik LM, Stancik DM, Schmidt B, Barnhart DM, Yoncheva YN, Slonczewski JL. pH-dependent expression of periplasmic proteins and amino acid catabolism in *Escherichia coli*. Journal of Bacteriology. 2002;**184**(15):4246-4258

[12] Tojo S, Hirooka K, Fujita Y. Expression of kinA and kinB of *Bacillus subtilis*, necessary for sporulation initiation is under positive stringent transcription control. Journal of Bacteriology. 2013

[13] Devis S, Kiehler S, Haggett L, Fujita M. Evidence that

autophosphorylation of the major sporulation kinase in *Bacillus subtilis* is able to occur in *trans*. Journal of Bacteriology. 2015;**197**(16):2675-2684

[14] McLoon AL, Guttenplan SB, Kearns DB, Kolter R, Losick R. Tracing the domestication of a biofilm-forming bacterium. Journal of Bacteriology. 2011;**193**:2027-2034

[15] Hamdallah I, Torok N, Bischof KM, Majdalani N, Chadalavada S, Mdluli N, et al. Experimental evolution of *Escherichia coli* K-12 at high pH and with RpoS induction. Applied and Environmental Microbiology. 2018;**84**(15):1-15

[16] Murray EJ, Stanley-Wall NR. The sensitivity of *Bacillus subtilis* to diverse antimicrobial compounds is influenced by Abh. Arch Microbiology. 2010;**192**:1059-1067

[17] Stein T. *Bacillus subtilis* antibiotics: Structures, syntheses and specific functions. Molecular Microbiology. 2005;**56**:845-857

[18] Chumsakul O, Takahashi H, Oshima T, Hishimoto T, Kanaya S, Ogasawara N, et al. Genome-wide binding profiles of the *Bacillus subtilis* transition state regulator AbrB and its homolog Abh reveals their interactive role in transcriptional regulation. Nucleic Acids Research. 2010;**39**(2):414-428

[19] Banse AV, Chastanet A, Rahn-Lee L, Hobbs EC, Losick R. Parallel pathways of repression and antirepression governing the transition to stationary phase in *Bacillus subtilis*. Proceedings of the National Academy of Sciences of the United States of America. 2008;**105**:15547-15552

[20] Elhariry H. Biofilm formation by endospore-froming bacilli on plastic surface under some food-related and environmental stress conditions. Journal of Biotechnology and Biochemistry. 2008;**3**(2):69-78

[21] Fujita K, Lazarovici P, Guroff G. Regulation of the differentiation of PC12 Pheochromocytoma cells. Environmental Health Perspectives. 2017;**80**:127-142

[22] Strauch MA et al. Abh and AbrB control of *Bacillus subtilis* antimicrobial gene expression. Journal of Bacteriology. 2007;**189**:7720-7732

[23] Sudiarta P, Fukushima T, Sekiguchi J. *Bacillus subtilis* CwlP of the SP-beta prophage has two novel peptidoglycan hydrolase domains, Muramidase and cross-linkage digesting D,D-endopeptidase. Journal of Biological Chemistry. 2010 http://www.jbc.org/content/early/2010/10/27/jbc.M110.156273.full.pdf

[24] Lee J, Zhang XS, Hegde M, Bentley WE, Jayaraman A, Wood TK. Indole cell signaling occurs primarily at low temperatures in *Escherichia coli*. The ISME Journal. 2008;**2**:1007-1023

[25] Christ NA, Bochmann S, Gottstein D, Duchardt-Ferner E, Hellmich UA, Düsterhus S, et al. The first structure of a lantibiotic immunity protein, SpaI from *Bacillus subtilis*, reveals a novel fold. Journal of Biological Chemistry. 2012;**M112**:401620. Available from: http://www.jbc.org/content/early/2012/08/17/jbc.M112.401620.full.pdf

[26] Kouwe T, Maarten van Dijl J. Applications of thiol-disulfide oxidoreductases for optimized in vivo production of functionally active proteins in *bacillus*. Applied Microbiology and Biotechnology. 2009;**85**:45-52

[27] Helmann JD. Deciphering a complex genetic regulatory network: The *Bacillus subtilis* σ^W protein and intrinsic resistance to antimicrobial compounds. Science Progress. 2006;**89**:243-266

[28] Sharma G, Dang S, Gupta S, Gabrani R. Antibacterial activity, cytotoxicity, and the mechanism of action of Bacteriocin from *Bacillus subtilis* GAS101. Medical Principles and Practice. 2018;**27**:186-192

[29] Butcher BG, Helmann JD. Identification of *Bacillus subtilis* W-dependent genes that provide intrinsic resistance to antimicrobial compounds produced by bacilli. Molecular Microbiology. 2006;**60**:765-782

[30] Zhang X, Garcıa-Contreras R, Wood TK. YcfR (BhsA) influences *Escherichia coli* biofilm formation through stress response and surface hydrophobicity. Journal of Bacteriology. 2007;**189**(8):3051-3062

[31] Heydorn A, Nielsen A, Hentzer M, Sternberg C, Givskov M, Ersbøll B, et al. Quantification of biofilm structures by thenovel computer program COMSTAT. Microbiology. 2000;**146**:2395-2407

[32] Nagorska K, Hinc K, Strauch MA, Obuchowski M. Influence of the _B stress factor and *yxaB*, the gene for a putative exopolysaccharidesynthase under σ^B control, on biofilm formation. Journal of Bacteriology. 2008;**190**:3546-3556

[33] Abdel-Mawgoud A, Aboulwafa M, Hassouna N. Optimization of Surfactin production by *Bacillus subtilis* Isolate BS5. Applied Biochemistry and Biotechnology. 2008;**150**:305-325

[34] Guttenplan SB, Blair KM, Kearns DB. The EpsE flagellar clutch is bifunctional and synergizes with EPS biosynthesis to promote *Bacillus subtilis* biofilm formation. PLoS Genetics. 2010;**6**:10-23

[35] Romero D, Aguilar C, Losick R, Kolter R. Amyloid fibers provide structural integrity to *Bacillus subtilis* biofilms. Proceedings of the National Academy of Sciences of the United States of America. 2010;**107**:2230-2234

[36] Illades-Aguiar B, Setlow P. Autoprocessing of the protease that degrades small, acid-soluble proteins of spores of bacillus species is triggered by low pH, dehydration, and dipicolinic acid. Journal of Bacteriology. 1994;**176**(22):7032-7037

Chapter 5

Factors Affecting Biofilm Formation and the Effects of These Factors on Bacteria

Tugba Kilic

Abstract

Biofilm structures are communities that emerge from microorganisms adhering to a surface and living in an extracellular polymer matrix (biofilm matrix). Biofilm formation is affected by various factors, such as strain type, the presence of other bacteria, extracellular polymeric substances, cell adhesion molecules, environmental conditions (such as temperature, pH, salt, relative humidity, oxygen availability, and nutrients), surface properties (such as carrier interface, hydrophobicity, wettability, and roughness), bacterial genome, hydrodynamic conditions, physicochemical properties, cell-to-cell signaling (quorum sensing), bacterial motility. Biofilm can form on the surfaces of devices used in the food and medical sectors (such as stainless steel, glass, and polyurethane) and cause device-related infections. This study presents the factors affecting biofilm formation and on which surfaces the biofilm structure is formed, especially in the food and medical sectors. Identifying the internal and external factors that influence the biofilm life cycle allows for the identification of current strategies for promoting the formation of beneficial biofilms and eliminating harmful biofilms.

Keywords: adhesion, bacteria, biofilm, biofilm-associated infections, extracellular polymeric substances, quorum sensing, surface

1. Introduction

Biofilms are bacterial communities embedded in a matrix formed by the adherence of planktonic cells to a surface and the synthesis of extracellular polymeric substances (EPS) by these attached cells [1]. The biofilm structure forms the living space of 95% of bacteria [2]. EPS in the biofilm layer constitutes the biofilm matrix [3]. The EPS matrix involves primarily extracellular polysaccharides (exPs) and contains smaller amounts of other biopolymers, including extracellular proteins (exPr), extracellular DNA (eDNA), and extracellular lipids (exLp). The macromolecular content of EPS varies depending on the diversity of microorganism species and the growth conditions of the cell [1, 3, 4]. These different EPS matrix components come together and interact. The EPS matrix is affected by various intrinsic (strain type, genotype, etc.)

and extrinsic factors (surface properties, environmental conditions, fluctuations in nutrients, physicochemicals, etc.) [5, 6]. These internal and external factors combine to produce a dynamic and heterogeneous microenvironment [5]. Moreover, microbial adhesion to surfaces is a complex process involving physicochemical, exPs, and exPr factors [7]. This inherent complexity can make the isolation and characterization of matrix components difficult [5].

Planktonic cells can attach to a surface. In this initial phase, the attachment is easily reversed but becomes strong and irreversible. Cell growth and division form a biofilm layer found everywhere life can exist [8]. Biofilm formation occurs naturally due to the balance between various chemical, physical, and biological processes [9]. Bacteria can be planktonic (free-living), but in most natural ecosystems, they prefer to grow as biofilms (sessile) at interfaces. This may be due to the nutrient concentration of the interface or adaptation to harsh conditions [8]. Biofilms in natural environments often maintain homeostasis under fluctuating and harsh environmental conditions [10]. Furthermore, biofilm formation is a survival mechanism for microorganisms and an adaptation strategy to adverse environmental conditions [6]. In addition, the EPS matrix plays an important role in bacterial physiology and ecology. These properties include structural protection, cellular interaction, nutrient utilization, horizontal gene transfer, and adaptation of bacterial populations to the environment. The matrix content varies depending on the bacterial species and the interface where the biofilm is formed. Cell migration to this interface can occur by passive mechanisms or by internal interactions of planktonic bacteria [1]. Biofilm-forming bacteria have advantages such as a greater abundance of nutrient molecules, protection from antibiotics, disinfectants, and dynamic environments, synergistic growth and survival in nutrient-deficient conditions, modification of their metabolic activities, stabilization of enzymes, promotion of ion exchange and a protective barrier formed by the EPS matrix they generate [11, 12].

Some biofilms contain only a single species, while others contain many species [13]. However, biofilms formed by multiple bacterial species are more common in the natural environment due to their ecological advantage. Mixed-species biofilms are generally more resistant to antibiofilm agents than monospecies biofilms [6]. In mixed-species biofilms, each type of component may produce different polymers. The physicochemical properties of such a biofilm matrix may differ significantly from those of purified components. Additionally, EPS components from two or more species may interact synergistically, increasing bacterial adhesion [5]. Production of EPS, such as surface-associated polysaccharides and proteins, may give a microorganism a competitive advantage in a mixed microbial community [9]. Moreover, dual-species biofilms can gain unique properties compared to their respective monoculture colonies [14]. The function and chemical compound of exPs may vary depending on the bacterial species or strain [1].

Microbial contamination on different surfaces can adversely affect human health and the environment. It can lead to significant problems in various technologies, such as food, medical, and service sectors [15, 16]. Contamination can occur at any stage of food processing industries, such as through contact of contaminated food with surfaces or food equipment. In addition, contaminants can contaminate surfaces and devices such as surgical instruments, ventricular-assisted devices, vascular catheters, urinary tracheal intubation, catheters, respiratory systems, endoscopes, orthopedic implants, pacemakers, mechanical heart valves, and needles. These contaminants can cause both food-related and healthcare-associated infections [17–19]. Understanding the relationship between surface conditions and microbial adhesion enables the improvement of new strategies to prevent bacteria and spores from adhering [15].

To prevent contamination and offer solutions different from current strategies against infections, revealing the factors that microorganisms need to form biofilms is a substantial step. If the mechanisms of surface attachment between planktonic and biofilm life forms, specific to the microorganism species, can be comprehensively explained, then we will be one step closer to the discovery of effective, cheap, and environmentally friendly biofilm prevention agents. In this context, this study aims to reveal which factors affect a microorganism's ability to form biofilms and discuss biofilms' importance in the food and medical sectors.

2. Factors affecting biofilm formation

Biofilms are considered responsible for food spoilage, epidemics, and damage to food processing equipment. Therefore, it is necessary to be well-informed about all the factors that affect the development or growth of bacteria (**Figure 1**), including the attachment surface, environmental conditions, associated bacterial cells, and electrostatic charging of the surfaces [28]. Bacterial extracellular surface components and environmental signals are vital for autoaggregation and biofilm formation. Due to their strategic location on the cell surface, outer membrane proteins, lipopolysaccharides, and proteinaceous structures such as pili and fimbriae are known to influence bacterial adhesion and autoaggregation phenotype [1, 29].

Microorganisms usually adhere fast to surfaces in which they come into contact [11]. In the biofilm life cycle, initial attachment occurs rapidly *via* physicochemical interactions between the surface and bacteria. Within a short time, gene expression changes, and biofilm structure growth begins as cells are physically attached to the surface by the EPS [17, 30]. Furthermore, the nonspecific adhesion of microorganisms to surfaces is a physicochemical phenomenon and results from electrostatic and non-electrostatic interactions between the surface of the solid and the bacteria. When electrostatic double layers connected by charged groups on each surface come into

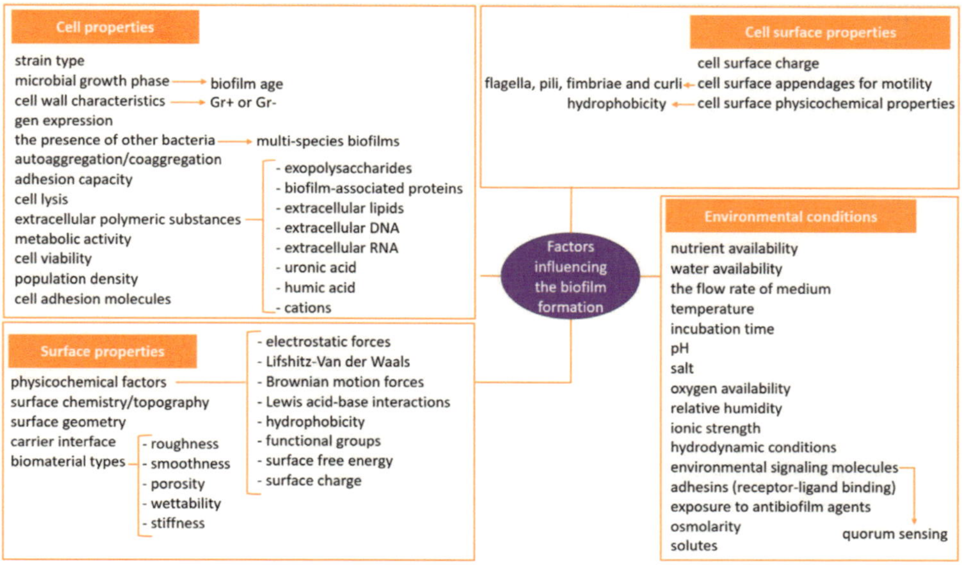

Figure 1.
Factors affecting biofilm formation [1, 5, 9, 19–27].

contact, electrostatic forces are generated between the microorganism's surface and the receiving surface. Covalent bonding, Van der Waals forces, acid-base and metallic interactions, and ionic bonding are the forces that play a role in non-electrostatic interactions [11]. To reduce or prevent microbial adhesion, it is important to know the physicochemical surface properties of microorganisms, such as Lewis acid-base or electron acceptor/electron donor character [31]. Liquids and polymer surfaces can contain three types of hydrogen-bonding molecules: (a) proton acceptors (electron donors or bases) (polystyrene and polycarbonate etc.), (b) proton donors (electron acceptors or acids) (polypropylene and polyvinyl chloride etc.), and (c) proton acceptors and donors (polyamides, polyimides, and polyvinyl alcohol etc.) [32]. In addition, bacteria may initially attach to the surface *via* flagella, pili, and fimbriae [33]. However, in a study, a swimming motility test revealed no relationship between the initial adhesion and motility of *Listeria monocytogenes*. In contrast, the cellular hydrophobicity of *L. monocytogenes* was shown to be an important feature in the initial adhesion to polyvinyl chloride and biofilm formation [34].

Depending on the type of interaction, the attachment to the surface may be transient or permanent. Under environmental conditions, bacterial cells may become irreversibly attached to the surface *via* surface adhesins. While adhesion to abiotic surfaces is generally mediated by nonspecific interactions, adhesion to biotic surfaces typically requires a specific receptor-adhesin interaction [30]. Zeta potential measurements have shown that most bacteria have a negative charge, so they will bind quickly and tightly to positively charged surfaces [35]. A hydrophobic surface, such as plastic, has a lower repulsive force than a hydrophilic surface, such as glass and metal. The decreased repulsive forces correspond to increased adhesion forces [13]. Moreover, microbial cells encounter repulsive hydrodynamic forces near the surface in a liquid environment. Bacteria often use cell surface organelles such as flagella or pili to overcome these repulsive barriers. When bacteria adhere to the surface, binding can be increased *via* adhesins, and irreversible binding can be triggered [30]. Motility *via* flagella can occur through free cells "swimming" in aqueous environments or bacterial populations "swarming" on solid, moist surfaces. If the bacteria do not have motility organelles, surface proteins play a role in initial attachment to the surface [1].

Microorganisms can communicate with each other. Cell communication is usually achieved by diverse chemical signaling molecules (autoinducers) produced and released by bacteria. In this process, called Quorum sensing (QS), bacteria communicate with each other *via* autoinducers to regulate their gene expression in response to fluctuations in bacterial cell population density [10]. QS is vital in regulating biofilm formation and its virulence [13]. QS regulates all the stages of biofilm formation [33]. Furthermore, QS modulates various cellular functions, including pathogenesis, obtaining nutrients, conjugation, motility, and secondary metabolite production [35]. Two types of QS systems are recognized in bacteria: intraspecific and interspecific communication. Intraspecific and interspecific interactions between microorganisms can be either antagonistic (such as competition for nutrients or inhibition of growth) or synergistic. Bioluminescence, virulence factor expression, antimicrobial resistance, sporulation, and maturation of microorganisms depends on complex interactions [36]. QS molecules, called autoinducers, consist of *N*-acyl homoserine lactones (AHLs), oligopeptides, and autoinducer-2. AHLs and oligopeptides are QS molecules in intraspecies communication in Gram-negative and Gram-positive bacteria, respectively. Autoinducer-2 is an interspecies communication signal in Gram-positive and Gram-negative bacteria [37]. It has been demonstrated that the QS system is required for full virulence of many important pathogenic organisms such as *Pseudomonas aeruginosa*, *Staphylococcus aureus*, *Burkholderia pseudomallei*, *Burkholderia cenocepacia*, and *Vibrio cholerae* [38]. The *las* system is a QS system that controls different physiological functions in response to cell density in many bacteria. *P. aeruginosa* requires the *las* QS signaling system to form biofilm. This system controls the synthesis of the intercellular signaling molecule *N*-(3-oxododecanoyl)-L-homoserine lactone [20]. The *Burkholderia cepacia* complex (Bcc) comprises opportunistic bacterial pathogens. These species cause cystic fibrosis and immunosuppression. These bacteria can use two chemical languages: AHLs and *cis*-2-unsaturated fatty acids [39].

Bacteria that form biofilms compete for nutrients and habitat. This competition can result in the production of toxins that aim to inhibit or kill neighboring cells. Additionally, bacteria can adapt to nutrient depletion and other environmental stresses by regulating their metabolism, gene expression, and protein synthesis, often resulting in reduced cell division rates and metabolic activity. Differential growth rates and gene transcription among biofilms result in distinct phenotypes that determine their characteristics [40]. Monospecies biofilm communities often consist of phenotypically distinct subpopulations. The differentiation of biofilm cells may depend on the environmental conditions surrounding the cells. Different concentrations of oxygen, nutrients, ions, and chemicals create various microhabitats that provide favorable conditions for bacterial colonization [10]. Furthermore, biofilm formation is a multifactorial process that involves the properties of the bacterial cell and the biological, chemical, and physical properties of the biomaterials relative to their surface. The microbial adhesion factors are not yet fully understood [41]. However, it is known that environmental factors such as temperature and pH affect biofilm formation and can facilitate bacterial adhesion. Environmental factors regulate biofilm formation in several pathways. Mature biofilms adapt to environmental conditions to obtain the best nutrients for survival and reproduction [33]. Nutrient deficiencies or low nutrient conditions stress microorganisms and trigger biofilm formation. However, if nutrient levels are consistently low, biofilms cannot mature [13].

Biofilm formation is a bacterial stress response to environmental conditions. In one study, the effects of different temperatures, pH, salt, glucose, and lactose concentrations on the biofilm cells of *Lactococcus lactis* subsp. *lactis* KGPMF23 and *Lactobacillus fermentum* KGPMF29 were examined. All tested glucose (0.5, 1.5, 2.5, 3.5%) and lactose (0.5, 1.5, 2.5, 3.5%) concentrations showed stimulatory effects on biofilm formation at 37°C. The biofilm formation ability of KGPMF23 was stimulated at 4 and 6.5% salt, while the biofilm formation ability of KGPMF29 was stimulated at all salt concentrations (4, 6.5, and 8%) [42]. Various factors such as temperature, time, substrate type, origin, and nutrient availability affect *L. monocytogenes* biofilm formation [43]. In *Bacillus subtilis*, the alternative sigma factor sigma B is activated by stress factors such as temperature, salt, and starvation [14]. The virulence of *Staphylococcus epidermidis*, such as its ability to produce gelatinase and slime, depends on the host and environmental factors [44]. *S. epidermidis* and *S. aureus* biofilms are governed by significant fluctuations in the pH of the medium under adverse conditions [45].

EPS comprises approximately 75–95% of the biofilm volume, with bacteria comprising 5–25% [45]. EPS secreted by individual cells provides advantages to microorganism communities, such as structural integrity and protection from environmental stress [40]. Moreover, the EPS matrix supports microbial growth and development [29]. EPS can vary across species and growth conditions and stimulates chemical communication, formation, and secretion between cells in the microbial community

[35]. In addition, EPS can be a nutrient source and electron donor/acceptor for microorganisms. The network of hollow channels between cells enables the exchange of oxygen, nutrients, and wastes [29]. EPS, and in the negative case, it prevents surface colonization due to the toxic effect of some metal ion species such as Cr [3]. The quantity of EPS varies depending on the age of the biofilms, the type of microorganisms, and the environmental conditions [46]. Changes in environmental conditions may cause the phenotype to change from planktonic to biofilm form. Furthermore, environmental conditions can affect bacterial and surface properties. exPs production serves a role in biofilm protection against environmental stress factors [9]. When a bacterial cell attaches to a surface, a series of physiological changes begin and can lead to the overproduction of exPs. These exPs help cells attach to the colonized surface and facilitate the spatial organization of different species within a biofilm [5]. Biofilm formation depends on the chemical environment. *Pseudomonas* strains can generate different exPs in soil or the human body. Furthermore, changes in biofilm composition have been observed with changing growth stages, alteration of carbon source, water availability, and toxins [47]. *S. aureus* and *S. epidermidis* are the predominant contaminants of vascular catheters, and the critical component for surface attachment is polysaccharide intercellular adhesin (PIA) [20]. Some adhesive factors such as aggregation-associated protein (Aap)/biofilm-associated protein (Bap), eDNA, and PIA can stabilize the biofilm. Although exPs are important and often essential components of the biofilm matrix, recent evidence suggests that surface proteins play a leading role in developing microbial communities [21, 33]. The exPr that comprises the EPS matrix is a mixture of secreted exPr, protein subunits of cell appendages (pili and flagella, etc.), cell surface adhesions, and outer membrane vesicle proteins. They interact with exPs and nucleic acid components to help stabilize the EPS matrix, promote surface colonization, and maintain the integrity and architecture of the biofilm [19]. Biofilm-associated proteins are Bap (*S. aureus*, and *B. cepacia*), Mus 20 (*Pseudomonas putida*), VP1443 (*Vibrio parahaemolyticus*) [21].

Biofilms are assemblages of surface-associated microbial cells [29]. Moreover, bacteria adhere to almost all natural and synthetic surfaces and are vital to survival (**Table 1**) [48]. Plastic-associated biofilms may have negative effects due to the accumulation of pathogens on the surface and the transfer of resistance genes such as antibiotics and metals [22]. Plastics, such as polycarbonate, polypropylene, polystyrene, polyamides, polyester, polyvinyl chloride, and polyethylene, are synthetic organic polymers, with 100 million tons produced annually worldwide and increasing daily production [29, 59]. In addition, stainless steels are commonly used in the food and beverage manufacturing and processing industries. Different surface properties can determine bacterial adhesion. A study evaluated the surface roughness of stainless steel by 3D polishing, brushing, grinding, and electropolishing. The results showed that the rate of adhering bacteria increased with increasing surface roughness. Bacteria adhere more to rougher surfaces because of increased interaction between the increased efficient surface area and the increased number of cracks, gaps, and spaces [15]. *S. epidermidis* adhesion to the surface may be related to the stiffness of the polymer substrate. However, the mechanisms that mediate cell surface interaction and the importance of physical properties in cell adhesion may be difficult to understand [35].

Stainless steel can be an ideal surface for bacteria to adhere to; still, it is the material most commonly used to make containers, pipes, valves, and different types of equipment in the food processing industry [60] because stainless steel is significantly more biocleanable than glass. Additionally, biofilm-associated microorganisms

Food sector	
Glass [17, 28]	Aluminum [43]
Stainless steel [17, 49, 50]	Polyurethane [51]
Ceramic [41, 51]	Polyvinyl chloride [34]
Rubber [17, 28, 43, 52]	Polystyrene [50]
Teflon [51]	Polypropylene [28, 43]
Wood [51]	Polycarbonate [43]
Medical sector	
Glass [7, 44]	Polyurethane [20]
Stainless steel [53]	Polypropylene [54]
Titanium [55]	Polyethylene [56]
Acrylic [7]	Polyethylene terephthalate [56]
Silicone [20]	Polymethyl methacrylate [57]
Cellulose [58]	Polydimethylsiloxane [53]
Teflon [58]	Polytetrafluoroethylene [57]
Polyamide [54]	Poly2-hydroxyethyl methacrylate [58]

Table 1.
Surface types are used in the food and medical sectors.

growing on a stainless steel surface can be killed by lower disinfectant concentrations than those on polymer surfaces. On stainless steel surfaces, it is important to consider the quality and age of the steel, the surface roughness, and the cleaning conditions used [11]. *L. monocytogenes* can adhere to food-contact surfaces (polystyrene, glass, stainless steel, etc.) and form biofilms [15]. In one study, the surface roughness of materials, including aluminum, rubber, polypropylene, and polycarbonate, varied greatly (0.7–3.5 $\log_{10}$ Ra) and was reported to have a positive correlation with biofilm formation ($r_s = 0.573$) [43]. *S. epidermidis* is one of the main causes of medical device-related infections, including prosthetic infections [44]. It has been found that most *S. epidermidis* strains produce more biofilm on acrylic surfaces than on glass. Therefore, a hydrophobic surface has been found to support biofilm formation on most clinical isolates of *S. epidermidis* [7].

Microbial hydrophobicity is the attractive energy between apolar or slightly polar cells immersed in an aqueous phase. In biological systems, hydrophobic interactions are generally the strongest noncovalent forces, often mediating surface adhesion [7]. Because most interface systems have multiple parameters, it is difficult to evaluate the results of most adhesion tests based solely on hydrophobicity [17]. While spreading, wetting, and adhesion are effective in the interaction of polymer surfaces with liquids (solid polymer-liquid interface), contact adhesion, hardness and scratching, friction, and wear are effective in the interaction with solids (solid polymer-solid interface). A reversible free energy change per unit area of the new interface occurs [32]. Surface-free energy correlates more with the binding force than the number of bacteria attached per unit of surface area [17].

Changes in hydrodynamic conditions can affect the structure of biofilm matrix cells. The shear rate affects the erosion rates of cells in the biofilm matrix [5]. Two mechanisms can lead to cell detachment from the biofilm: increased external shear forces or decreased internal strength [9]. The role of wettability is essential in the attachment of planktonic cells to the hydrophobic and hydrophilic biofilm carrier surface. Wettability can help overcome the electrostatic repulsion during the initial attachment between cells with different affinities (hydrophobicity-hydrophilicity) and the surface. In addition, the wettability of the biofilm colony is a result of multiple interactions with EPS, such as ionic protein, exPs, humic acid, uronic acid, eDNA, and cations. EPS contains both hydrophilic and hydrophobic components. As the biofilm matures, the role of EPS in determining the surface properties and microbial attachment-detachment interactions becomes more dominant. As a result, EPS changes the surface properties and improves cellular attachment. In addition, wettability can affect the initial biofilm attachment rate and the durability of established biofilms. In addition, roughness can increase the wettability of the surface. Rough surfaces are effective in the initial attachment and detachment of cells. Therefore, selecting the optimum roughness is important for balancing the biofilm formation and detachment rate [46]. The importance of fluid hydrodynamics for resistance to external shear forces in *P. putida* and *P. aeruginosa* biofilms has been actively studied. Observations indicated that biofilm maturation and distribution are regulated somewhat by shear forces and microenvironmental hydrodynamics [45]. One study reported that cell surface hydrophobicity increased with temperature [50]. On the other hand, it was determined that *S. epidermidis* hydrophobicity had little or no effect on surface adhesion [7].

3. Application areas

Biofilm is a significant concern in several applications, from biomedical implants and devices to food packaging and industrial equipment [61]. *Escherichia coli*, *P. aeruginosa*, *S. aureus*, *Streptococcus pneumoniae*, and *Salmonella typhimurium* can cause food poisoning and nosocomial infections [2]. *P. aeruginosa* is found in humans, animals, abiotic surfaces, food, and medical devices, and its ability to infect increases when it forms a biofilm [16].

3.1 Food sector

In the food industry, sedimentation due to gravity, the dominant mechanism in storage or fermentation tanks, turbulence of the suspension liquid in large pipeline systems, and Brownian motion are factors that initially affect the attachment of microorganisms to a surface [11]. Biofilms have been found on equipment and tools in milk processing plants, including bends in pipes, gaskets, floors, and milk-handling devices [49].

Adequate nutrients on food and food processing surfaces create ideal conditions for microbial growth and attachment [62]. In the food industry, the binding surface properties (hydrophobicity, electrostatic charging, interface roughness, topography, etc.) affect the overall hygiene of the surface as they affect biofilm formation [28]. Microscope analysis has determined that smooth stainless steel surfaces can be damaged by mechanical cleaning and that bacteria and organic residues can adhere to small cracks and scratches formed on the surfaces [50]. Type 304 stainless steel is the most widely used food-contact material in the food industry because it is easy to clean and resistant to extreme corrosion at different processing temperatures [28].

Biofilms can form on processing environment surfaces and food, causing cross-contamination and post-process contamination. Thus, microbial colonization can be found on food surfaces, packaging material surfaces, milk storage tanks and heat exchange equipment [17]. *S. aureus* is a pathogenic bacterium that forms biofilms on food processing surfaces [50]. Moreover, *Streptococcus thermophilus* is a well-known contaminant strain of heat exchanger plates in the dairy industry [63]. *Bacillus cereus* spores in raw milk could remain in heat exchange equipment and grow out, contaminating the product [17]. Furthermore, the commonly isolated pathogens were *L. monocytogenes*, *Salmonella* spp., *E. coli*, *Vibrio* spp., *Campylobacter jejuni*, and *Clostridium perfringens* in the food sector. During milk processing, thermophilic streptococcal strains can adhere to pasteurizers' heat exchanger plates and lead to pasteurized product contamination, adversely affecting their taste [64].

3.2 Medial sector

Typical biologically important interfaces include the cell surface-synthetic biomaterial, EPS matrix-biomolecule, EPS matrix-cell, hydrated tissue-air (lung), and mineral-protein (bone) [58]. Biofilm may form on biological implants and drug-delivery devices [62, 65]. Biofilm formation after protein adsorption on biological implants reduces the effectiveness of the devices and may lead to harmful side effects such as thrombosis. Biofilm may form at the interface between bone and the implant surface. Moreover, infection around orthopedic implants and in chronic osteomyelitis is associated with developing bacterial biofilm, a barrier to antibiotics. One solution to this problem could be delivering antibacterial drugs by local carriers. The ideal vehicle should provide high local antibiotic concentrations above the minimal inhibitory concentrations for most common pathogens without causing systemic toxicity [65].

The biofilm cells that develop on carrier surfaces are more resistant than planktonic cells in terms of survival mechanisms [46]. In addition, biofilm-associated bacteria may exhibit different characteristics than planktonic cells, such as different physiology, immune system, and high antibiotic resistance, making biofilms a source of chronic and persistent infection [9]. It was observed that *P. aeruginosa*, which formed a biofilm on the catheter surface, was still viable after 1000 μg/mL tobramycin exposure for 12 hours. Two mechanisms can explain antibiotic resistance. First, the biofilm matrix absorbs and degrades antibiotics, forming a strong barrier and limiting their penetration. Second, bacteria within the biofilm can slow down their metabolism when exposed to antibiotics, thus reducing their uptake and sensitivity to antibiotics [66].

The most common bacterial microorganisms that cause biofilm infections are *S. epidermidis*, *S. aureus*, *P. aeruginosa*, *Haemophilus* spp., *Acinetobacter* spp., and Enterobacteriaceae [67]. Moreover, most microorganisms that cause hospital infections are biofilm producers, and due to this ability, they can adhere to abiotic surfaces and cause initial catheter infections and later bloodstream infections. Hospital-acquired infections are associated with medical insertion devices such as intravenous catheters [16]. Infections caused by microbial biofilms include intravascular catheter, prosthetic joint, and implant (such as knee and hip) infections [67, 68]. Intravenous catheter infections frequently lead to bloodstream infections, which can be a significant cause of death and healthcare costs. Furthermore, multispecies biofilms can cause infections in sterile body parts, such as urinary tract infections in patients with urinary tract catheters or ventilator-associated pneumonia in intubated patients [67].

Biofilm is a substantial problem in the medical sector because it forms on medical implants within human tissue and causes many serious chronic infections. Due to their adapted biofilm phenotypes, *S. aureus* and *S. epidermidis* are among the most important bacteria causing device-associated infections [16, 62]. Methicillin-resistant *S. aureus*'s ability to form biofilms on biotic and abiotic surfaces is the primary cause of its antibiotic resistance and pervasiveness [68]. Generally, staphylococci are the most common cause of infections associated with indwelling medical devices [67]. Moreover, coagulase-negative staphylococci can cause endovascular and catheter-related bloodstream infections. The most important virulence factor of *S. epidermidis* is its ability to adhere to devices and form biofilms [7]. Moreover, *S. epidermidis* is a significant infectious agent in patients with peritoneal dialysis catheters [44].

4. Conclusions

Identifying the regulatory mechanisms required for biofilm formation and characterizing the properties of biofilm matrix components are important for biofilm studies [14]. The exact result of some parameters, such as roughness and hydrophobicity, can vary greatly under different laboratory conditions. The lack of clear results may be due to the different methods and bacterial strains [28]. Despite these handicaps, developing methods to prevent biofilm growth and/or formation by harmful bacteria allows the detailed elucidation of the five-stage biofilm life cycle mechanism [2, 23].

The increased use of materials resistant to bacterial adhesion in the food industry can improve food safety [60]. In addition, strong hydrophobic and low-energy surfaces are preferred for biofilm control in industries due to their stability and lower interaction with living cells. Materials with surface energy between 20 and 30 mN/m are reported to be suitable antibiofilm materials [59]. One of the most promising strategies to prevent or delay biofilm formation in medical and industrial environments is to use antiadhesive coatings that release contact killers or biocidal substances. Since medical and industrial biofilms usually develop in areas with fluid movement, studying the environmental conditions during bacterial-surface interactions during initial adhesion is an important step [69]. Knowing the nature of polymers is important for applications such as organic coatings to prevent corrosion [59]. Moreover, different strategies to prevent biofilm include antibiofilm surface coatings as an environmentally friendly alternative. Nontoxic polydimethylsiloxane coatings can create self-cleaning surfaces [70].

Protein-resistant coatings can be used to inhibit bacterial attachment. These coatings can be designed to release biocidal agents (antibiotics, quaternary ammonium salts, silver, etc.) into the surrounding aqueous environment. However, alternative strategies, such as using polycations, enzymes, biocides, nanomaterials, and photoactive agents, should be developed for antibiotic- and silver-resistant pathogen strains. The most widely known photoactive material is titanium dioxide (TiO_2), which has a self-cleaning effect. Different types of surfaces, such as glass and catheters, can be coated with TiO_2 [61]. Antibiotic doses effective against planktonic forms *in vitro* are ineffective against the same bacteria in biofilm forms. Therefore, a 200–1000-fold higher concentration of the same antibiotic may be required. Effective doses for biofilm removal may be toxic to the patient [65]. Particulate drug-delivery systems are considered a promising strategy to solve problems associated with antibiotic treatments in biofilm environments [71].

The EPS matrix contains organic molecules as well as inorganic compounds such as metal ions and minerals [14]. Removing metal ions reduces the surface's chemical reactivity, rendering it less susceptible to bacterial attachment [60]. A common method of biofilm inhibition involves disrupting cellular function with substrate-associated metals. Nanoparticles such as silver are interesting for thermodynamically mediated biofilm inhibition and are more effective when used with a secondary antimicrobial component [2]. In a study, an innovative approach to direct live cell migration on patterned quasi-liquid surfaces was applied and presented as a promising strategy to prevent biofilm formation and combat biofilm-associated infections. This study induced living bacterial cells to aggregate on adhesive patterns [66].

To develop strategic measures such as increasing the use of antifouling surfaces in biofilm control studies, the factors affecting biofilm structure should be addressed individually, and the interaction mechanisms between them should be revealed on a strain-specific basis. In addition, whether there is a difference between the two life forms containing planktonic and biofilm cells in terms of EPS content or other factors should be evaluated in detail. Determining how similar biofilm matrix polymers are to planktonic cell polymers and which polymers are biofilm-specific will bring us one step closer to new biofilm control strategies. Considering biofilm control strategies' positive and negative aspects, the most effective method for humans and the environment should be selected according to bacterial species.

Author details

Tugba Kilic
Department of Medical Services and Techniques, Program of Medical Laboratory Techniques, Gazi University, Vocational School of Health Services, Ankara, Turkey

*Address all correspondence to: tugbakilic@gazi.edu.tr

References

[1] Bogino PC, de las Mercedes Oliva M, Sorroche FG, Giordano W. The role of bacterial biofilms and surface components in plant-bacterial associations. International Journal of Molecular Sciences. 2013;**14**(8):15838-15859. DOI: 10.3390/ijms140815838

[2] Cavitt TB, Carlisle JG, Dodds AR, Faulkner RA, Garfield TC, Ghebranious VN, et al. Thermodynamic surface analyses to inform biofilm resistance. Iscience. 2020;**23**(11):101702. DOI: 10.1016/j.isci.2020.101702

[3] Beech IB. Corrosion of technical materials in the presence of biofilms—Current understanding and state-of-the art methods of study. International Biodeterioration and Biodegradation. 2004;**53**(3):177-183. DOI: 10.1016/S0964-8305(03)00092-1

[4] Jakubovics NS, Shields RC, Rajarajan N, Burgess JG. Life after death: The critical role of extracellular DNA in microbial biofilms. Letters in Applied Microbiology. 2013;**57**(6):467-475. DOI: 10.1111/lam.12134

[5] Allison DG. The biofilm matrix. Biofouling. 2003;**19**(2):139-150. DOI: 10.1080/0892701031000072190

[6] Sharan M, Vijay D, Dhaka P, Bedi JS, Gill JPS. Biofilms as a microbial hazard in the food industry: A scoping review. Journal of Applied Microbiology. 2022;**133**(4):2210-2234. DOI: 10.1111/jam.15766

[7] Cerca N, Pier GB, Vilanova M, Oliveira R, Azeredo J. Quantitative analysis of adhesion and biofilm formation on hydrophilic and hydrophobic surfaces of clinical isolates of *Staphylococcus epidermidis*. Research in Microbiology. 2005;**156**(4):506-514. DOI: 10.1016/j.resmic.2005.01.007

[8] Beveridge TJ, Makin SA, Kadurugamuwa JL, Li Z. Interactions between biofilms and the environment. FEMS Microbiology Reviews. 1997;**20**(3-4):291-303. DOI: 10.1111/j.1574-6976.1997.tb00315.x

[9] Alotaibi GF, Bukhari MA. Factors influencing bacterial biofilm formation and development. American Journal of Biomedical Science and Research. 2021;**12**(6):617-626. DOI: 10.34297/AJBSR.2021.12.001820

[10] Dufour D, Leung V, Lévesque CM. Bacterial biofilm: Structure, function, and antimicrobial resistance. Endodontic Topics. 2010;**22**(1):2-16. DOI: 10.1111/j.1601-1546.2012.00277.x

[11] Boulané-Petermann L. Processes of bioadhesion on stainless steel surfaces and cleanability: A review with special reference to the food industry. Biofouling. 1996;**10**(4):275-300. DOI: 10.1080/08927019609386287

[12] Aravinthan A, Arkatkar A, Juwarkar AA, Doble M. Synergistic growth of *Bacillus* and *Pseudomonas* and its degradation potential on pretreated polypropylene. Preparative Biochemistry & Biotechnology. 2016;**46**(2):109-115. DOI: 10.1080/10826068.2014.985836

[13] Samrot AV, Abubakar Mohamed A, Faradjeva E, Si Jie L, Hooi Sze C, Arif A, et al. Mechanisms and impact of biofilms and targeting of biofilms using bioactive compounds—A review. Medicina. 2021;**57**(8):839. DOI: 10.3390/medicina57080839

[14] Arnaouteli S, Bamford NC, Stanley-Wall NR, Kovács ÁT. *Bacillus subtilis*

biofilm formation and social interactions. Nature Reviews. Microbiology. 2021;**19**(9):600-614. DOI: 10.1038/s41579-021-00540-9

[15] Bohinc K, Dražić G, Abram A, Jevšnik M, Jeršek B, Nipič D, et al. Metal surface characteristics dictate bacterial adhesion capacity. International Journal of Adhesion and Adhesives. 2016;**68**:39-46. DOI: 10.1016/j.ijadhadh.2016.01.008

[16] Cangui-Panchi SP, Ñacato-Toapanta AL, Enríquez-Martínez LJ, Reyes J, Garzon-Chavez D, Machado A. Biofilm-forming microorganisms causing hospital-acquired infections from intravenous catheter: A systematic review. Current Research in Microbial Sciences. 2022;**3**:100175. DOI: 10.1016/j.crmicr.2022.100175

[17] Brooks JD, Flint SH. Biofilms in the food industry: Problems and potential solutions. International Journal of Food Science and Technology. 2008;**43**(12):2163-2176. DOI: 10.1111/j.1365-2621.2008.01839.x

[18] Abdallah M, Benoliel C, Drider D, Dhulster P, Chihib NE. Biofilm formation and persistence on abiotic surfaces in the context of food and medical environments. Archives of Microbiology. 2014;**196**(7):453-472. DOI: 10.1007/s00203-014-0983-1

[19] Rather MA, Gupta K, Mandal M. Microbial biofilm: Formation, architecture, antibiotic resistance, and control strategies. Brazilian Journal of Microbiology. 2021;**52**:1701-1718. DOI: 10.1007/s42770-021-00624-x

[20] Danese PN. Antibiofilm approaches: Prevention of catheter colonization. Chemistry & Biology. 2002;**9**(8):873-880. DOI: 10.1016/S1074-5521(02)00192-8

[21] Latasa C, Solano C, Penadés JR, Lasa I. Biofilm-associated proteins. Comptes Rendus Biologies. 2006;**329**(11):849-857. DOI: 10.1016/j.crvi.2006.07.008

[22] Bhagwat G, O'Connor W, Grainge I, Palanisami T. Understanding the fundamental basis for biofilm formation on plastic surfaces: Role of conditioning films. Frontiers in Microbiology. 2021;**12**:687118. DOI: 10.3389/fmicb.2021.687118

[23] Kilic T, Bali EB. Biofilm control strategies in the light of biofilm-forming microorganisms. World Journal of Microbiology and Biotechnology. 2023;**39**(5):131. DOI: 10.1007/s11274-023-03584-6

[24] Felz S, Vermeulen P, van Loosdrecht MC, Lin YM. Chemical characterization methods for the analysis of structural extracellular polymeric substances (EPS). Water Research. 2019;**157**:201-208. DOI: 10.1016/j.watres.2019.03.068

[25] Feng J, Ma L, Nie J, Konkel ME, Lu X. Environmental stress-induced bacterial lysis and extracellular DNA release contribute to *Campylobacter jejuni* biofilm formation. Applied and Environmental Microbiology. 2018;**84**(5):e02068-17. DOI: 10.1128/AEM.02068-17

[26] Zikalala NE, Zikalala SA, Azizi S, Kamika IA, Nxumalo EN, Zinatizadeh AA, et al. The role of inorganic and carbon nanomaterials in surface modification to attain antibiofouling polymeric membranes for water treatment—A review. Industrial and Engineering Chemistry Research. 2023;**62**(24):9354-9380. DOI: 10.1021/acs.iecr.3c00400

[27] Kalia VC, Patel SK, Lee JK. Bacterial biofilm inhibitors: An overview.

Ecotoxicology and Environmental Safety. 2023;**264**:115389. DOI: 10.1016/j.ecoenv.2023.115389

[28] Carrascosa C, Raheem D, Ramos F, Saraiva A, Raposo A. Microbial biofilms in the food industry—A comprehensive review. International Journal of Environmental Research and Public Health. 2021;**18**(04):2014. DOI: 10.3390/ijerph18042014

[29] Moyal J, Dave PH, Wu M, Karimpour S, Brar SK, Zhong H, et al. Impacts of biofilm formation on the physicochemical properties and toxicity of microplastics: A concise review. Reviews of Environmental Contamination and Toxicology. 2023;**261**(1):8. DOI: 10.1007/s44169-023-00035-z

[30] Berne C, Ducret A, Hardy GG, Brun YV. Adhesins involved in attachment to abiotic surfaces by Gram-negative bacteria. Microbiology Spectrum. 2015;**3**(4):1-45. DOI: 10.1128/microbiolspec.MB-0018-2015

[31] Bellon-Fontaine MN, Rault J, Van Oss CJ. Microbial adhesion to solvents: A novel method to determine the electron-donor/electron-acceptor or Lewis acid-base properties of microbial cells. Colloids and Surfaces. B, Biointerfaces. 1996;**7**(1-2):47-53. DOI: 10.1016/0927-7765(96)01272-6

[32] Briggs D, Rance DG, Briscoe BJ. Surface properties. In: Allen J, Bevington JC, editors. Comprehensive Polymer Science. Vol. 2. Oxford: Pergamon; 1989. pp. 707-732. DOI: 10.1016/B978-0-08-096701-1.00060-4

[33] Zhao X, Zhao F, Wang J, Zhong N. Biofilm formation and control strategies of foodborne pathogens: Food safety perspectives. RSC Advances. 2017;**7**(58):36670-36683. DOI: 10.1039/C7RA02497E

[34] Takahashi H, Suda T, Tanaka Y, Kimura B. Cellular hydrophobicity of *Listeria monocytogenes* involves initial attachment and biofilm formation on the surface of polyvinyl chloride. Letters in Applied Microbiology. 2010;**50**(6):618-625. DOI: 10.1111/j.1472-765X.2010.02842.x

[35] Renner LD, Weibel DB. Physicochemical regulation of biofilm formation. MRS Bulletin. 2011;**36**(5):347-355. DOI: 10.1557/mrs.2011.65

[36] Mohana Sheela G, Prathyusha AMVN, Neelapu NRR, Bramhachari PV. Intra and inter-species communication in microbes: Living with complex and sociable neighbors. In: Bramhachari PV, editor. Implication of Quorum Sensing System in Biofilm Formation and Virulence. Singapore: Springer; 2018. pp. 7-16. DOI: 10.1007/978-981-13-2429-1

[37] Liu L, Zeng X, Zheng J, Zou Y, Qiu S, Dai Y. AHL-mediated quorum sensing to regulate bacterial substance and energy metabolism: A review. Microbiological Research. 2022;**262**:127102. DOI: 10.1016/j.micres.2022.127102

[38] Diggle SP, Crusz SA, Cámara M. Quorum sensing. Current Biology. 2007;**17**(21):R907-R910. DOI: 10.1016/j.cub.2007.08.045

[39] Suppiger A, Schmid N, Aguilar C, Pessi G, Eberl L. Two quorum sensing systems control biofilm formation and virulence in members of the *Burkholderia cepacia* complex. Virulence. 2013;**4**(5):400-409. DOI: 10.4161/viru.25338

[40] Dsouza FP, Dinesh S, Sharma S. Understanding the intricacies of

microbial biofilm formation and its endurance in chronic infections: A key to advancing biofilm-targeted therapeutic strategies. Archives of Microbiology. 2024;**206**(2):85. DOI: 10.1007/s00203-023-03802-7

[41] Kreve S, Dos Reis AC. Effect of surface properties of ceramic materials on bacterial adhesion: A systematic review. Journal of Esthetic and Restorative Dentistry. 2022;**34**(3):461-472. DOI: 10.1111/jerd.12799J

[42] Muruzović MŽ, Mladenović KG, Čomić LR. In vitro evaluation of resistance to environmental stress by planktonic and biofilm form of lactic acid bacteria isolated from traditionally made cheese from Serbia. Food Bioscience. 2018;**23**:54-59. DOI: 10.1016/j.fbio.2018.03.005

[43] Dygico LK, Gahan CG, Grogan H, Burgess CM. The ability of *Listeria monocytogenes* to form biofilm on surfaces relevant to the mushroom production environment. International Journal of Food Microbiology. 2020;**317**:108385. DOI: 10.1016/j.ijfoodmicro.2019.108385

[44] Chaieb K, Chehab O, Zmantar T, Rouabhia M, Mahdouani K, Bakhrouf A. In vitro effect of pH and ethanol on biofilm formation by clinical ica-positive *Staphylococcus epidermidis* strains. Annales de Microbiologie. 2007;**57**:431-437. DOI: 10.1007/BF03175085

[45] Biswas T, Ahmed M, Mondal S. Mixed species biofilm: Structure, challenge and its intricate involvement in hospital associated infections. Microbial Pathogenesis. 2024;**195**:106866. DOI: 10.1016/j.micpath.2024.106866

[46] Al-Amshawee S, Yunus MYBM, Lynam JG, Lee WH, Dai F, Dakhil IH. Roughness and wettability of biofilm carriers: A systematic review. Environmental Technology and Innovation. 2020;**21**:101233. DOI: 10.1016/j.eti.2020.101233

[47] Delolme C, Spadini L, Muris M, Causse B, Gaudet JP. Comparison of the acid–base reactivity of free-living *Pseudomonas putida* cells and biofilm. Chemical Geology. 2011;**289**(1-2):48-54. DOI: 10.1016/j.chemgeo.2011.07.007

[48] Chen Y, Harapanahalli AK, Busscher HJ, Norde W, van der Mei HC. Nanoscale cell wall deformation impacts long-range bacterial adhesion forces on surfaces. Applied and Environmental Microbiology. 2014;**80**(2):637-643. DOI: 10.1128/AEM.02745-13

[49] Cherif-Antar A, Moussa–Boudjemâa B, Didouh N, Medjahdi K, Mayo B, Flórez AB. Diversity and biofilm-forming capability of bacteria recovered from stainless steel pipes of a milk-processing dairy plant. Dairy Science and Technology. 2016;**96**:27-38. DOI: 10.1007/s13594-015-0235-4

[50] Di Ciccio P, Vergara A, Festino AR, Paludi D, Zanardi E, Ghidini S, et al. Biofilm formation by *Staphylococcus aureus* on food contact surfaces: Relationship with temperature and cell surface hydrophobicity. Food Control. 2015;**50**:930-936. DOI: 10.1016/j.foodcont.2014.10.048

[51] Zore A, Bezek K, Jevšnik M, Abram A, Runko V, Slišković I, et al. Bacterial adhesion rate on food grade ceramics and Teflon as kitchen worktop surfaces. International Journal of Food Microbiology. 2020;**332**:108764. DOI: 10.1016/j.ijfoodmicro.2020.10876

[52] Teixeira P, Lopes Z, Azeredo J, Oliveira R, Vieira MJ. Physico-chemical surface characterization of a bacterial population isolated from a milking machine. Food Microbiology.

2005;**22**(2-3):247-251. DOI: 10.1016/j.fm.2004.03.010

[53] Mishra A, Aggarwal A, Khan F. Medical device-associated infections caused by biofilm-forming microbial pathogens and controlling strategies. Antibiotics. 2024;**13**(7):623. DOI: 10.3390/antibiotics13070623

[54] Teo AJ, Mishra A, Park I, Kim YJ, Park WT, Yoon YJ. Polymeric biomaterials for medical implants and devices. ACS Biomaterials Science & Engineering. 2016;**2**(4):454-472. DOI: 10.1021/acsbiomaterials.5b00429

[55] Crawford RJ, Webb HK, Truong VK, Hasan J, Ivanova EP. Surface topographical factors influencing bacterial attachment. Advances in Colloid and Interface Science. 2012;**179**:142-149. DOI: 10.1016/j.cis.2012.06.015

[56] Paxton NC, Allenby MC, Lewis PM, Woodruff MA. Biomedical applications of polyethylene. European Polymer Journal. 2019;**118**:412-428. DOI: 10.1016/j.eurpolymj.2019.05.037

[57] Kasemo B. Biological surface science. Surface Science. 2002;**500**(1-3):656-677. DOI: 10.1016/S0039-6028(01)01809-X

[58] Castner DG, Ratner BD. Biomedical surface science: Foundations to frontiers. Surface Science. 2002;**500**(1-3):28-60. DOI: 10.1016/S0039-6028(01)01587-4

[59] Artham T, Sudhakar M, Venkatesan R, Nair CM, Murty KVGK, Doble M. Biofouling and stability of synthetic polymers in sea water. International Biodeterioration & Biodegradation. 2009;**63**(7):884-890. DOI: 10.1016/j.ibiod.2009.03.003

[60] Arnold JW, Bailey GW. Surface finishes on stainless steel reduce bacterial attachment and early biofilm formation: Scanning electron and atomic force microscopy study. Poultry Science. 2000;**79**(12):1839-1845. DOI: 10.1093/ps/79.12.1839

[61] Banerjee I, Pangule RC, Kane RS. Antifouling coatings: Recent developments in the design of surfaces that prevent fouling by proteins, bacteria, and marine organisms. Advanced Materials. 2011;**23**(6):690-718. DOI: 10.1002/adma.201001215

[62] Abebe GM. The role of bacterial biofilm in antibiotic resistance and food contamination. International Journal of Microbiology. 2020;**2020**(1):1-10. DOI: 10.1155/2020/1705814

[63] Boulangé-Petermann L, Rault J, Bellon-Fontaine MN. Adhesion of *Streptococcus thermophilus* to stainless steel with different surface topography and roughness. Biofouling. 1997;**11**(3):201-216. DOI: 10.1080/08927019709378331

[64] Bos R, Van der Mei HC, Busscher HJ. Physico-chemistry of initial microbial adhesive interactions–its mechanisms and methods for study. FEMS Microbiology Reviews. 1999;**23**(2):179-230. DOI: 10.1111/j.1574-6976.1999.tb00396.x

[65] Babiak I, Pędzisz P, Janowicz J, Małdyk P. Antimicrobial biomaterials in the prevention and local treatment of infection in orthopedics. Chirurgia Narzadów Ruchu i Ortopedia Polska. 2018;**83**(6):221-228. DOI: 10.31139/chnriop.2018.83.6.44

[66] Chen F, Boylan D, Khan FZ, Shan L, Monga D, Zimmern PE, et al. Patterning bacterial cells on quasi-liquid surfaces for biofilm morphological control. Advanced Functional Materials. 2024;**34**:2407099. DOI: 10.1002/adfm.202407099

[67] Ciofu O, Moser C, Jensen PØ, Høiby N. Tolerance and resistance of microbial biofilms. Nature Reviews. Microbiology. 2022;**20**(10):621-635. DOI: 10.1038/s41579-022-00682-4

[68] Cascioferro S, Carbone D, Parrino B, Pecoraro C, Giovannetti E, Cirrincione G, et al. Therapeutic strategies to counteract antibiotic resistance in MRSA biofilm-associated infections. ChemMedChem. 2021;**16**(1):65-80. DOI: 10.1002/cmdc.202000677

[69] Alves P, Moreira JM, Miranda JM, Mergulhão FJ. Analysing the initial bacterial adhesion to evaluate the performance of antifouling surfaces. Antibiotics. 2020;**9**(7):421. DOI: 10.3390/antibiotics9070421

[70] Cagnola GN, Cabrera JN, Negri RM, D'Accorso NB, Lizarraga L, Pettinari MJ. Biofilm formation of two different marine bacteria on modified PDMS surfaces is affected by surface roughness and topography. Current Microbiology. 2023;**80**(8):256. DOI: 10.1007/s00284-023-03370-5

[71] Da Costa D, Exbrayat-Héritier C, Rambaud B, Megy S, Terreux R, Verrier B, et al. Surface charge modulation of rifampicin-loaded PLA nanoparticles to improve antibiotic delivery in *Staphylococcus aureus* biofilms. Journal of Nanbiotechnology. 2021;**19**:1-17. DOI: 10.1186/s12951-020-00760-w

Chapter 6

Persisters of Bacterial Biofilms

Peng Li and Siqi Yao

Abstract

Bacterial biofilms are associated with increased ability to withstand antibiotics, making it extremely difficult to treat biofilm-related infections. This chapter focuses on a unique subpopulation of bacterial biofilms, persisters, which are highly tolerant to lethal doses of antibiotics. It has been recognized that antibiotic-tolerant biofilm persisters are closely linked with recalcitrance and relapse of infectious diseases. Biofilms contribute to physiological heterogeneity of the community and offer a protective environment suitable for the formation and survival of persisters. Current evidence suggests that biofilm persisters adopt a series of molecular mechanisms to generate antibiotic tolerance. They may enter into a dormant state with reduced growth and metabolic activities, while maintaining essential biological processes such as stress responses and efflux pumps. When exposed to high concentrations of antibiotics, the majority of biofilms can be killed and only persisters survive. This raises the hypothesis that persisters are the responsible subpopulation for the antibiotic tolerance of biofilms. Therefore, targeting biofilm persisters represents a promising strategy for combatting biofilm-related infections. This chapter presents evidence supporting the clinical relevance of bacterial biofilms persisters, the uncovered mechanisms behind their antibiotic tolerance, and the development of approaches to combat bacterial biofilm infections by targeting persisters.

Keywords: persisters, antibiotic tolerance, biofilm, bacteria, infection

1. Introduction

Bacteria can live as independent free-floating cells or organize into aggregates as biofilms, and biofilm is the preferred lifestyle of bacteria [1]. Bacterial biofilms are complex community of aggregated bacteria embedded in self-produced matrix of extracellular polymeric substance (EPS). Biofilms derived from single or multiple species of bacteria account for the majority of chronic infections and represent a critical threat to human health. These biofilm infections can result from either sessile bacteria attached on various biotic/abiotic surfaces or non-surface associated aggregates formed in tissues/secretions [2]. Accumulating evidence has shown that biofilms exhibit enhanced adaptability to external stresses such as antibiotics and host immune system compared to planktonic cells [3]. In clinical settings, bacterial biofilms, located in tissues or on medical devices (e.g., catheters, prosthetics, valves, artificial joints and dentures), are extremely difficult to treat with antibiotics and become a major cause for persistent infections and therapeutic failure [4]. For a long time, researchers and clinicians have attempted to figure out the mechanisms

IntechOpen

behind the increased antibiotic resistance of biofilms even though they are formed by susceptible species. It has been recognized that the ability of biofilms to withstand antibiotics involves genetic antibiotic resistance occurring within biofilms, and more importantly phenotypic antibiotic tolerance corresponding to the biofilm lifestyle. Multiple hypotheses have been proposed to account for the phenotypic antibiotic tolerance of biofilms, such as protection of EPS, reduced growth/metabolic rate, efflux pumps, quorum sensing (QS), stress response, and formation of antibiotic-tolerant persisters [5, 6]. Among these concepts, persisters are expected to become a keystone for uncovering the exact mechanism.

Bacterial persisters refer to small subpopulations of cells that are highly tolerant to lethal doses of antibiotics and other harsh environmental conditions [7, 8]. Different from antibiotic resistant mutant, persisters are phenotypic variants of a susceptible population and their antibiotic tolerance is nonheritable and reversible. Upon antibiotic treatment, the majority of a bacterial population is killed rapidly followed by a significant decrease of killing rate, leaving persisters alive. When antibiotic treatment is interrupted, persisters are able to resuscitate and form a new population as sensitive to the antibiotic as the original one. The phenomenon was first discovered in 1942 by Hobby et al. who found that penicillin failed to kill about 1% of *Staphylococcus aureus* cells [9]. The concept of persisters was coined in 1944 by Bigger based on a similar observation [10]. However, the discovery did not draw much attention, and the importance of persisters was ignored for decades until they were identified in biofilms and linked with recalcitrant infections. Current evidence shows that biofilm persisters play a critical role in the recalcitrance and recurrence of infectious diseases [11]. The survival of persisters represents a "bet-hedging" strategy which facilitates adaptation of bacteria to unpredictable environmental challenges [12, 13]. Interestingly, akin to the ability of biofilms to withstand antibiotics, it has been demonstrated that similar strategies are used by persisters to engender antibiotic tolerance, suggesting persisters are the responsible population for intrinsic biofilm resistance. This chapter systematically summarizes the identification and clinical relevance of bacterial biofilms persisters, the mechanisms exploited by persisters to form and survive in bacterial biofilms, and the strategies to combat bacterial biofilm infections by targeting persisters.

2. Identification of bacterial biofilm persisters

It was previously assumed that rapidly growing planktonic bacteria cause acute infections, whereas slowly growing biofilms cause chronic infections [14]. Recent findings have shown that bacterial biofilms are also associated with acute infections [15]. Biofilm-related infections are insensitive to treatment with currently available antibiotics despite bacterial susceptibility, posing a severe threat to global health. Single or multiple species bacterial biofilms have been found in various organs and tissues of the body, and they can lead to persistent infections in the presence of predisposing factors. Moreover, the dispersal of biofilms is capable of causing infections in new niches. It is estimated that, about 80% of bacterial infections are associated with biofilm formation [16]. Bacterial biofilms are responsible for a series of notorious infectious diseases, including lung infection in cystic fibrosis, periodontitis, endocarditis, otitis media, osteomyelitis, chronic wound infections, and urogenital infections [17]. With the widespread use of medical devices, there is an increasing concern on medical device-related biofilm infections in clinical practice. Dependent on the bacteria species adherent on the devices, local inflammatory reactions or severe infections may be induced around the foreign bodies. Such infections are highly challenging to treat with antibiotics and removal of the infected devices is frequently the only option [18].

Bacterial biofilms can be 10–1000 times more resistant to antibiotics compared to their planktonic counterparts. Due to the high antibiotic tolerance, the treatment of biofilm infections requires prolonged therapy with higher concentrations of antibiotics in clinical practice [19]. Although most of cells in biofilms can be killed when exposed to high doses of antibiotics, a small subpopulation of antibiotic-tolerant persisters remain survival. The immune system is believed to work together with antibiotics and eliminate pathogens that escape antibiotic treatment. However, the three-dimensional biofilm structure serves as a protective barrier and shields the encased bacteria from clearance by host cells [3]. Therefore, when antibiotic therapy ceases or the concentration of antibiotics reduces, persisters can regrow and repopulate the biofilms, leading to recurrence and persistence of the biofilm infections. The identification of persisters in biofilms explains the puzzling therapeutic failures associated with biofilm infections despite the absence of antibiotic-resistant mutants. At the beginning of the twentieth century, the research team of Kim Lewis revealed the presence of persisters in *Pseudomonas aeruginosa* biofilms and put forward the hypothesis that antibiotic tolerance of biofilms is largely dependent on the persister subpopulation [20, 21]. Since then, persisters have been identified in biofilms of various predominant pathogens such as *Escherichia coli* [22], *Candida albicans* [23], *Mycobacterium tuberculosis* [24], and *Staphylococcus aureus* [25].

3. Clinical relevance of bacterial biofilms persisters

Despite the discovery of biofilm persisters in various labs, a direct link between persisters and clinical infections was missing for a long time. *P. aeruginosa* is an opportunistic pathogen that can cause severe infections in immunocompromised individuals, and most notably, it can lead to persistent biofilm infections in the lungs of patients with cystic fibrosis. Mulcahy et al. examined 35 longitudinal isolates of *P. aeruginosa* collected between the ages of 8 and 96 months in a single patient receiving prolonged antibiotic treatments. The late four isolates obtained at 92 and 96 months were high-persister (*hip*) strains that exhibited a dramatic increase in the persister level compared to the earlier isolates. Further analysis revealed that *hip* strains emerged in 10 out of 14 additional cystic fibrosis cases [26]. A similar investigation demonstrated that cancer patients with long-term oral carriage of *C. albicans* and daily chlorhexidine treatment possessed strains capable of producing higher level of persisters in the *C. albicans* biofilms, whereas no *hip* strains was isolated from patients with transient *Candida* carriage [27]. The two pioneering studies directly correlate persisters with clinical infections and implicate biofilm persisters in recalcitrance of chronic infections to antimicrobial therapy. And, the findings are in line with the selection of a *E. coli hip* mutant *hipA7 in vitro* by repetitive application of ampicillin at high doses [28]. *E. coli* is the predominant pathogen for urinary tract infections, and multidrug-tolerant *hipA7* mutants were isolated in patients with such infections, indicating persisters are important players for the recurrence of the infections [29]. In patients with recurrent bloodstream infections caused by *E. coli*, 36% isolates (4/11) collected during relapse had higher persister formation ability with reference to the initial infection isolate [30]. In a lager cohort of 39 patients suffering from cystic fibrosis, 460 longitudinal isolates of *P. aeruginosa* were subject to persister phenotype assay. In total, 19% of the isolates distributed in 56% of the patients were classified as *hip* variants. Interestingly, in a mixed biofilm model formed by *hip* variant and non-*hip* strain, the *hip* variant survived better than non-*hip* strain upon antibiotic dosing for patients. The emergence of *hip* variant contributes to strain fitness and treatment failure in cystic fibrosis airways [31]. Taken together, the identification of *hip* isolates from patient cohorts with recurrent infections has corroborated the critical role of persisters in refractory infectious diseases.

In addition, comparative genomic methods have been used to examine the genotypes of isolates from initial and recurrent episodes of infection in the same patient. Emerging evidence has indicated that recurrence of bacterial infections mainly results from relapse by initial infecting strain instead of reinfection by another strain [32]. For example, whole-genome comparison of *Burkholderia pseudomallei* isolates from patients with recurrent melioidosis revealed that the genotypes were clonal, while the chance of reinfection with the same clone was very low after months or years [33]. Therefore, it is believed that persisters are the culprit for infection relapse when there are no detectable antibiotic-resistant mutants. Importantly, the selection of *hip* mutants by prolonged antibiotic treatments raises the concern of eventual emergence of resistant mutants. Increasing evidence has shown that persisters are a group of adaptively evolving cells which promote the acquisition of genetically heritable antibiotic resistance [34–36].

Besides rendering antibiotic tolerance and resistance, it is noteworthy that persisters have evolved other strategies to persist in the host and cause therapeutic failure. Certain bacteria can enter host cells and survive intracellularly. The internalization of *M. tuberculosis*, *Salmonella*, and *S. aureus* is accompanied by intracellular persister formation and induction of antibiotic tolerance [37–39]. Persisters of the keystone periodontal pathogen, *Porphyromonas gingivalis*, maintained the ability to invade human gingival epithelial cells [40]. The intracellular persisters use host cells as sanctuary and constitute a reservoir for relapsing infections.

4. Mechanisms behind antibiotic tolerance of bacterial persisters

Persisters represent a transient and reversible state of low abundance bacteria in a whole population, making it extremely difficult to isolate and characterize them. Extensive studies have been carried out to investigate the elusive molecular mechanisms behind the formation and survival of persisters. Although the current understanding of persisters remains limited, increasing evidence has linked antibiotic tolerance of persisters with dormancy and multiple active mechanisms, such as different stress responses, efflux pumps, and QS.

Based on an elegant single-cell study by Balaban and colleagues [41], it is generally assumed that persisters can arise spontaneously in a growing bacterial population by stochastic phenotypic switch or emerge in response to environmental triggers (e.g., starvation). In the same study, it was shown that persisters are nongrowing or slowly growing cells and exist before antibiotic treatment. Given that antibiotics mainly target actively growing bacteria, slow growth could protect bacteria against antibiotic activities. Moreover, decreased metabolism and intracellular ATP level are associated with the formation and survival of persisters [7]. Therefore, a prevailing hypothesis is that persisters enter into a dormant state with drastically reduced growth and metabolic activities [42]. Toxin-antitoxin (TA) modules consisting of toxins and cognate antitoxin are closely associated with bacterial dormancy and persistence [43]. Toxins are stable proteins implicated in inhibition of essential cellular process such as DNA replication and protein translation. Antitoxins are unstable proteins or RNAs that interrupt the function of toxins. Under normal conditions, toxins and antitoxins are maintained in balance, and cell growth is not affected. When exposed to stresses, antitoxins are selectively degraded, leading to activation of toxins and subsequent cellular dormancy. Single cell analysis of *E. coli* revealed that persister formation was associated with stochastic expression of TA operon [29]. The dynamic regulation of TA systems contributes to switch between growth and dormancy of bacteria, possibly mediating their entry and exit of the persister state [44].

Although dormancy provides a paradigm to explain antibiotic tolerance, it should be noted the majority of dormant cells in a population are not persisters, and persisters can originate from growing and metabolic active cells [45, 46]. Increasing evidence suggests that mechanisms of persister formation are redundant and a series of active biological processes are organized along with dormancy to engender antibiotic tolerance. In nature, bacteria routinely encounter a myriad of stresses and have evolved corresponding protective stress responses to promote their survival. Under amino acid starvation and other nutrient limitation conditions, bacteria trigger (p)ppGpp signaling to induce stringent response. When exposed to DNA damaging pressure such as oxidative stress and fluoroquinolones, SOS response is initiated as a DNA repair system. In the presence of high levels of reactive oxygen species, adaptive oxidative stress responses are activated. Numerous studies have shown that these stress responses play important roles in bacterial persistence [7, 47]. The use of efflux pumps to reduce intracellular antibiotic level is a classical approach to induce antibiotic resistance, while recent studies show that enhanced drug efflux can also promote antibiotic tolerance [48, 49]. Furthermore, bacteria exploit the communication network QS to establish phenotypic heterogeneity and strengthen their adaptation to complex environments. Notably, various QS molecules are found to have a regulatory role in antibiotic tolerance of persisters [50–52].

5. Contribution of biofilm formation to bacterial persistence

Biofilm formation serves as a survival strategy for bacteria to cope with diverse environments, and biofilms are likely to generate higher level of persisters compared to planktonic cells [24, 53, 54]. Within the complex structure of biofilms, chemical gradients of nutrients, oxygen, and metabolic products are established, creating different micro-niches. Bacteria residing at various locations of biofilms exhibit remarkable physiological and phenotypic heterogeneity [55]. The availability of nutrients and oxygen is limited in the interior regions of biofilms. Therefore, cells in the deep layers of biofilms are associated with reduced growth and metabolic activities, entering into a dormant state. In fact, the formation of persisters in biofilms can be promoted by dormancy, TA modules, stringent response, and SOS response as suggested in planktonic cells [56–61]. In addition, control of oxidative stress is linked with antibiotic tolerance of bacterial biofilm persisters [53, 57]. The frequency of persisters is significantly reduced in biofilms formed by mutants of *Pseudomonas aeruginosa* deficient in Anr-mediated hypoxia stress, RpoS regulated stationary-phase growth, and stringent response, respectively [54].

The development and maturation bacterial biofilms are associated with the production of EPS matrix. The presence of matrix acts as a barrier to limit penetration

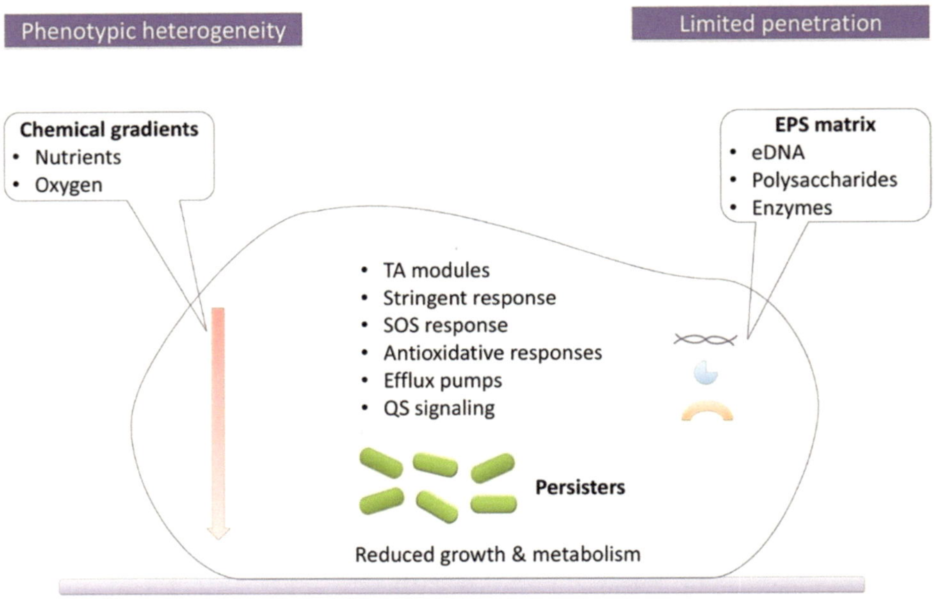

Figure 1.
The mechanisms exploited by persisters to form and survive in bacterial biofilms. Biofilm community provides an environment suitable for the formation and survival of persisters. Owing to the chemical gradients of nutrients and oxygen, biofilms are composed of heterogeneous subpopulations with different growth rates and metabolic activities. The EPS matrix contains components that can sequester antibiotics and impair antibiotic diffusion, such as extracellular DNA (eDNA), polysaccharides, and β-lactamases. This builds up microenvironments characterized by limited nutrients, oxygen, and antibiotics alone or in combination, which prepare fractional cells for the formation of persisters by inducing dormancy along with essential biological processes. When exposed to antibiotics, persisters in biofilms exploit redundant mechanisms to obtain antibiotic tolerance including TA modules, stringent response, SOS response, antioxidative response, efflux pumps, and QS signaling.

of antibiotics and other toxic substances into biofilms. For example, the negatively charged biofilm matrix components such as extracellular DNA and polysaccharide can bind to positively charged antibiotics like aminoglycosides via ionic interaction, thereby hindering antibiotic penetration [62]. Other than sequestration of antibiotics, EPS matrix contains enzymes such as β-lactamases that can inactivate antibiotics before they reach bacterial cells [63]. Therefore, the delayed and insufficient antibiotic delivery results in exposure of bacteria within biofilms to relatively low concentration of antibiotics [64]. It is of concern that sublethal levels of antibiotics enable bacteria to form more persisters tolerate to multiple antibiotics [65–68]. The reduced rate of antibiotic diffusion in biofilms may cause a dilemma that antibiotics are at levels insufficient to kill the bacteria but suitable to induce antibiotic tolerance. Taken together, bacterial biofilms provide a protective environment for formation and survival of persisters, and the potential mechanisms are depicted in **Figure 1**.

6. Control of bacterial biofilm infections by targeting persisters

The presence of multidrug-tolerant persisters in biofilms has been recognized as the predominant cause for antibiotic treatment failure and relapse of bacterial infections. It is becoming clear that the key of controlling bacterial biofilms translates to the ability to prevent persister formation or elimination of the persister subpopulation. Therefore, the development of agents targeting persisters represents a promising strategy for effective management of biofilm infections. Based on the growing knowledge about biofilms, persisters and antibiotic tolerance, a series of novel approaches have been developed to combat bacterial biofilm persisters.

As persisters mainly enter into a dormant state, it is expected that metabolic stimuli may restore the antibiotic susceptibility by resuscitating persisters. Therefore, various metabolites have been tested for the ability to sensitize biofilm persisters to antibiotics. A fatty acid signaling molecule, *cis*-2-decenoic acid, was able to awake persisters by elevating respiratory activity and protein synthesis. Combinational treatment with *cis*-2-decenoic acid and ciprofloxacin caused significant reduction of persister levels in planktonic and biofilm populations of *P. aeruginosa* and *E. coli* [69]. The use of metabolic adjuvant L-arginine resulted in 99% increase in the susceptibility of planktonic and biofilm persisters of *S. aureus*, *E. coli*, and *P. aeruginosa* to gentamicin *in vitro* through modifying membrane pH gradient. The L-arginine and gentamicin cocktail completely eradicated *S. aureus* and *E. coli* biofilms in a mouse model of catheter-related infection [70]. Metabolic stimuli by glycolysis intermediates (e.g., glucose, mannitol, fructose, and pyruvate) induced killing of *E. coli* and *S. aureus* persisters by gentamicin. The combination of metabolites with gentamicin markedly reduced biofilm and persister viability *in vitro*, and the effect was confirmed in a mouse urinary tract catheter infection model [71]. A similar study showed addition of mannitol significantly increased tobramycin sensitivity of *P. aeruginosa* biofilms and persisters [72]. Notably, the metabolite-enabled killing by aminoglycosides was due to enhanced aminoglycoside uptake by induction of proton-motive force, whereas such effect did not apply to β-lactams or fluoroquinolones [71].

QS signaling is closely related to biofilm formation and bacterial persistence. BF8, an inhibitor of QS, was shown to suppress antibiotic tolerance of both planktonic and biofilm persisters in *P. aeruginosa* and *E. coli*, although the exact mechanism of action was unclear [73, 74]. The formation of colistin-tolerant *P. aeruginosa* biofilm persisters relies on cell migration and QS. Combined use of erythromycin and colistin could promote the elimination of the biofilm persisters via inhibition of motility and QS by erythromycin [75].

Semisynthesis is an essential approach to develop novel antibiotics. A semisynthetic antibiotic (V-r8) conjugated vancomycin with a cell-penetrating molecular transporter d-octaarginine which could enhance the access of the antibiotic in the EPS matrix of biofilm and cellular uptake. It was reported that V-r8 exhibited potent killing efficacy against methicillin-resistant *S. aureus* (MRSA) biofilms and their persister cells *in vitro* and caused 97% reduction of biofilm-associated MRSA in a mouse wound infection model [76]. Another conjugate (V-IDR1018) constructed by vancomycin and innate defense regulator IDR1018 showed superior activity against MRSA biofilms and persisters both *in vitro* and *in vivo* [77].

Furthermore, an array of agents has been screened to eradicate biofilm persisters. Kim W and colleagues had developed multiple compounds to attack biofilm persisters by targeting bacterial membrane. Synthetic retinoids, CD437 and CD1530, were able to eradicate persisters formed in MRSA biofilms alone or in combination with gentamicin by disrupting membrane lipid bilayers and inducing membrane permeabilization. The effects were further confirmed in a MRSA mouse deep-seated thigh infection model shown by dramatic decrease of bacterial burden [78]. Similarly, a clinically approved anthelmintic drug bithionol killed stationary-phase MRSA planktonic and biofilm persisters alone or combined with gentamicin by disrupting membrane lipid bilayers [79]. Another membrane-active agent NH125 and its analogs were identified and found to have potent biofilm eradication and rapid persister killing efficacy *in vitro* [80–82]. ADEP4, as a potent activator of an important bacterial protease ClpP, can cause uncontrolled protein degradation and subsequent cell death. The combination of ADEP4 and rifampicin was shown to successfully eradicate *S. aureus* biofilm persisters *in vitro* and clear a deep-seated murine thigh infection *in vivo* [25]. However, the recipe failed to manage *S. aureus* biofilm infections in a mouse skin infection model [83]. FDA-approved anti-cancer drugs mitomycin C and cisplatin were found to effectively eliminate planktonic and biofilm persisters of *E. coli*, *S. aureus* and *P. aeruginosa* via cross-linking DNA [84, 85]. Biofilm persisters derived from different bacteria could be effectively eradicated by polymeric nanoemulsions loaded with dual hydrophobic antimicrobials (eugenol and triclosan). Moreover, the nanoemulsion eliminated 99% of pathogens in a murine model of mature wound biofilm infections by MRSA [86]. In addition, halogenated phenazines showed the ability to remove biofilms of several superbugs and kill the inherent persisters by inducing rapid iron starvation [87, 88].

7. Conclusions

The discovery of persisters in bacterial biofilms is indeed a major breakthrough in the realm of infection. Additional to antibiotic resistance, antibiotic tolerance incurred by bacterial biofilms and their persisters has been recognized as the underlying reason for recalcitrance and relapse of infectious diseases. It is inspiring that extensive studies have started to shed light on the molecular mechanisms behind biofilm persisters and put forward the development of novel approaches against them. Accumulating evidence has indicated that biofilm offer a protective environment for persister formation and persisters are the responsible population for antibiotic tolerance of biofilms. Targeting persisters is therefore a promising strategy to control biofilm-related infections. Nevertheless, bacterial persistence involves complex and redundant mechanisms, which are largely unexplored. Notably, current insights on biofilm persisters are mainly based on *in vitro* studies, whereas the conditions in the host would be more intricate. There is still a lack of direct evidence that persisters can resume growth and repopulate biofilms in the host to cause relapse of infections. Due to the frequent failure of current therapeutic methods, novel approaches are urgently needed to effectively and safely combat persister-based biofilm infections. Further studies are therefore highly warranted to uncover the mystery of persisters and overcome the challenges of biofilm infections.

Acknowledgements

We acknowledge the support by the National Natural Science Foundation of China for Peng Li (grant no. 81700975) and for Siqi Yao (grant no. 82301077).

Author details

Peng Li[1*] and Siqi Yao[2]

1 Department of Periodontology, Peking University School and Hospital of Stomatology, National Center for Stomatology, National Clinical Research Center for Oral Diseases, National Engineering Research Center of Oral Biomaterials and Digital Medical Devices, Beijing Key Laboratory of Digital Stomatology, NHC Key Laboratory of Digital Stomatology, NMPA Key Laboratory for Dental Materials, Beijing, China

2 Department of Stomatology, Beijing Tongren Hospital, Capital Medical University, Beijing, China

*Address all correspondence to: lp_nathan@hotmail.com

References

[1] Penesyan A, Paulsen IT, Kjelleberg S, Gillings MR. Three faces of biofilms: A microbial lifestyle, a nascent multicellular organism, and an incubator for diversity. npj Biofilms and Microbiomes. 2021;**7**(1):80. DOI: 10.1038/s41522-021-00251-2

[2] Sauer K, Stoodley P, Goeres DM, Hall-Stoodley L, Burmolle M, Stewart PS, et al. The biofilm life cycle: Expanding the conceptual model of biofilm formation. Nature Reviews. Microbiology. 2022;**20**(10):608-620. DOI: 10.1038/s41579-022-00767-0

[3] Ciofu O, Moser C, Jensen PO, Hoiby N. Tolerance and resistance of microbial biofilms. Nature Reviews. Microbiology. 2022;**20**(10):621-635. DOI: 10.1038/s41579-022-00682-4

[4] Zhao A, Sun J, Liu Y. Understanding bacterial biofilms: From definition to treatment strategies. Frontiers in Cellular and Infection Microbiology. 2023;**13**:1137947. DOI: 10.3389/fcimb.2023.1137947

[5] Liu HY, Prentice EL, Webber MA. Mechanisms of antimicrobial resistance in biofilms. NPJ Antimicrobials and Resistance. 2024;**2**(1):27. DOI: 10.1038/s44259-024-00046-3

[6] Hall CW, Mah TF. Molecular mechanisms of biofilm-based antibiotic resistance and tolerance in pathogenic bacteria. FEMS Microbiology Reviews. 2017;**41**(3):276-301. DOI: 10.1093/femsre/fux010

[7] Niu H, Gu J, Zhang Y. Bacterial persisters: Molecular mechanisms and therapeutic development. Signal Transduction and Targeted Therapy. 2024;**9**(1):174. DOI: 10.1038/s41392-024-01866-5

[8] Fisher RA, Gollan B, Helaine S. Persistent bacterial infections and persister cells. Nature Reviews. Microbiology. 2017;**15**(8):453-464. DOI: 10.1038/nrmicro.2017.42

[9] Hobby GL, Meyer K, Chaffee E. Observations on the mechanism of action of penicillin. Proceedings of the Society for Experimental Biology and Medicine. 1942;**50**:281-285

[10] Bigger JW. Treatment of staphylococcal infections with penicillin. Lancet. 1944;**244**(6320):497-500

[11] Yan J, Bassler BL. Surviving as a community: Antibiotic tolerance and persistence in bacterial biofilms. Cell Host & Microbe. 2019;**26**(1):15-21. DOI: 10.1016/j.chom.2019.06.002

[12] Veening JW, Smits WK, Kuipers OP. Bistability, epigenetics, and bet-hedging in bacteria. Annual Review of Microbiology. 2008;**62**:193-210. DOI: 10.1146/annurev.micro.62.081307.163002

[13] Grimbergen AJ, Siebring J, Solopova A, Kuipers OP. Microbial bet-hedging: The power of being different. Current Opinion in Microbiology. 2015;**25**:67-72. DOI: 10.1016/j.mib.2015.04.008

[14] Bjarnsholt T, Alhede M, Alhede M, Eickhardt-Sorensen SR, Moser C, Kuhl M, et al. The in vivo biofilm. Trends in Microbiology. 2013;**21**(9):466-474. DOI: 10.1016/j.tim.2013.06.002

[15] Kolpen M, Jensen PO, Faurholt-Jepsen D, Bjarnsholt T. Prevalence of biofilms in acute infections challenges a longstanding paradigm. Biofilms. 2022;**4**:100080. DOI: 10.1016/j.bioflm.2022.100080

[16] Sharma D, Misba L, Khan AU. Antibiotics versus biofilm: An emerging battleground in microbial communities. Antimicrobial Resistance and Infection Control. 2019;**8**:76. DOI: 10.1186/s13756-019-0533-3

[17] Perry EK, Tan MW. Bacterial biofilms in the human body: Prevalence and impacts on health and disease. Frontiers in Cellular and Infection Microbiology. 2023;**13**:1237164. DOI: 10.3389/fcimb.2023.1237164

[18] Donne J, Dewilde S. The challenging world of biofilm physiology. Advances in Microbial Physiology. 2015;**67**:235-292. DOI: 10.1016/bs.ampbs.2015.09.003

[19] Hoiby N, Bjarnsholt T, Moser C, Bassi GL, Coenye T, Donelli G, et al. ESCMID guideline for the diagnosis and treatment of biofilm infections 2014. Clinical Microbiology and Infection. 2015;**21**(Suppl 1):S1-S25. DOI: 10.1016/j.cmi.2014.10.024

[20] Brooun A, Liu S, Lewis K. A dose-response study of antibiotic resistance in Pseudomonas aeruginosa biofilms. Antimicrobial Agents and Chemotherapy. 2000;**44**(3):640-646. DOI: 10.1128/AAC.44.3.640-646.2000

[21] Spoering AL, Lewis K. Biofilms and planktonic cells of Pseudomonas aeruginosa have similar resistance to killing by antimicrobials. Journal of Bacteriology. 2001;**183**(23):6746-6751. DOI: 10.1128/JB.183.23.6746-6751.2001

[22] Keren I, Shah D, Spoering A, Kaldalu N, Lewis K. Specialized persister cells and the mechanism of multidrug tolerance in *Escherichia coli*. Journal of Bacteriology. 2004;**186**(24):8172-8180. DOI: 10.1128/JB.186.24.8172-8180.2004

[23] Li P, Seneviratne CJ, Alpi E, Vizcaino JA, Jin L. Delicate metabolic control and coordinated stress response critically determine antifungal tolerance of *Candida albicans* biofilm persisters. Antimicrobial Agents and Chemotherapy. 2015;**59**(10):6101-6112. DOI: 10.1128/AAC.00543-15

[24] Ojha AK, Baughn AD, Sambandan D, Hsu T, Trivelli X, Guerardel Y, et al. Growth of mycobacterium tuberculosis biofilms containing free mycolic acids and harbouring drug-tolerant bacteria. Molecular Microbiology. 2008;**69**(1):164-174. DOI: 10.1111/j.1365-2958.2008.06274.x

[25] Conlon BP, Nakayasu ES, Fleck LE, LaFleur MD, Isabella VM, Coleman K, et al. Activated ClpP kills persisters and eradicates a chronic biofilm infection. Nature. 2013;**503**(7476):365-370. DOI: 10.1038/nature12790

[26] Mulcahy LR, Burns JL, Lory S, Lewis K. Emergence of *Pseudomonas aeruginosa* strains producing high levels of persister cells in patients with cystic fibrosis. Journal of Bacteriology. 2010;**192**(23):6191-6199. DOI: 10.1128/JB.01651-09

[27] Lafleur MD, Qi Q, Lewis K. Patients with long-term oral carriage harbor high-persister mutants of *Candida albicans*. Antimicrobial Agents and Chemotherapy. 2010;**54**(1):39-44. DOI: 10.1128/AAC.00860-09

[28] Moyed HS, Bertrand KP. hipA, a newly recognized gene of *Escherichia coli* K-12 that affects frequency of persistence after inhibition of murein synthesis. Journal of Bacteriology. 1983;**155**(2):768-775. DOI: 10.1128/jb.155.2.768-775.1983

[29] Schumacher MA, Balani P, Min J, Chinnam NB, Hansen S, Vulic M, et al. HipBA-promoter structures reveal the basis of heritable multidrug tolerance.

Nature. 2015;**524**(7563):59-64. DOI: 10.1038/nature14662

[30] Parsons JB, Sidders AE, Velez AZ, Hanson BM, Angeles-Solano M, Ruffin F, et al. In-patient evolution of a high-persister *Escherichia coli* strain with reduced in vivo antibiotic susceptibility. Proceedings of the National Academy of Sciences of the United States of America. 2024;**121**(3):e2314514121. DOI: 10.1073/pnas.2314514121

[31] Bartell JA, Cameron DR, Mojsoska B, Haagensen JAJ, Pressler T, Sommer LM, et al. Bacterial persisters in long-term infection: Emergence and fitness in a complex host environment. PLoS Pathogens. 2020;**16**(12):e1009112. DOI: 10.1371/journal.ppat.1009112

[32] Moldoveanu AL, Rycroft JA, Helaine S. Impact of bacterial persisters on their host. Current Opinion in Microbiology. 2021;**59**:65-71. DOI: 10.1016/j.mib.2020.07.006

[33] Hayden HS, Lim R, Brittnacher MJ, Sims EH, Ramage ER, Fong C, et al. Evolution of *Burkholderia pseudomallei* in recurrent melioidosis. PLoS ONE. 2012;**7**(5):e36507. DOI: 10.1371/journal.pone.0036507

[34] Levin-Reisman I, Ronin I, Gefen O, Braniss I, Shoresh N, Balaban NQ. Antibiotic tolerance facilitates the evolution of resistance. Science. 2017;**355**(6327):826-830. DOI: 10.1126/science.aaj2191

[35] Windels EM, Michiels JE, Fauvart M, Wenseleers T, Van den Bergh B, Michiels J. Bacterial persistence promotes the evolution of antibiotic resistance by increasing survival and mutation rates. The ISME Journal. 2019;**13**(5):1239-1251. DOI: 10.1038/s41396-019-0344-9

[36] Liu J, Gefen O, Ronin I, Bar-Meir M, Balaban NQ. Effect of tolerance on the evolution of antibiotic resistance under drug combinations. Science. 2020;**367**(6474):200-204. DOI: 10.1126/science.aay3041

[37] Helaine S, Cheverton AM, Watson KG, Faure LM, Matthews SA, Holden DW. Internalization of Salmonella by macrophages induces formation of nonreplicating persisters. Science. 2014;**343**(6167):204-208. DOI: 10.1126/science.1244705

[38] Adams KN, Takaki K, Connolly LE, Wiedenhoft H, Winglee K, Humbert O, et al. Drug tolerance in replicating mycobacteria mediated by a macrophage-induced efflux mechanism. Cell. 2011;**145**(1):39-53. DOI: 10.1016/j.cell.2011.02.022

[39] Peyrusson F, Varet H, Nguyen TK, Legendre R, Sismeiro O, Coppee JY, et al. Intracellular Staphylococcus aureus persisters upon antibiotic exposure. Nature Communications. 2020;**11**(1):2200. DOI: 10.1038/s41467-020-15966-7

[40] Wang C, Cheng T, Li X, Jin L. Metronidazole-treated *Porphyromonas gingivalis* persisters invade human gingival epithelial cells and perturb innate responses. Antimicrobial Agents and Chemotherapy. 2020;**64**(6):e02529-19. DOI: 10.1128/AAC.02529-19

[41] Balaban NQ, Merrin J, Chait R, Kowalik L, Leibler S. Bacterial persistence as a phenotypic switch. Science. 2004;**305**(5690):1622-1625. DOI: 10.1126/science.1099390

[42] Wood TK, Knabel SJ, Kwan BW. Bacterial persister cell formation and dormancy. Applied and Environmental Microbiology. 2013;**79**(23):7116-7121. DOI: 10.1128/AEM.02636-13

[43] Ronneau S, Helaine S. Clarifying the link between toxin-antitoxin modules

and bacterial persistence. Journal of Molecular Biology. 2019;**431**(18):3462-3471. DOI: 10.1016/j.jmb.2019.03.019

[44] Page R, Peti W. Toxin-antitoxin systems in bacterial growth arrest and persistence. Nature Chemical Biology. 2016;**12**(4):208-214. DOI: 10.1038/nchembio.2044

[45] Orman MA, Brynildsen MP. Dormancy is not necessary or sufficient for bacterial persistence. Antimicrobial Agents and Chemotherapy. 2013;**57**(7):3230-3239. DOI: 10.1128/AAC.00243-13

[46] Goormaghtigh F, Van Melderen L. Single-cell imaging and characterization of *Escherichia coli* persister cells to ofloxacin in exponential cultures. Science Advances. 2019;**5**(6):eaav9462. DOI: 10.1126/sciadv.aav9462

[47] Yuan S, Shen Y, Quan Y, Gao S, Zuo J, Jin W, et al. Molecular mechanism and application of emerging technologies in study of bacterial persisters. BMC Microbiology. 2024;**24**(1):480. DOI: 10.1186/s12866-024-03628-3

[48] Pu Y, Zhao Z, Li Y, Zou J, Ma Q, Zhao Y, et al. Enhanced efflux activity facilitates drug tolerance in dormant bacterial cells. Molecular Cell. 2016;**62**(2):284-294. DOI: 10.1016/j.molcel.2016.03.035

[49] Martini CL, Coronado AZ, Melo MCN, Gobbi CN, Lopez US, de Mattos MC, et al. Cellular growth arrest and efflux pumps are associated with antibiotic persisters in streptococcus pyogenes induced in biofilm-like environments. Frontiers in Microbiology. 2021;**12**:716628. DOI: 10.3389/fmicb.2021.716628

[50] Moker N, Dean CR, Tao J. *Pseudomonas aeruginosa* increases formation of multidrug-tolerant persister cells in response to quorum-sensing signaling molecules. Journal of Bacteriology. 2010;**192**(7):1946-1955. DOI: 10.1128/JB.01231-09

[51] Leung V, Levesque CM. A stress-inducible quorum-sensing peptide mediates the formation of persister cells with noninherited multidrug tolerance. Journal of Bacteriology. 2012;**194**(9):2265-2274. DOI: 10.1128/JB.06707-11

[52] Vega NM, Allison KR, Khalil AS, Collins JJ. Signaling-mediated bacterial persister formation. Nature Chemical Biology. 2012;**8**(5):431-433. DOI: 10.1038/nchembio.915

[53] Van Acker H, Sass A, Bazzini S, De Roy K, Udine C, Messiaen T, et al. Biofilm-grown *Burkholderia cepacia* complex cells survive antibiotic treatment by avoiding production of reactive oxygen species. PLoS ONE. 2013;**8**(3):e58943. DOI: 10.1371/journal.pone.0058943

[54] Stewart PS, Franklin MJ, Williamson KS, Folsom JP, Boegli L, James GA. Contribution of stress responses to antibiotic tolerance in *Pseudomonas aeruginosa* biofilms. Antimicrobial Agents and Chemotherapy. 2015;**59**(7):3838-3847. DOI: 10.1128/AAC.00433-15

[55] Obando MC, Serra DO. Dissecting cell heterogeneities in bacterial biofilms and their implications for antibiotic tolerance. Current Opinion in Microbiology. 2024;**78**:102450. DOI: 10.1016/j.mib.2024.102450

[56] Bernier SP, Lebeaux D, DeFrancesco AS, Valomon A, Soubigou G, Coppee JY, et al. Starvation, together with the SOS response, mediates high biofilm-specific tolerance to the fluoroquinolone ofloxacin.

PLoS Genetics. 2013;**9**(1):e1003144. DOI: 10.1371/journal.pgen.1003144

[57] Nguyen D, Joshi-Datar A, Lepine F, Bauerle E, Olakanmi O, Beer K, et al. Active starvation responses mediate antibiotic tolerance in biofilms and nutrient-limited bacteria. Science. 2011;**334**(6058):982-986. DOI: 10.1126/science.1211037

[58] Amato SM, Brynildsen MP. Nutrient transitions are a source of persisters in *Escherichia coli* biofilms. PLoS ONE. 2014;**9**(3):e93110. DOI: 10.1371/journal.pone.0093110

[59] Kim J, Hahn JS, Franklin MJ, Stewart PS, Yoon J. Tolerance of dormant and active cells in *Pseudomonas aeruginosa* PA01 biofilm to antimicrobial agents. The Journal of Antimicrobial Chemotherapy. 2009;**63**(1):129-135. DOI: 10.1093/jac/dkn462

[60] Wang X, Wood TK. Toxin-antitoxin systems influence biofilm and persister cell formation and the general stress response. Applied and Environmental Microbiology. 2011;**77**(16):5577-5583. DOI: 10.1128/AEM.05068-11

[61] Harrison JJ, Wade WD, Akierman S, Vacchi-Suzzi C, Stremick CA, Turner RJ, et al. The chromosomal toxin gene yafQ is a determinant of multidrug tolerance for *Escherichia coli* growing in a biofilm. Antimicrobial Agents and Chemotherapy. 2009;**53**(6):2253-2258. DOI: 10.1128/AAC.00043-09

[62] Ciofu O, Tolker-Nielsen T. Tolerance and resistance of *Pseudomonas aeruginosa* biofilms to antimicrobial agents-how *P. aeruginosa* can escape antibiotics. Frontiers in Microbiology. 2019;**10**:913. DOI: 10.3389/fmicb.2019.00913

[63] Hoiby N, Bjarnsholt T, Givskov M, Molin S, Ciofu O. Antibiotic resistance of bacterial biofilms. International Journal of Antimicrobial Agents. 2010;**35**(4):322-332. DOI: 10.1016/j.ijantimicag.2009.12.011

[64] Jefferson KK, Goldmann DA, Pier GB. Use of confocal microscopy to analyze the rate of vancomycin penetration through *Staphylococcus aureus* biofilms. Antimicrobial Agents and Chemotherapy. 2005;**49**(6):2467-2473. DOI: 10.1128/AAC.49.6.2467-2473.2005

[65] Dorr T, Lewis K, Vulic M. SOS response induces persistence to fluoroquinolones in *Escherichia coli*. PLoS Genetics. 2009;**5**(12):e1000760. DOI: 10.1371/journal.pgen.1000760

[66] Johnson PJ, Levin BR. Pharmacodynamics, population dynamics, and the evolution of persistence in *Staphylococcus aureus*. PLoS Genetics. 2013;**9**(1):e1003123. DOI: 10.1371/journal.pgen.1003123

[67] Dorr T, Vulic M, Lewis K. Ciprofloxacin causes persister formation by inducing the TisB toxin in Escherichia coli. PLoS Biology. 2010;**8**(2):e1000317. DOI: 10.1371/journal.pbio.1000317

[68] Knudsen GM, Fromberg A, Ng Y, Gram L. Sublethal concentrations of antibiotics cause shift to anaerobic metabolism in listeria monocytogenes and induce phenotypes linked to antibiotic tolerance. Frontiers in Microbiology. 2016;**7**:1091. DOI: 10.3389/fmicb.2016.01091

[69] Marques CN, Morozov A, Planzos P, Zelaya HM. The fatty acid signaling molecule cis-2-decenoic acid increases metabolic activity and reverts persister cells to an antimicrobial-susceptible state. Applied and Environmental Microbiology. 2014;**80**(22):6976-6991. DOI: 10.1128/AEM.01576-14

[70] Lebeaux D, Chauhan A, Letoffe S, Fischer F, de Reuse H, Beloin C, et al. pH-mediated potentiation of aminoglycosides kills bacterial persisters and eradicates in vivo biofilms. The Journal of Infectious Diseases. 2014;**210**(9):1357-1366. DOI: 10.1093/infdis/jiu286

[71] Allison KR, Brynildsen MP, Collins JJ. Metabolite-enabled eradication of bacterial persisters by aminoglycosides. Nature. 2011;**473**(7346):216-220. DOI: 10.1038/nature10069

[72] Barraud N, Buson A, Jarolimek W, Rice SA. Mannitol enhances antibiotic sensitivity of persister bacteria in Pseudomonas aeruginosa biofilms. PLoS ONE. 2013;**8**(12):e84220. DOI: 10.1371/journal.pone.0084220

[73] Pan J, Bahar AA, Syed H, Ren D. Reverting antibiotic tolerance of *Pseudomonas aeruginosa* PAO1 persister cells by (Z)-4-bromo-5-(bromomethylene)-3-methylfuran-2(5H)-one. PLoS ONE. 2012;**7**(9):e45778. DOI: 10.1371/journal.pone.0045778

[74] Pan J, Xie X, Tian W, Bahar AA, Lin N, Song F, et al. (Z)-4-Bromo-5-(bromomethylene)-3-methylfuran-2(5H)-one sensitizes *Escherichia coli* persister cells to antibiotics. Applied Microbiology and Biotechnology. 2013;**97**(20):9145-9154. DOI: 10.1007/s00253-013-5185-2

[75] Chua SL, Yam JK, Hao P, Adav SS, Salido MM, Liu Y, et al. Selective labelling and eradication of antibiotic-tolerant bacterial populations in *Pseudomonas aeruginosa* biofilms. Nature Communications. 2016;**7**:10750. DOI: 10.1038/ncomms10750

[76] Antonoplis A, Zang X, Huttner MA, Chong KKL, Lee YB, Co JY, et al. A dual-function antibiotic-transporter conjugate exhibits superior activity in sterilizing MRSA biofilms and killing persister cells. Journal of the American Chemical Society. 2018;**140**(47):16140-16151. DOI: 10.1021/jacs.8b08711

[77] Etayash H, Alford M, Akhoundsadegh N, Drayton M, Straus SK, Hancock REW. Correction to "multifunctional antibiotic-host defense peptide conjugate kills bacteria, eradicates biofilms, and modulates the innate immune response". Journal of Medicinal Chemistry. 2022;**65**(3):2710-2711. DOI: 10.1021/acs.jmedchem.1c02112

[78] Kim W, Zhu W, Hendricks GL, Van Tyne D, Steele AD, Keohane CE, et al. A new class of synthetic retinoid antibiotics effective against bacterial persisters. Nature. 2018;**556**(7699):103-107. DOI: 10.1038/nature26157

[79] Kim W, Zou G, Hari TPA, Wilt IK, Zhu W, Galle N, et al. A selective membrane-targeting repurposed antibiotic with activity against persistent methicillin-resistant Staphylococcus aureus. Proceedings of the National Academy of Sciences of the United States of America. 2019;**116**(33):16529-16534. DOI: 10.1073/pnas.1904700116

[80] Kim W, Conery AL, Rajamuthiah R, Fuchs BB, Ausubel FM, Mylonakis E. Identification of an antimicrobial agent effective against methicillin-resistant *Staphylococcus aureus* persisters using a fluorescence-based screening strategy. PLoS ONE. 2015;**10**(6):e0127640. DOI: 10.1371/journal.pone.0127640

[81] Abouelhassan Y, Basak A, Yousaf H, Huigens RW 3rd. Identification of N-arylated NH125 analogues as rapid eradicating agents against MRSA persister cells and potent biofilm killers of Gram-positive pathogens. Chembiochem. 2017;**18**(4):352-357. DOI: 10.1002/cbic.201600622

[82] Basak A, Abouelhassan Y, Zuo R, Yousaf H, Ding Y, Huigens RW. Antimicrobial peptide-inspired NH125 analogues: Bacterial and fungal biofilm-eradicating agents and rapid killers of MRSA persisters. Organic & Biomolecular Chemistry. 2017;**15**(26):5503-5512. DOI: 10.1039/c7ob01028a

[83] Yee R, Yuan Y, Tarff A, Brayton C, Gour N, Feng J, et al. Eradication of *Staphylococcus aureus* biofilm infection by persister drug combination. Antibiotics. 2022;**11**(10):1278. DOI: 10.3390/antibiotics11101278

[84] Kwan BW, Chowdhury N, Wood TK. Combatting bacterial infections by killing persister cells with mitomycin C. Environmental Microbiology. 2015;**17**(11):4406-4414. DOI: 10.1111/1462-2920.12873

[85] Chowdhury N, Wood TL, Martinez-Vazquez M, Garcia-Contreras R, Wood TK. DNA-crosslinker cisplatin eradicates bacterial persister cells. Biotechnology and Bioengineering. 2016;**113**(9):1984-1992. DOI: 10.1002/bit.25963

[86] Nabawy A, Makabenta JM, Schmidt-Malan S, Park J, Li CH, Huang R, et al. Dual antimicrobial-loaded biodegradable nanoemulsions for synergistic treatment of wound biofilms. Journal of Controlled Release. 2022;**347**:379-388. DOI: 10.1016/j.jconrel.2022.05.013

[87] Garrison AT, Abouelhassan Y, Norwood VM, Kallifidas D, Bai F, Nguyen MT, et al. Structure-activity relationships of a diverse class of halogenated phenazines that targets persistent, antibiotic-tolerant bacterial biofilms and mycobacterium tuberculosis. Journal of Medicinal Chemistry. 2016;**59**(8):3808-3825. DOI: 10.1021/acs.jmedchem.5b02004

[88] Yang H, Abouelhassan Y, Burch GM, Kallifidas D, Huang G, Yousaf H, et al. A highly potent class of halogenated phenazine antibacterial and biofilm-eradicating agents accessed through a modular Wohl-Aue synthesis. Scientific Reports. 2017;**7**(1):2003. DOI: 10.1038/s41598-017-01045-3

Section 2

Natural Phytochemicals against Biofilm Formation

Chapter 7

Essential Oils in Battle against MRSA Biofilms: Mechanisms, Challenges, and Future Prospects

Sai Sristi Panda, Maheswary Datchanamoorthy, Leela Kakithakara Vajravelu and W. Richard Thilagaraj

Abstract

Methicillin-resistant *Staphylococcus aureus* (MRSA) poses a significant public health threat, particularly due to its ability to form biofilms that enhance its virulence and resistance to conventional antibiotic treatments. This chapter provides a comprehensive overview of MRSA strains, distinguishing between community-associated (CA-MRSA) and healthcare-associated (HA-MRSA) strains and their implications for infection management. We delve into the molecular mechanisms underlying biofilm formation, emphasizing the roles of the polysaccharide intercellular adhesin (PIA) and the mecA gene, which contribute to the enhanced biofilm production in MRSA compared to methicillin-sensitive *Staphylococcus aureus* (MSSA). Importantly, we investigate the potential of essential oils as innovative biofilm disruptors, highlighting their diverse antibacterial properties and the specific active compounds that contribute to their efficacy against MRSA biofilms. The chapter also addresses the challenges of integrating essential oils into clinical practice, including their safety, effectiveness, and the potential for resistance development. By enhancing our understanding of essential oils in biofilm management, we aim to provide insights that could lead to improved strategies for preventing biofilm-associated infections and enhancing treatment outcomes.

Keywords: essential oils, phytochemicals, quorum-sensing inhibition, natural biofilm disruptors, plant-derived antimicrobials

1. Introduction

Methicillin-resistant *Staphylococcus aureus* (MRSA) represents a significant public health challenge due to its resistance to commonly used antibiotics, particularly beta-lactams like methicillin. The two primary categories of MRSA strains are community-associated MRSA (CA-MRSA) and healthcare-associated MRSA (HA-MRSA). HA-MRSA strains typically emerge in healthcare settings and are associated with severe infections, leading to increased morbidity and mortality rates. In contrast,

CA-MRSA strains are increasingly prevalent in community settings, often linked to skin and soft tissue infections, and exhibit a remarkable capacity for rapid transmission among healthy individuals [1].

2. Biofilm formation by MRSA and MSSA and its significances

The formation of biofilms is a critical factor in the pathogenicity of both MRSA and MSSA, contributing to chronic infections and complicating treatment strategies. Biofilm production in *Staphylococcus aureus* is primarily facilitated by the polysaccharide intercellular adhesin (PIA), encoded by the ica operon [2]. The mecA gene, which promotes methicillin resistance in MRSA, has been demonstrated to enhance biofilm development by inhibiting the accessory gene regulator (AGR) quorum-sensing system, responsible for regulating virulence factors and biofilm formation [3]. Alterations in regulatory pathways result in a higher propensity for biofilm formation in MRSA compared to MSSA, as evidenced by studies indicating that a significant percentage of MRSA isolates are strong biofilm producers [4].

2.1 Differences between MRSA and MSSA biofilms

While both MRSA and MSSA can form biofilms, there are notable differences in their biofilm-forming capabilities and associated virulence factors. Studies indicate that MRSA strains generally exhibit a higher biofilm production rate compared to MSSA strains [3, 5]. This is attributed to the unique genetic and phenotypic characteristics of MRSA, including the presence of specific adhesins and regulatory systems that promote biofilm formation [6, 7]. For example, the agr system, while downregulated in MRSA, is more active in MSSA, leading to different biofilm dynamics [6].

Furthermore, the composition of the biofilm matrix may differ between MRSA and MSSA, influencing their susceptibility to antibiotics and host immune responses [2, 6]. Research has shown that the biofilm matrix of MRSA is more robust, providing enhanced protection against antimicrobial agents and immune clearance compared to that of MSSA [2, 8, 9]. This distinction is critical for developing targeted therapies that can effectively disrupt biofilms and enhance treatment outcomes.

2.2 Strategies for biofilm disruption

Considering the difficulties associated with biofilm formation, numerous ways have been investigated to disrupt biofilms and improve the effectiveness of antibiotic therapies. This encompasses enzymatic therapies, such as DNase, which can destroy extracellular DNA in the biofilm matrix, thereby disrupting the structure and rendering bacteria more vulnerable to antibiotics [10, 11]. Additionally, novel antimicrobial agents and combinations of existing antibiotics with biofilm-disrupting agents are being investigated to improve treatment outcomes for biofilm-associated infections [1, 9, 12].

Recent studies have also explored the potential of photothermal therapy and nanotechnology to target biofilms effectively. For instance, the use of photothermal agents that can generate localized heat has shown promise in eradicating biofilms formed by MRSA [1]. Moreover, the development of nanoparticles that can penetrate biofilm layers and deliver antimicrobial agents directly to the bacterial cells is an exciting area of research that may lead to more effective treatment modalities [2].

3. What is so special in MRSA biofilms?

One of the defining features of MRSA biofilms is their composition shown in **Figure 1**, which includes polysaccharides, proteins, and extracellular DNA (eDNA).

The polysaccharide intercellular adhesin (PIA) is a critical component that facilitates biofilm formation by promoting cell-to-cell adhesion. Interestingly, MRSA can form biofilms independently of the ica operon, which is typically required for biofilm formation in methicillin-sensitive *Staphylococcus aureus* (MSSA) [3, 4]. This ability allows MRSA to establish biofilms in various environments, including on medical devices, which significantly increases the risk of persistent infections. The protective nature of biofilms is attributed to their EPS matrix, which acts as a barrier against antimicrobial agents and immune cells. Research indicates that bacteria within biofilms can demonstrate resistance to antibiotics that is up to 1000 times greater than that of their planktonic counterparts [5]. This resistance arises not only from the physical obstruction of the biofilm matrix but also from metabolic alterations inside the biofilm that modify the bacteria's vulnerability to antibiotics.

4. Why do we need to investigate MRSA biofilms?

Methicillin-resistant *Staphylococcus aureus* (MRSA) poses a considerable public health concern owing to its capacity to form biofilms, which enhance its virulence and treatment resistance [6]. The study of MRSA biofilms is essential for formulating viable therapeutic approaches and comprehending the mechanisms that drive MRSA infections.

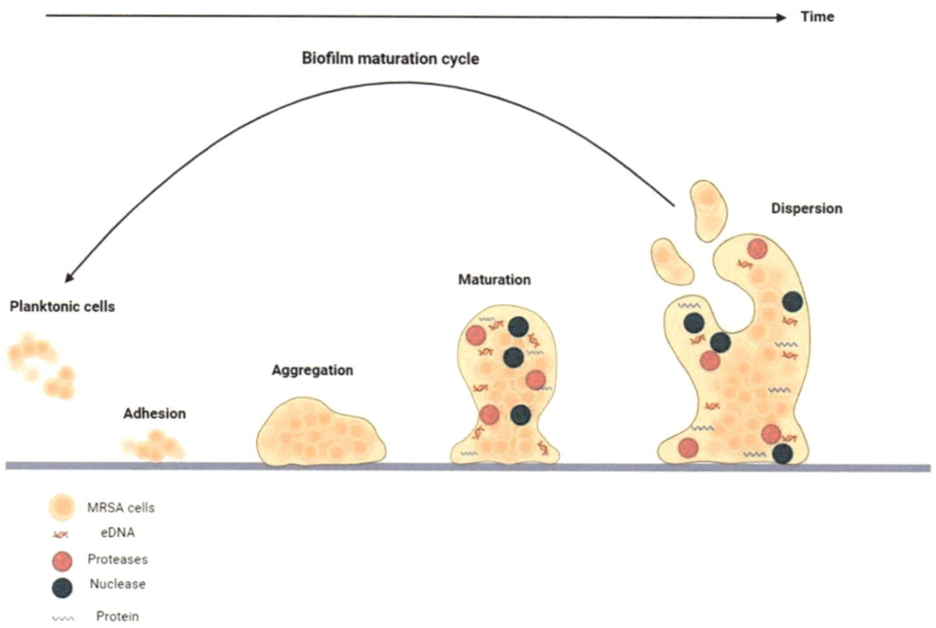

Figure 1.
Biofilm formation cycle.

4.1 Challenges in treating MRSA biofilms

The treatment of MRSA infections becomes complicated by biofilms, which can render traditional drugs ineffective. Studies demonstrate that biofilm-associated bacteria can display resistance to drugs that is up to 1000 times greater than that of their planktonic counterparts [7, 8]. This resistance can be attributed to multiple mechanisms, including the diminished penetration of antibiotics through the biofilm matrix and the modified metabolic state of the bacteria within the biofilm [8, 9].

Recent studies have highlighted the need for novel therapeutic approaches to combat MRSA biofilms. For example, the use of combination therapies, such as antibiotics paired with antibiofilm agents, has shown promise in enhancing the efficacy of treatment against biofilm-associated MRSA [10]. Additionally, the development of new materials and coatings that can prevent biofilm formation on medical devices is an area of active research [11, 12].

4.2 Novel therapeutic strategies

Investigating MRSA biofilms has led to the exploration of various novel therapeutic strategies. One promising approach involves the use of natural compounds that exhibit antibiofilm properties. For instance, compounds like geraniol and cinnamaldehyde have demonstrated the ability to inhibit biofilm formation and enhance the effectiveness of traditional antibiotics [2, 13, 14]. These natural products could serve as adjunct therapies to improve treatment outcomes for MRSA infections.

Moreover, the integration of nanotechnology in the development of drug delivery systems has shown potential in targeting MRSA biofilms. Nanoparticles can be engineered to deliver antibiotics directly to the biofilm, increasing local concentrations and improving efficacy [11]. This targeted approach may help overcome the challenges posed by biofilm-associated antibiotic resistance.

5. Control of MRSA biofilms-strategies and approaches

MRSA biofilms are characterized by their complex architecture, which includes extracellular polymeric substances (EPS) such as polysaccharides, proteins, and extracellular DNA (eDNA) [13, 15]. These components not only provide structural integrity but also contribute to the biofilm's resistance to antimicrobial agents. The development of biofilms is governed by multiple genetic elements, especially the icaADBC operon, which is essential for intercellular adhesion and biofilm maturation [16, 17]. Understanding these mechanisms is essential for developing effective treatment strategies.

5.1 Antibiotic combinations and novel agents

One of the most promising approaches to combat MRSA biofilms involves the use of antibiotic combinations. For instance, the combination of vancomycin and Zhenqi granules has shown improved efficacy against MRSA biofilms compared to vancomycin alone [6]. Similarly, the use of zinc imidazole framework nanoparticles has been reported to disperse MRSA biofilms by inhibiting arginine biosynthesis and down-regulating adhesion-related proteins [15].

Moreover, the incorporation of natural compounds has gained attention. For example, geraniol has been shown to inhibit biofilm formation and enhance the therapeutic effect of vancomycin *in vivo* [13]. Additionally, the methanolic extract of *Hemidesmus indicus* root has been reported to augment the antibacterial and antibiofilm activity of conventional antibiotics like amoxicillin and clindamycin against MRSA [18]. These natural compounds may offer alternative strategies to enhance the efficacy of existing antibiotics.

5.2 Targeting biofilm matrix components

Targeting the biofilm matrix itself is another effective strategy. The degradation of eDNA, a critical component of the biofilm matrix, has been shown to significantly reduce biofilm formation and facilitate eradication [13]. Enzymatic treatments, such as the application of DNase I, can disrupt the biofilm structure and enhance the susceptibility of MRSA to antibiotics [13]. Furthermore, the use of nanoparticles that release reactive oxygen species has been proposed to degrade the biofilm matrix and enhance antibiotic penetration [19].

5.3 Probiotics and antimicrobial peptides

The role of probiotics and antimicrobial peptides in controlling MRSA biofilms is an emerging area of research. Probiotic strains, such as *Bacillus subtilis*, have demonstrated the ability to neutralize MRSA biofilms through their bacteriocin production [20]. Additionally, synthetic antimicrobial peptides have shown promise in disrupting biofilm formation and enhancing the host immune response against MRSA [8]. These approaches leverage the natural mechanisms of microbial competition and host defense to combat biofilm-associated infections.

5.4 Photothermal and photodynamic therapies

Innovative therapies, such as photothermal and photodynamic therapies, are being explored for their potential to eradicate MRSA biofilms. Near-infrared light-activatable nanoparticles have been shown to combat established MRSA biofilms while simultaneously reducing inflammation [21]. Photodynamic therapy employs light-activated chemicals to produce reactive oxygen species, effectively compromising biofilm integrity and augmenting antibiotic effectiveness [6, 22]. This discrepancy can be attributed to multiple factors, including the diminished penetration of antibiotics through the biofilm matrix and the modified metabolic state of bacteria residing within biofilms. These conditions may result in a quiescent or persister phenotype that exhibits reduced susceptibility to antibiotic intervention [14].

Moreover, the genetic basis for biofilm formation in MRSA involves multiple regulatory systems, including the accessory gene regulator (agr) and the intercellular adhesion (ica) locus. These systems modulate the expression of virulence factors and biofilm-related genes, enhancing the bacteria's ability to form biofilms and resist antibiotic treatment [23, 24]. The mecA gene, responsible for methicillin resistance, also indirectly influences biofilm formation by affecting the expression of other genes involved in virulence and adhesion (**Table 1**) [24, 30].

Antibiotic name	Mechanism of action	Effectiveness against biofilms	Limitations	Advantages	References
Vancomycin	Inhibits cell wall synthesis by binding to D-Ala-D-Ala terminus of peptidoglycan precursors.	First-line treatment for MRSA; limited penetration into biofilm matrix; requires high concentrations for effectiveness.	The emergence of vancomycin-intermediate and resistant strains complicates treatment options.	Established efficacy against a wide range of Gram-positive bacteria; well-studied and widely used.	[11, 25]
Daptomycin	Binds to bacterial membrane, causing depolarization and cell death.	Effective against early-stage biofilms; bypasses some biofilm defenses.	Less effective against mature biofilms; best used in combination with other antibiotics.	Rapid bactericidal activity; effective against resistant strains of MRSA.	[12]
Linezolid	Inhibits protein synthesis by preventing initiation complex formation.	Good tissue penetration; effective for severe biofilm-related infections (e.g., bone, joint).	Long-term use is limited by side effects like thrombocytopenia and neuropathy; reserved for severe cases.	Oral and intravenous formulations available; effective against multi-drug-resistant bacteria.	[26]
Ceftaroline	Higher affinity for PBP2a, a penicillin-binding protein associated with MRSA resistance.	Viable option for MRSA infections but has limited effectiveness against biofilm-associated infections due to structural barriers.	Requires higher doses for effective concentrations, increasing the risk of adverse side effects.	Broad spectrum of activity against both MRSA and other Gram-positive pathogens.	[27]
Tigecycline	Inhibits protein synthesis, offering broad spectrum activity against resistant strains.	Potential option against MRSA biofilms; less vulnerable to common resistance mechanisms.	Limited penetration into biofilm matrix; often requires combination therapies for effectiveness.	Effective against a wide range of bacteria, including those resistant to other antibiotics.	[28]
Rifampicin	Disrupts RNA synthesis by binding to DNA-dependent RNA polymerase.	Valuable in combination therapy for biofilm-related MRSA infections, particularly with medical implants.	Rapid resistance development when used alone; requires careful monitoring due to hepatotoxicity.	Effective at penetrating biofilms and inhibiting bacterial metabolism; synergistic effects in combination therapy.	[16, 29]

Table 1.
Comparative analysis of antibiotics for MRSA biofilm treatment.

6. Antibiotic strategies against MRSA biofilms

The treatment of MRSA biofilms requires innovative strategies due to their inherent resistance mechanisms. Traditional antibiotics, such as beta-lactams and vancomycin, often fail to effectively penetrate and eradicate biofilm-associated bacteria. However, recent research has explored various approaches to enhance the efficacy of these antibiotics against MRSA biofilms. For instance, the use of combination therapies, where antibiotics are paired with biofilm-disrupting agents, has shown promise in overcoming the protective barriers of biofilms [4, 31, 32].

Furthermore, novel antimicrobial peptides and natural compounds are being investigated for their ability to inhibit biofilm formation and enhance the effectiveness of conventional antibiotics. For instance, melittin, a peptide derived from bee venom, has demonstrated significant antibiofilm activity when used in conjunction with penicillin and oxacillin against multidrug-resistant MRSA [8, 33]. Similarly, the incorporation of nanoparticles into antibiotic formulations has been shown to improve the delivery and efficacy of antibiotics against biofilm-associated MRSA [24, 30].

7. Essential oils on MRSA biofilms

Methicillin-resistant *Staphylococcus aureus* (MRSA) poses a significant threat in clinical environments due to its capacity to form biofilms, which serve to shield the bacteria from both the host's immune response and antibiotic therapies. Essential oils (Eos) have emerged as promising agents against MRSA biofilms, exhibiting antimicrobial properties that can disrupt biofilm formation and enhance the efficacy of conventional antibiotics. This chapter synthesizes recent findings on how EOs affect MRSA biofilms, focusing on their mechanisms of action, effectiveness, and potential applications in clinical settings. Different constituents of essential oils are mentioned in **Figure 2** that exhibit antimicrobial properties against MRSA.

7.1 Mechanisms of action of essential oils against MRSA biofilms

Essential oils exert their antimicrobial effects through various mechanisms, primarily targeting the bacterial cell membrane. For instance, studies have shown that components like carvacrol and thymol can disrupt the integrity of the bacterial membrane, leading to increased permeability and cell lysis [34, 35]. The disruption of membrane integrity is crucial as it allows for the leakage of intracellular components, which is detrimental to bacterial survival.

Moreover, the interaction of EOs with bacterial membranes can alter membrane potential and adenosine triphosphate (ATP) synthesis, further compromising bacterial viability [34]. This is particularly relevant for MRSA, which relies on its membrane integrity for maintaining homeostasis and resisting external stressors. The ability of EOs to modulate membrane properties enhances their effectiveness against biofilms, which are notoriously difficult to penetrate due to their dense extracellular matrix [3]. The mechanism of action of essential at glace is shown in **Figure 3**.

7.2 Inhibition of biofilm formation

Recent studies have shown that essential oils can markedly impede biofilm formation in MRSA. For example, Kim et al. reported that *Pinus koraiensis* essential oil

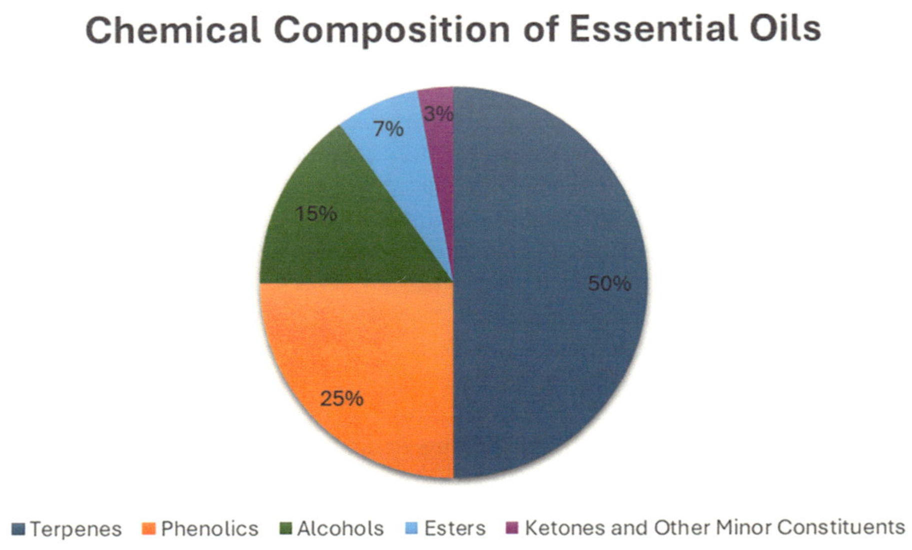

Figure 2.
A pie chart illustrating the major chemical constituents (e.g., terpenes, phenolics, aldehydes) found in various essential oils that exhibit antimicrobial properties against MRSA.

inhibited biofilm formation by up to 96.1% at optimal concentrations [26]. Similarly, Ghazal et al. found that *Origanum majorana* extracts and its essential oil components effectively inhibited biofilm formation in MRSA, with inhibition rates ranging from 36% to 86% [36]. This inhibition is crucial as biofilm formation is a key factor in the persistence of MRSA infections.

The mechanisms underlying the inhibition of biofilm formation by EOs may involve the downregulation of virulent genes associated with biofilm development. For instance, thymol has been shown to inhibit the expression of the sarA gene in MRSA, which is critical for biofilm formation [27]. This suggests that EOs not only disrupt existing biofilms but also prevent the initial stages of biofilm development by targeting specific genetic pathways.

7.3 Synergistic effects on antibiotics

The combination of EOs with conventional antibiotics has shown promising results in enhancing antimicrobial efficacy against MRSA. For instance, studies have indicated that carvacrol can enhance the activity of antibiotics like oxacillin by increasing membrane permeability, thereby allowing greater penetration of the antibiotic into the bacterial cell [34, 35]. This synergistic effect is particularly important in the context of MRSA, which is often resistant to multiple antibiotics.

Sreepian et al. demonstrated that citrus essential oils combined with gentamicin exhibited synergistic effects against MRSA, suggesting that the lipophilic nature of these oils facilitates their interaction with the bacterial membrane, enhancing the overall antimicrobial activity [37]. Such combinations could provide a viable strategy for overcoming antibiotic resistance in MRSA infections.

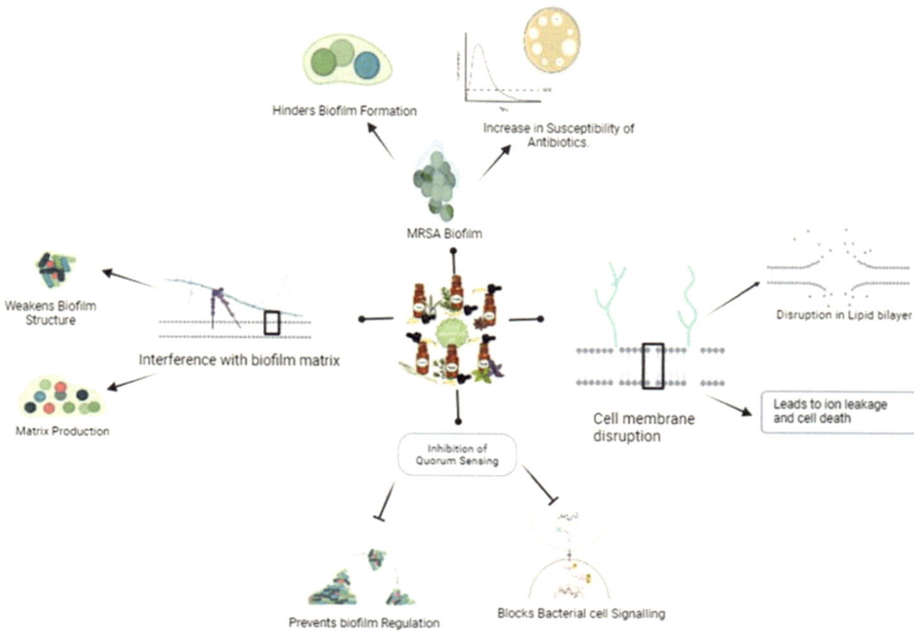

Figure 3.
Mechanism of action of essential oil.

7.4 Chemical composition of essential oils

The antimicrobial activity of EOs is largely attributed to their complex chemical composition, which includes various phenolic compounds, terpenes, and aldehydes. For example, the essential oil from *Croton conduplicatus* has been shown to affect the membrane integrity of MRSA strains, facilitating the action of other antimicrobial agents [3]. The presence of compounds like p-cymene and citral in EOs has been linked to their ability to disrupt biofilm formation and enhance the susceptibility of MRSA to antibiotics [29].

Furthermore, the specific composition of EOs can influence their effectiveness against MRSA biofilms. For instance, the study by Liu et al. highlighted that the essential oil extracted from *Carum carvi* L. seeds exhibited significant antibacterial properties, suggesting that the specific metabolites present in EOs play a critical role in their antimicrobial efficacy [25]. This underscores the importance of understanding the chemical profiles of EOs to optimize their use in clinical applications. The application of EOs in clinical settings offers a promising alternative to combat MRSA infections, particularly in the context of biofilm-related complications. The ability of EOs to inhibit biofilm formation and enhance the efficacy of existing antibiotics positions them as valuable adjuncts in the treatment of MRSA infections [38].

8. Antimicrobial efficacies of essential oils against drug-resistant strains

The increasing prevalence of drug-resistant bacterial strains poses a significant challenge to global health. Traditional antibiotics are becoming less effective, necessitating the exploration of alternative antimicrobial agents. Essential oils (EOs), derived from various plants, have garnered attention for their potential antimicrobial properties. This chapter synthesizes recent findings on the antimicrobial efficacies of EOs against drug-resistant strains, highlighting their mechanisms of action, effectiveness, and potential applications in combating antibiotic resistance.

8.1 Mechanisms of action of essential oils

Essential oils exhibit antimicrobial activity through various mechanisms, primarily targeting the bacterial cell membrane. The disruption of membrane integrity leads to increased permeability, resulting in cell lysis and death. For instance, the essential oils of *Curcuma longa* and *Syzygium aromaticum* have been shown to disrupt the cytoplasmic membrane of multiple drug-resistant bacteria, effectively inhibiting their growth [39]. Additionally, the multi-target nature of EOs allows them to affect various cellular processes, which is a significant advantage over conventional antibiotics that typically target a single pathway [40].

The chemical composition of EOs plays a crucial role in their antimicrobial efficacy. Compounds such as phenols, terpenes, and aldehydes contribute to their bioactivity. For example, *Thymus fallax* essential oil has demonstrated strong antibacterial and antibiofilm activities against oral pathogens, attributed to its high phenolic content [41, 42]. Furthermore, the synergistic effects of combining EOs with conventional antibiotics have been explored, revealing enhanced antimicrobial activity against resistant strains [43].

8.2 Efficacy against specific drug-resistant strains

Recent studies have highlighted the effectiveness of various EOs against specific drug-resistant strains. For instance, *Cinnamomum cassia* essential oil has shown potent activity against vancomycin-resistant *Enterococci*, with significant reductions in bacterial viability observed *in vitro* [36]. Similarly, *Melaleuca alternifolia* (Tea Tree Oil) has been effective against methicillin-resistant *Staphylococcus aureus* (MRSA), demonstrating its potential as an alternative treatment option [44].

Furthermore, essential oils obtained from citrus species, such as *citrus sinensis*, have demonstrated extensive antibacterial efficacy against both Gram-positive and Gram-negative bacteria, including resistant strains such as *Pseudomonas aeruginosa* and *Klebsiella pneumoniae* [37, 45]. The essential oil from *Zingiber cassumunar* has also been reported to inhibit extensively drug-resistant *Acinetobacter baumannii* within 1 hour of treatment, showcasing its rapid action against resistant pathogens [46].

8.3 Synergistic effects with conventional antibiotics

The combination of EOs with conventional antibiotics has been shown to enhance antimicrobial efficacy, particularly against resistant strains. For example, the combination of lavender and fennel essential oils with amoxicillin has demonstrated synergistic effects, significantly improving the antibacterial activity against resistant bacteria [47]. This synergism is attributed to the ability of EOs to disrupt bacterial membranes, making them more susceptible to antibiotics [43].

Additionally, studies have indicated that the incorporation of EOs into antimicrobial films can enhance their effectiveness. For instance, clove and cinnamon essential oils incorporated into poly(butylene adipate-co-terephthalate) films showed promising antimicrobial properties against various pathogens, suggesting potential applications in food preservation and packaging [48].

8.4 Potential applications in food preservation and healthcare

The antimicrobial properties of EOs extend beyond clinical applications; they also hold promise in food preservation. EOs can be utilized as natural preservatives to inhibit the growth of foodborne pathogens, thereby extending food life and ensuring food safety. For instance, *Trachyspermum ammi* essential oil has demonstrated significant antibacterial activity against *Streptococcus mutans*, a common foodborne pathogen [49, 50]. Furthermore, the use of EOs in food packaging materials has been explored, with studies indicating their effectiveness in reducing microbial contamination [51].

In healthcare, EOs can serve as adjunct therapies in managing infections caused by drug-resistant bacteria. Their ability to inhibit biofilm formation, a common trait of resistant strains, makes them valuable in treating chronic infections [52]. The incorporation of EOs into wound dressings has also been investigated, with promising results in promoting healing and preventing infections [53].

9. Future perspectives and clinical implications

Research has demonstrated that essential oils derived from plants such as *Curcuma longa* and *Syzygium aromaticum* exhibit potent antimicrobial activity against MRSA, with effective concentrations reported as low as 25 μL/mL [39]. Similarly, eucalyptus oil has been shown to enhance its antibacterial effects when encapsulated, reducing its volatility and increasing its stability against environmental factors [54]. The systematic review of eucalyptus oil's efficacy against MRSA highlights its potential as a natural alternative to conventional antibiotics, particularly in the face of rising antibiotic resistance [54]. Furthermore, essential oils like thyme and cinnamon have been reported to significantly inhibit the expression of biofilm-related genes in MRSA, thereby reducing biofilm formation [55].

The synergistic effects of combining essential oils with conventional antibiotics have also been a focal point of recent research. For instance, the combination of gentamicin with lavender essential oil has shown promising results in enhancing antibacterial activity against MRSA strains [56]. This synergy not only improves the efficacy of existing antibiotics but also offers a strategic approach to overcoming the challenges posed by antibiotic resistance. The interaction of essential oils with antibiotics can enhance membrane permeability and disrupt biofilm integrity, leading to increased susceptibility of MRSA to treatment [57].

Proteomic studies have also provided insights into the mechanisms by which MRSA biofilms respond to treatment with essential oils and antibiotics. These studies reveal that essential oils can modulate the expression of genes associated with biofilm formation and virulence, thereby enhancing the susceptibility of MRSA to antibiotic treatment [55]. For example, essential oils have been shown to affect the expression of genes related to biofilm matrix production, which is crucial for the structural integrity of biofilms [58]. This modulation of gene expression, combined with the physical disruption of biofilms, underscores the potential of essential oils as adjunctive therapies in the treatment of MRSA infections.

10. Conclusion

In conclusion, the integration of essential oils into the therapeutic arsenal against MRSA biofilms presents a promising avenue for enhancing infection management. Future research should focus on elucidating the molecular interactions between essential oils and MRSA, employing advanced techniques such as molecular docking and genomic analysis to identify the specific pathways and mechanisms affected by these compounds. Clinical trials are crucial to evaluate the safety, efficacy, and optimal dosing regimens of essential oils in human subjects, particularly among patients with chronic MRSA infections. Given the challenges posed by MRSA's multidrug resistance, especially with the rise of vancomycin-intermediate and vancomycin-resistant strains, the role of biofilms in complicating treatment regimens is critical. Essential oils may offer a novel approach to disrupt these biofilms, thereby enhancing the effectiveness of existing antibiotics and reducing the incidence of recurrent infections. Continued exploration of alternative treatment modalities, including the synergistic use of essential oils with traditional antibiotics, phage therapy, and nanoparticle-based interventions, will be essential. Ultimately, a multidisciplinary approach that combines rigorous research, clinical evaluation, and innovative therapeutic strategies will be vital in combating the clinical and community impacts of MRSA.

Acknowledgements

The authors acknowledge the efforts of management, SRM Institute of Science and Technology, Kattankulathur, Tamil Nadu, India, 603203 for their assistance.

The author acknowledges the use of Quillbot and Scite.ai for language polishing of the manuscript.

Conflict of interest

The authors declare no conflict of interest.

Author details

Sai Sristi Panda[1], Maheswary Datchanamoorthy[2], Leela Kakithakara Vajravelu[2] and W. Richard Thilagaraj[1]*

1 Department of Biotechnology, School of Bioengineering, SRM Institute of Science and Technology (SRM IST), Chennai, India

2 Department of Microbiology, SRM Medical College Hospital and Research Centre, SRM IST, Chennai, India

*Address all correspondence to: richardw@srmist.edu.in

References

[1] Zhang L, Wen B, Feng X, Xia Y, Li L, Cheng Y, et al. The Combined Administration of Vancomycin and Zhenqi Granules can Improve the Treatment of MRSA and Its Biofilms [Internet]. In Review. 2024. Available from: https://www.researchsquare.com/article/rs-4588113/v1

[2] Banerjee B, Gowda P, Ananda KT. Biofilm formation and antibiotic resistance of *S. aureus* strains isolated from chronic traumatic wounds. Journal of Pure and Applied Microbiology. 2022;**16**(1):424-429

[3] Maharjan S, Ansari M, Maharjan P, Rai KR, Sabina KC, Kattel HP, et al. Phenotypic detection of methicillin resistance, biofilm production, and inducible clindamycin resistance in *Staphylococcus aureus* clinical isolates in Kathmandu, Nepal. Tropical Medicine and Health. 2022;**50**(1):71

[4] Kaushik A, Kest H, Sood M, Steussy B, Thieman C, Gupta S. Biofilm producing methicillin-resistant *Staphylococcus aureus* [MRSA] infections in humans: Clinical implications and management. Pathogens. 2024;**13**(1):76

[5] Ahmad P. Phenotypic and molecular detection of biofilm formation in methicillin-resistant *Staphylococcus aureus* isolated from different clinical source in Erbil city. Mediterranean Journal of Hematology and Infectious Diseases. 2023;**15**(1):e2023016

[6] Hernández-Cuellar E, Tsuchiya K, Valle-Ríos R, Medina-Contreras O. Differences in biofilm formation by methicillin-resistant and methicillin-susceptible *Staphylococcus aureus* strains. Diseases. 2023;**11**(4):160

[7] Mashaly G, Badr D. Adhesins encoding genes and biofilm formation as virulence determinants in methicillin resistant *Staphylococcus aureus* causing hospital acquired infections. Egyptian Journal of Medical Microbiology. 2022;**31**(3):125-133

[8] Yu J, Han W, Xu Y, Shen L, Zhao H, Zhang J, et al. Biofilm-producing ability of methicillin-resistant *Staphylococcus aureus* clinically isolated in China. BMC Microbiology. 2024;**24**(1):241

[9] Elsawy L, Shohayeb M, El-Banna T, EL-Bouseary MM. Antibiotic resistance and β-lactamase production and biofilm formation by MRSA isolated from Dakahlia Governorate, Egypt. Delta University Scientific Journal. 2023;**6**(2):123-130

[10] Gu K, Ouyang P, Hong Y, Dai Y, Tang T, He C, et al. Geraniol inhibits biofilm formation of methicillin-resistant *Staphylococcus aureus* and increases the therapeutic effect of vancomycin in vivo. Frontiers in Microbiology. 2022;**13**:960728

[11] Chen Q, Dong Z, Yao X, Sun H, Pan X, Liu J, et al. Bactericidal and biofilm eradication efficacy of a fluorinated benzimidazole derivative, TFBZ, against methicillin-resistant *Staphylococcus aureus*. Frontiers in Pharmacology. 2024;**15**:1342821

[12] Ndukwe ARN, Hawas S, Qin J, Wiedbrauk S, Totsika M, Boase NRB, et al. Simple and efficient synthesis of 3-Aryl-2-oxazolidinone scaffolds enabling increased potency toward biofilms. Molecular Pharmaceutics. 2023;**20**(7):3484-3493

[13] Correia AAV, De Almeida Campos LA, De Queiroz Macêdo HLR,

De Lacerda CD, Agreles MAA, Xavier DE, et al. Antibacterial and antibiofilm potential of bacterial cellulose hydrogel containing vancomycin against multidrug-resistant *Staphylococcus aureus* and *Staphylococcus epidermidis*. Biology. 2024;**13**(5):354

[14] Manimaran M, Teo YY, Kah JCY, Beishenaliev A, Loke YL, Foo YY, et al. PDADMAC/alginate-coated gold nanorod for eradication of *Staphylococcus aureus* biofilms. International Journal of Nanomedicine. 2024;**19**:3697-3714

[15] Katsipis G, Pantazaki AA. Serrapeptase impairs biofilm, wall, and phospho-homeostasis of resistant and susceptible *Staphylococcus aureus*. Applied Microbiology and Biotechnology. 2023;**107**(4):1373-1389

[16] Wang W, Zhong Q, Cheng K, Tan L, Huang X. Molecular characteristics, antimicrobial susceptibility, biofilm-forming ability of clinically invasive *Staphylococcus aureus* isolates. Infection and Drug Resistance. 2023;**16**:7671-7681

[17] Peter IU, Okolo IO, Uzoeto HO, Edemekong CI, Thompson MD, Chukwu EB, et al. Identification and antibiotic resistance profile of biofilm-forming methicillin resistant *Staphylococcus aureus* [MRSA] causing infection among orthopedic wound patients. Asian Journal of Research in Medical and Pharmaceutical Sciences. Oct 2022;**12**:45-55

[18] Wu S, Liu Y, Lei L, Zhang H. An antisense yycF RNA modulates biofilm organization of methicillin-resistant *Staphylococcus aureus* and pathogenicity in a rat model of osteomyelitis. Antibiotics. 2021;**10**(5):603

[19] Wei G, He Y. Antibacterial and antibiofilm activities of novel cyclic peptides against methicillin-resistant *Staphylococcus aureus*. International Journal of Molecular Sciences. 2022;**23**(14):8029

[20] Purwoningsih E, Arfijanto MV, Widodo ADW. N-acetyl cysteine in combination with vancomycin or linezolid for biofilm eradication of methicillin-resistant *Staphylococcus aureus* [MRSA]. International Journal of Health Sciences. Sep 2022;**6**:803-810

[21] Deusenbery C, Carneiro O, Oberkfell C, Shukla A. Synergy of antibiotics and antibiofilm agents against methicillin-resistant *Staphylococcus aureus* biofilms. ACS Infectious Diseases. 2023;**9**(10):1949-1963

[22] Mao C, Zhu W, Xiang Y, Zhu Y, Shen J, Liu X, et al. Enhanced near-infrared photocatalytic eradication of MRSA biofilms and osseointegration using oxide perovskite-based P–N heterojunction. Advancement of Science. 2021;**8**(15):2002211

[23] Li J, Lu T, Chu Y, Zhang Y, Zhang J, Fu W, et al. Cinnamaldehyde targets SarA to enhance β-lactam antibiotic activity against methicillin-resistant *Staphylococcus aureus*. mLife. 2024;**3**(2):291-306

[24] Tian X, Liu B, Wu H, Cai R, Yang Y, Zhou C, et al. Zinc imidazole framework-8 nanoparticles disperse MRSA biofilm by inhibiting arginine biosynthesis and down-regulating adhesion-related proteins. Advanced Materials Interfaces. 2024;**11**(14):2300957

[25] Liu C, Cheng F, Aisa HA, Maiwulanjiang M. Comprehensive study of components and antimicrobial properties of essential oil extracted from *Carum carvi* L. Seeds. Antibiotics. 2023;**12**(3):591

[26] Kim JH, Kim YH, Park BI, Choi NY, Kim KJ. *Pinus koraiensis* essential oil attenuates the pathogenicity of superbacteria by suppressing virulence gene expression. Molecules. 2023;**29**(1):37

[27] Zhang L, Yang W, Chu Y, Wen B, Cheng Y, Mahmood T, et al. The inhibition effect of linezolid with reyanning mixture on MRSA and its biofilm is more significant than that of linezolid alone. Frontiers in Pharmacology. 2022;**12**:766309

[28] Yang M, Özdemir Z, Kim H, Nah S, Andris E, Li X, et al. Acid-responsive nanoporphyrin evolution for near-infrared fluorescence-guided photo-ablation of biofilm. Advanced Healthcare Materials. 2022;**11**(14):2200529

[29] Wei W, Li H, Yin C, Tang F. Research progress in the application of in situ hydrogel system in tumor treatment. Drug Delivery. 2020;**27**(1):460-468

[30] Sannat C, Hirpurkar SD, Shakya S, Dutta GK, Roy M, Jolhe DK, et al. Methanolic extract of *Hemidesmus indicus* root augments the antibacterial and antibiofilm activity of amoxicillin and clindamycin against methicillin-resistant *Staphylococcus aureus* of bovine origin. Letters in Applied Microbiology. 2022;**75**(6):1579-1589

[31] Chen X, Li W, Li X, Li K, Zhang G, Hong W. Photodynamic cationic ultrasmall copper oxide nanoparticles-loaded liposomes for alleviation of MRSA biofilms. International Journal of Nanomedicine. 2023;**18**:5441-5455

[32] Sudan S, Li J. Dispersal of pathogen-associated multispecies biofilm by novel probiotic *Bacillus subtilis* in a contact-dependent manner. Journal of Applied Microbiology. 2022;**133**(4):2501-2515

[33] Yuan Z, Lin C, Dai L, He Y, Hu J, Xu K, et al. Near-infrared light-activatable dual-action nanoparticle combats the established biofilms of methicillin-resistant *Staphylococcus aureus* and its accompanying inflammation. Small. 2021;**17**(13):2007522

[34] Kabotso DEK, Neglo D, Kwashie P, Agbo IA, Abaye DA. GC/MS composition and resistance modulatory inhibitory activities of three extracts of lemongrass: Citral modulates the activities of five antibiotics at sub-inhibitory concentrations on methicillin-resistant *Staphylococcus aureus*. Chemistry & Biodiversity. 2022;**19**(9):e202200296

[35] Chan YL, Chee CF, Tang SN, Tay ST. Unveilling genetic profiles and correlations of biofilm-associated genes, quorum sensing, and antibiotic resistance in *Staphylococcus aureus* isolated from a Malaysian Teaching Hospital. European Journal of Medical Research. 2024;**29**(1):246

[36] Ghazal TSA, Schelz Z, Vidács L, Szemerédi N, Veres K, Spengler G, et al. Antimicrobial, multidrug resistance reversal and biofilm formation inhibitory effect of *Origanum majorana* extracts, essential oil and monoterpenes. Plants. 2022;**11**(11):1432

[37] Sreepian A, Popruk S, Nutalai D, Phutthanu C, Sreepian PM. Antibacterial activities and synergistic interaction of citrus essential oils and limonene with gentamicin against clinically isolated methicillin-resistant *Staphylococcus aureus*. Scientific World Journal. 2022;**2022**:1-12

[38] Long L, Sulaiman JE, Xiao Y, Cheng A, Wang R, Malit JJ, et al. Mode of action of elasnin as biofilm formation eradicator of methicillin-resistant *Staphylococcus aureus*. Frontiers in Microbiology. 2022;**13**:967845

[39] Jalalifar S, Razavi S, Mirzaei R, Irajian G, Pooshang BK. A hope for ineffective antibiotics to return to treatment: Investigating the anti-biofilm potential of melittin alone and in combination with penicillin and oxacillin against multidrug resistant-MRSA and -VRSA. Frontiers in Microbiology. 2024;**14**:1269392

[40] Al-Tawalbeh D, Alkhawaldeh Y, Sawan H, Al-Mamoori F, Al-Samydai A, Mayyas A. Assessment of carvacrol-antibiotic combinations' antimicrobial activity against methicillin-resistant *Staphylococcus aureus*. Frontiers in Microbiology. 2024;**14**:1349550

[41] Wang Y, Liu X, Song L, Chen K, Shi C, Peng C, et al. Antibacterial and antibiofilm activities of protocatechualdehyde and its synergy with ampicillin against methicillin-resistant *Staphylococcus aureus*. Frontiers in Microbiology. 2024;**15**:1366400

[42] Thanh NPT, Kim XV, Kim MTN, Tran TT. Extracting and evaluating the antibacterial activity of carvacrol from *Plectranthus amboinicus* essential oil against *Staphylococcus aureus* and MRSA. IOP Conference Series: Earth and Environmental Science. 2024;**1340**(1):012030

[43] Oliveira GDD, Rocha WRVD, Rodrigues JFB, Alves HDS. Synergistic and antibiofilm effects of the essential oil from *Croton conduplicatus* [Euphorbiaceae] against methicillin-resistant *Staphylococcus aureus*. Pharmaceuticals. 2022;**16**(1):55

[44] Kim BC, Kim H, Lee HS, Kim SH, Cho DH, Jung HJ, et al. 4-Chloro-2-isopropyl-5-methylphenol exhibits antimicrobial and adjuvant activity against methicillin-resistant *Staphylococcus aureus*. Journal of Microbiology and Biotechnology. 2022;**32**(6):730-739

[45] Piasecki B, Biernasiuk A, Skiba A, Skalicka-Woźniak K, Ludwiczuk A. Composition, anti-MRSA activity and toxicity of essential oils from *Cymbopogon* species. Molecules. 2021;**26**(24):7542

[46] Alinezhad Z, Hashemi M, Afshari A, Shakeri G. Combatting methicillin-resistant *Staphylococcus aureus* [MRSA] in the food industry by harnessing the power of nature: A systematic review. Archives of Veterinary Medicine. 2023;**16**(2):5-51

[47] Zeshan MQ et al. Antimicrobial activity of essential oils of *Curcuma longa* and *Syzygium aromaticum* against multiple drug-resistant pathogenic bacteria. Tropical Biomedicine. 2023;**40**(2):174-182

[48] Alam A, Foudah AI, Salkini MA, Raish M, Sawale J. Herbal fennel essential oil nanogel: Formulation, characterization and antibacterial activity against *Staphylococcus aureus*. Gels. 2022;**8**(11):736

[49] Moshaverinia M, Sahmeddini S, Lavaee F, Zareshahrabadi Z, Zomorodian K. Antimicrobial and anti-biofilm activities of *Thymus fallax* essential oil against oral pathogens. BioMed Research International. 2022;**2022**(1):9744153

[50] Nouri Gharajalar S, Hassanzadeh M, Mahmoudi R, et al. Antibacterial activity of *Trachyspermum ammi* essential oil against *Streptococcus mutans* isolated from human dental plaques. Journal of Medical Microbiology and Infectious Diseases. 2022;**10**(4):192-198

[51] Naz A, Haider S, Ali SM. Antimicrobial activity, alone and

in conjunction with cefuroxime. International Journal of Pharmacy & Integrated Health Sciences [Internet]. 2023;**4**(1). Available from: http://ijpihs.pk/index.php/IJPIHS/article/view/55:41-48 [Accessed: December 4, 2024]

[52] Taufiq MMJ, Darah I. Effects of cultural conditions in enhancing the production of anti-MRSA activity of *Lasiodiplodia pseudotheobromae* IBRL OS-64, an endophytic fungus isolated from leaf of *Ocimum sanctum* L. in submerged fermentation system. Journal of Pure and Applied Microbiology. 2019;**13**(4):2517-2531

[53] de Rapper SL, Viljoen A, Van Vuuren S. Optimizing the antimicrobial synergism of *Melaleuca alternifolia* [tea tree] essential oil combinations for application against respiratory related pathogens. Planta Medica. 2023;**89**(04):454-463

[54] Naveed R, Siddique AB, Hussain I, Ulhaq M, Aslam B, Mahmood MS. Antimicrobial activity of bioactive components of essential oils from *Citrus sinensis* against important pathogens. International Food Research Journal. 2021;**28**(1):189-198

[55] Hu H, Hua SY, Lin X, Lu F, Zhang W, Zhou L, et al. Hybrid biomimetic membrane coated particles-mediated bacterial ferroptosis for acute MRSA pneumonia. ACS Nano. 2023;**17**(12):11692-11712

[56] Quirino A, Giorgi V, Palma E, Marascio N, Morelli P, Maletta A, et al. *Citrus bergamia*: Kinetics of antimicrobial activity on clinical isolates. Antibiotics. 2022;**11**(3):361

[57] Karadağ AE, Çaşkurlu A, Demirci B, Demirci F. Binary synergistic combinations of lavender and fennel essential oils with amoxicillin. Planta Medica. 2023;**89**(08):800-807

[58] Moraes Filho LEPT, Andrade MF, Freitas LF, Palha MDLAPF, Vinhas GM. Development and characterization of poly[butylene adipate-co-terephthalate] [PBAT] antimicrobial films with clove and cinnamon essential oils. Journal of Food Processing & Preservation [Internet]. 2022;**46**(4). Available from: https://onlinelibrary.wiley.com/doi/10.1111/jfpp.16489:e16489–e16489 [Accessed: December 4, 2024]

Chapter 8

Natural Antimicrobials: The Anti-Biofilm Potential of Garlic and Thyme Essential Oils against *Salmonella typhimurium*

Alaa T. Qumsani

Abstract

Salmonella typhimurium is a pathogenic bacterium that presents significant challenges in food processing environments, primarily due to its ability to form biofilms, which confer resistance to traditional cleaning protocols and antimicrobial treatments. With the increasing prevalence of antibiotic-resistant strains, the exploration of natural antimicrobials, particularly garlic (*Allium sativum*) and thyme (*Thymus vulgaris*) essential oils, has become increasingly important. This chapter investigates the antibacterial and anti-biofilm properties of these essential oils, highlighting their ability to disrupt quorum sensing, inhibit biofilm formation, and suppress virulence factors. The potential applications of these oils as natural preservatives in food safety are discussed, presenting a promising natural approach to combating microbial contamination and enhancing food safety.

Keywords: *Salmonella typhimurium*, pathogenic bacterium, biofilm formation, antibiotic-resistant strains, garlic essential oil (*Allium sativum*), thyme essential oil (*Thymus vulgaris*), quorum sensing disruption, antibacterial properties, anti-biofilm activity, natural antimicrobials, food safety, natural preservatives

1. Introduction

In recent years, the issue of food safety has increasingly garnered attention from public health experts, consumers, and regulatory agencies, primarily due to the persistent threat posed by foodborne pathogens such as *Salmonella typhimurium* [1]. This particular strain of *Salmonella* is renowned for its ability to contaminate a wide array of food products, leading to significant health risks and economic losses [2]. The capacity of *S. typhimurium* to form robust biofilms enables it to adhere to surfaces within food processing environments, creating a protective matrix that facilitates its survival and resistance to cleaning and sanitizing efforts [3]. Consequently, biofilms not only complicate contamination control but also serve as reservoirs for persistent infections, ultimately leading to outbreaks with serious public health ramifications [4].

IntechOpen

Compounding this issue is the alarming rise in antibiotic resistance among bacterial strains, including *S. typhimurium*, which reduces the efficacy of conventional antibiotic treatments and highlights the urgent need for alternative interventions [5]. As the limitations of traditional antimicrobial strategies become evident, there is growing interest in exploring natural and holistic approaches to food safety that can mitigate the risks associated with antibiotic-resistant pathogens [6]. Natural antimicrobials, particularly those derived from plants, have attracted significant interest due to their ability to offer effective antibacterial properties with fewer side effects compared to synthetic alternatives [7].

This chapter explores the potential of garlic (*Allium sativum*) and thyme (*Thymus vulgaris*) essential oils as promising natural agents in the fight against biofilm formation and microbial contamination [8]. The unique phytochemical composition of these essential oils contributes to their multifaceted mechanisms of action, which include the suppression of virulence gene expression, disruption of bacterial communication pathways through quorum sensing, and interference with adherence mechanisms used by bacteria to colonies surfaces [9]. By investigating the efficacy and safety of these natural compounds, this chapter aims to shed light on their role as viable alternatives to traditional preservatives and antimicrobials in the food industry [10]. Ultimately, the exploration of garlic and thyme essential oils underscores the potential for sustainable and innovative strategies to enhance food safety, combat antibiotic-resistant pathogens, and promote a healthier food supply [11].

Salmonella typhimurium is a significant pathogen that poses serious challenges to public health, particularly in food safety [12]. Understanding the characteristics of *S. typhimurium* is crucial to addressing its impact on health and hygiene practices in food processing environments [13]. This bacterium is notorious for its ability to form biofilms, which are structured communities of bacteria enmeshed in a self-produced matrix of polymeric substances [14]. Biofilms not only enhance bacterial resistance to environmental stresses and disinfectants but also promote persistence on surfaces of food-processing equipment [15]. The formation of biofilms is a crucial factor that contributes to the survival and proliferation of *S. typhimurium* in various settings, facilitating its transmission through contaminated food products [16]. The presence of biofilms can lead to persistent contamination of food processing facilities, resulting in recurrent outbreaks of salmonellosis [17]. Moreover, the resilient nature of biofilms complicates eradication efforts, making routine cleaning and sanitization protocols less effective [18]. Understanding the biofilm-forming abilities of *S. typhimurium* is essential for developing targeted strategies to minimize its persistence in the food supply chain, thereby reducing the risk of salmonellosis outbreaks and addressing broader public health implications [19].

The antibacterial properties of garlic (*Allium sativum*) and thyme (*Thymus vulgaris*) essential oils have been extensively researched, revealing their effectiveness as natural antimicrobial agents against a variety of pathogens, including *Salmonella typhimurium* [20]. Garlic essential oil is particularly renowned for its rich composition of bioactive compounds, among which allicin is the most prominent [21]. Allicin, a sulfur-containing compound released when garlic is crushed or chopped, has been shown to possess potent antimicrobial activity [22]. Mechanistically, allicin exerts its antibacterial effects primarily by disrupting the integrity of bacterial cell membranes [23]. This disruption leads to increased permeability, allowing for uncontrolled influx and efflux of ions and other small molecules essential for bacterial survival, ultimately culminating in cell lysis [24]. Furthermore, garlic oil has been implicated in the suppression of virulence gene expression within *Salmonella* [25], interfering with regulatory pathways that control the expression of factors crucial for virulence, such as fimbriae and secreted toxins (**Figure 1**) [26].

In addition to garlic, thyme essential oil emerges as another significant natural antimicrobial with a distinct mechanism of action [27]. Rich in phenolic compounds such as thymol and carvacrol, thyme essential oil is recognized for its broad-spectrum antibacterial properties [28]. Thymol acts by disrupting bacterial cell membranes similarly to allicin but also targets the respiratory chain, leading to a decline in ATP production and overall energy disruption within bacterial cells [29]. Carvacrol complements this effect by interfering with biosynthetic pathways necessary for cell wall synthesis and functioning [30]. Importantly, thyme oil has been demonstrated to disrupt quorum sensing, a cell-to-cell communication process that bacteria use to coordinate behaviors such as biofilm formation and virulence factor expression [31]. By inhibiting quorum sensing, thyme essential oil effectively diminishes the ability of *Salmonella* to establish biofilms, crucial for its persistence in host environments and food processing settings [32].

Moreover, the combination of garlic and thyme essential oils provides a synergistic effect, enhancing their overall antimicrobial activity [33]. Research suggests that when used in conjunction, these essential oils may potentiate each other's effects, leading to reduced minimum inhibitory concentrations and enhanced efficacy against biofilm-forming pathogens [34]. This synergism is particularly valuable in food safety applications, where preventing biofilm formation is essential in reducing the risk of contamination and ensuring the safety of food products [35]. Additionally, both garlic and thyme essential oils possess anti-inflammatory properties, which can further mitigate the immune response triggered by foodborne pathogens [36], offering potential therapeutic benefits in managing gastrointestinal infections caused by *Salmonella* [37]. Overall, a comprehensive understanding of the antibacterial properties, mechanisms of action, and potential synergistic effects of garlic and thyme essential oils highlights their role as promising natural alternatives in combating antibiotic-resistant pathogens like *Salmonella typhimurium*, paving the way for innovative applications in the food industry [38].

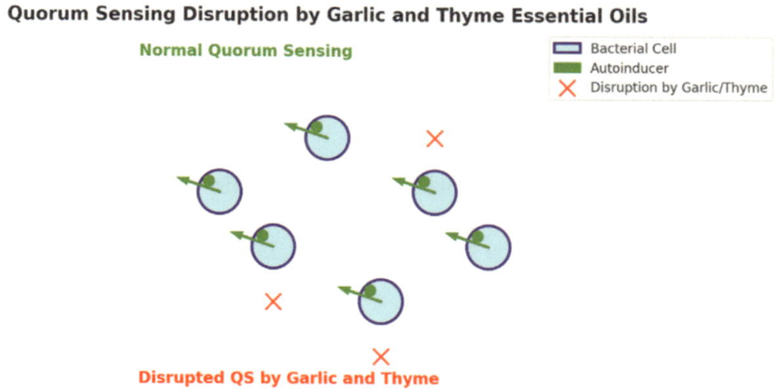

Figure 1.
Quorum sensing and its disruption by garlic and thyme: illustrates the quorum sensing (QS) mechanism in Salmonella typhimurium *and how garlic (allicin) and thyme (thymol, carvacrol) essential oils disrupt this process. On the left, bacterial cells communicate by releasing signaling molecules called autoinducers. As these accumulate, they activate biofilm formation and virulence factors. On the right, garlic and thyme essential oils interfere with this communication, disrupting membrane integrity, inhibiting quorum sensing, and reducing biofilm formation, offering a natural approach to combating bacterial contamination [26].*

The application of garlic (*Allium sativum*) and thyme (*Thymus vulgaris*) essential oils as natural preservatives in food safety is not only innovative but also represents a significant advancement in addressing contemporary challenges faced by the food industry [39]. In response to rising consumer demand for transparency in food labeling and increasing awareness of the potential adverse effects associated with synthetic preservatives, manufacturers are progressively exploring natural alternatives [40]. Garlic essential oil, rich in bioactive compounds such as allicin and diallyl sulfones, has garnered attention for its remarkable antimicrobial properties effective against a spectrum of foodborne pathogens, including *Salmonella typhimurium* [41]. Allicin, in particular, exhibits powerful antibacterial activity by disrupting bacterial cell membranes and inhibiting enzyme function, thereby minimizing the risk of infection associated with contaminated food products [42]. Conversely, thyme essential oil is characterized by high concentrations of thymol and carvacrol, which not only demonstrate strong antibacterial activity but also possess antioxidant properties that help preserve the flavor, color, and nutritional value of food items [43]. Integrating these essential oils into food products holds significant promise for inhibiting bacterial growth and biofilm formation, critical in extending the shelf life of perishable goods such as meats, dairy products, and fresh produce [44].

Furthermore, the application of garlic and thyme essential oils as natural preservatives aligns with the emerging trend of clean-label products sought by consumers increasingly wary of artificial additives [45]. These essential oils can play a dual role by acting as both antimicrobial and natural flavor enhancers, ensuring that food remains safe for consumption and appealing to consumers' palates [46]. Incorporating these essential oils into processing protocols can critically enhance current food safety practices [47]. For instance, they can be employed in coating technologies or incorporated into packaging materials, creating a barrier against microbial contamination and providing a proactive solution to the issue of foodborne pathogens [48].

Moreover, ongoing research continues to uncover the synergistic effects when garlic and thyme essential oils are combined with other natural preservatives or food processing techniques, suggesting a compounding effect that can further elevate their antimicrobial efficacy [49]. Such findings imply that using these essential oils could lead to more effective strategies in minimizing microbial loads not only during production but also throughout the supply chain, including storage and distribution [50]. The utilization of garlic and thyme essential oils positions the food industry to effectively combat the rising tide of antibiotic-resistant microorganisms, which pose severe public health challenges [51]. By embracing these natural antimicrobial agents, food producers can better align with broader sustainability goals while enhancing public health outcomes [52]. Overall, incorporating these essential oils into food safety not only addresses immediate safety concerns but also contributes to a long-term vision of promoting more sustainable, health-conscious practices in the food industry [53].

2. *Salmonella typhimurium* biofilm formation

Biofilms are structured bacterial communities that provide protection to bacteria from environmental stressors, including disinfectants and antibiotics [19]. *S. typhimurium* forms biofilms on various surfaces, making it difficult to remove from food processing environments [20, 21]. The extracellular polymeric substance (EPS) matrix that forms biofilms acts as a barrier that reduces the effectiveness of antimicrobial agents, allowing bacteria to survive [22–24].

Quorum sensing (QS) plays a critical role in biofilm formation by regulating gene expression in response to population density [25, 26]. Disruption of QS signaling has been shown to inhibit biofilm formation, making it a promising target for controlling *S. typhimurium* [27–29].

Essential oils, including those derived from garlic and thyme, have been shown to interfere with quorum sensing, thereby inhibiting biofilm formation and reducing bacterial virulence [30–32]. These findings suggest that natural antimicrobials could be an effective alternative to synthetic antimicrobials in controlling microbial contamination in food processing environments [33, 34].

3. Mechanisms of action of garlic essential oil

Garlic essential oil is known for its potent antimicrobial properties, primarily due to the presence of allicin, a sulfur-containing compound released when garlic is crushed [35–37]. Allicin disrupts bacterial cell membranes, increasing their permeability and leading to cell death [38–40]. In addition, allicin interferes with quorum sensing, which is essential for biofilm formation and bacterial virulence [41].

By inhibiting QS, garlic essential oil reduces the expression of biofilm-associated genes, such as those responsible for fimbriae and flagella production, which are necessary for bacterial adhesion and invasion [42, 43]. One study showed that garlic essential oil reduced biofilm formation by over 80% in *S. typhimurium* [44].

Other compounds in garlic essential oil, such as diallyl sulfide and diallyl disulfide, contribute to its broad-spectrum antimicrobial activity. These compounds have been shown to inhibit the growth of various foodborne pathogens, including *Escherichia coli* and *Staphylococcus aureus* [45–48]. The primary antimicrobial compounds in essential garlic oil are listed in **Table 1**.

4. Anti-biofilm activity of thyme essential oil

Thyme essential oil is another natural antimicrobial with significant antibacterial properties due to the presence of phenolic compounds such as thymol and carvacrol [49–51]. Thymol and carvacrol disrupt bacterial membranes, increasing permeability and leading to cell lysis [52, 53, 57]. These compounds also interfere with bacterial energy production and the synthesis of cell walls, further inhibiting bacterial growth [58].

Essential oil	Active compounds	Antimicrobial activity	Target pathogens
Garlic (*Allium sativum*)	Allicin, Diallyl sulfide, Diallyl disulfide	Disrupts bacterial cell membranes, inhibits quorum sensing	*Salmonella typhimurium*, *E. coli*, *S. aureus*
Thyme (*Thymus vulgaris*)	Thymol, Carvacrol, p-Cymene	Disrupts membrane integrity, inhibits cell wall synthesis	*S. typhimurium*, *Listeria monocytogenes*, *Bacillus cereus*

Table 1.
Antimicrobial compounds in garlic and thyme essential oils synergistic effects of garlic and thyme essential oils [54–56].

Combination	Minimum Inhibitory Concentration (MIC)	Reduction in biofilm formation	Mechanisms
Garlic + Thyme Essential Oils	Lower MIC compared to individual oils	>95%	Membrane disruption, quorum sensing inhibition, biofilm breakdown

Table 2.
Synergistic effects of garlic and thyme essential oils against Salmonella typhimurium *[70–72].*

Research has shown that thyme essential oil is effective at inhibiting biofilm formation in *S. typhimurium* by disrupting quorum sensing [59–61]. By reducing QS signaling, thyme essential oil inhibits the expression of biofilm-related genes, making it difficult for bacteria to form stable biofilms on food processing surfaces [62]. A study reported that thyme essential oil reduced biofilm formation by 70% in *S. typhimurium* [63].

Thyme essential oil has also been shown to inhibit the growth of other foodborne pathogens, such as *Listeria monocytogenes*, *Bacillus cereus*, and *Campylobacter jejuni* [54–56]. The main bioactive compounds in the thyme essential oil are summarized in **Table 1**.

When used together, garlic and thyme essential oils demonstrate a synergistic effect that enhances their antimicrobial efficacy [64, 65]. Studies have shown that combining these essential oils reduces the minimum inhibitory concentration (MIC) required to inhibit bacterial growth, making them more effective at lower concentrations [66, 67]. This is especially important in food safety applications, where minimizing the concentration of antimicrobials is crucial for maintaining food quality [68].

In one study, the combination of garlic and thyme essential oils reduced biofilm formation by over 95% in *S. typhimurium* [69]. The synergistic effect is attributed to the complementary mechanisms of allicin, thymol, and carvacrol. Allicin disrupts bacterial membranes and inhibits quorum sensing, while thymol and carvacrol weaken the bacterial cell wall, further enhancing the antimicrobial effect [70–72]. These results are summarized in **Table 2**.

5. Applications in food safety

Garlic and thyme essential oils offer significant potential as natural preservatives and surface decontaminants in food safety applications [73, 74]. These oils can be incorporated into food packaging materials or applied directly to food products to prevent microbial contamination and extend the shelf life of perishable goods [75]. Their natural antimicrobial properties make them attractive alternatives to synthetic preservatives, especially as consumers demand clean-label products [76, 77].

In food processing environments, garlic and thyme essential oils can be used to disinfect surfaces and equipment, thereby reducing the risk of contamination by *S. typhimurium* and other pathogens [78, 79]. The ability of these oils to reduce biofilm formation on food processing surfaces makes them particularly effective for preventing contamination in packaged and ready-to-eat foods [80]. These applications are summarized in **Table 3**.

Application	Essential oil used	Mode of action	Examples
Food Packaging	Garlic, Thyme	Antimicrobial coatings, encapsulation in packaging	Meat, dairy, fresh produce
Surface Decontamination	Garlic, Thyme	Direct application on surfaces to inhibit biofilm formation	Food processing equipment
Food Preservation	Garlic, Thyme	Reduces microbial contamination, extends shelf life	Packaged foods, ready-to-eat products

Table 3.
Summary of applications of essential oils in food preservation [80].

6. Conclusion

The persistent challenge posed by *S typhimurium*, particularly its capacity to form resilient biofilms within food processing environments, underscores a critical concern in modern food safety management [57]. This pathogenic bacterium not only jeopardizes public health through potential contamination of various food products but has also demonstrated an alarming ability to adapt and survive under harsh environmental conditions, complicating effective control measures and food safety protocols [58]. The rise of antibiotic-resistant strains has further exacerbated these challenges, rendering conventional treatment options less effective and raising urgent questions about mitigation strategies [59]. Therefore, exploring and developing alternative strategies that can effectively complement or replace antibiotic treatments is essential, focusing on naturally derived solutions that are safe, effective, and widely acceptable to consumers [60].

In light of these pressing concerns, this chapter highlights the substantial promise of natural antimicrobials, such as garlic (*Allium sativum*) and thyme (*Thymus vulgaris*) essential oils, in the ongoing battle against *Salmonella* biofilms [61]. These essential oils, long celebrated for their traditional medicinal properties, are increasingly recognized by the scientific community for their potent antibacterial activities against a range of pathogens, including multidrug-resistant strains [62]. The unique phytochemical compositions of garlic and thyme reveal sophisticated mechanisms of action that not only inhibit bacterial growth but also target and disrupt critical cellular processes essential for pathogenicity [63]. For instance, the ability of these essential oils to suppress virulence gene expression represents a promising avenue for reducing the pathogenic potential of Salmonella, while their interference with quorum sensing pathways serves to disrupt communication systems that bacteria rely on for biofilm formation and maturation [54]. Such multifaceted modes of action elevate garlic and thyme essential oils to significant relevance in natural food preservation research [55].

Moreover, the implications of incorporating these essential oils into food safety interventions extend beyond simple antibacterial effects; they pave the way for a more holistic approach to food safety that prioritizes natural solutions over synthetic alternatives, often met with increasing consumer skepticism and regulatory scrutiny [56]. As consumers today become more health-conscious and demand cleaner and safer food products, the strategic integration of garlic and thyme essential oils into food safety protocols can enhance the safety of food products and potentially revolutionize current industry practices by providing effective and sustainable alternatives to conventional preservatives [64]. However, harnessing the full potential of garlic and thyme essential oils requires further comprehensive research to elucidate their precise mechanisms of action, optimal application methods, and potential interactions with various food components or processing conditions [65]. Understanding these factors will provide a more nuanced comprehension of how these natural agents can be effectively utilized in food processing systems while ensuring consumer safety and maximizing efficacy [66].

To that end, continued investigation into the bioactive compounds present in garlic and thyme, as well as their synergistic effects with other natural preservatives, is essential in developing innovative food safety strategies that address both consumer expectations and foodborne pathogen challenges [67]. Ultimately, the strategic employment of garlic and thyme essential oils signifies not only a proactive and innovative approach to safeguarding public health but also represents a paradigm shift toward environmentally sustainable practices in food production [68]. By embracing such innovative methods, the food industry can proactively contribute to creating healthier food systems, safeguard consumer health, and play an important role in the broader global effort to combat antibiotic resistance in foodborne pathogens [69]. This multidimensional strategy holds the potential for improving food safety outcomes and reflects a profound commitment to nurturing the health of both consumers and the environment, ensuring that future generations can enjoy safe, wholesome food produced through sustainable means [70].

The persistence of *S. typhimurium* in food processing environments, particularly through biofilm formation, presents a major challenge to food safety. Garlic and thyme essential oils, with their potent antimicrobial and anti-biofilm properties, offer a natural and effective alternative to synthetic antimicrobials [81–83]. By disrupting quorum sensing, inhibiting biofilm formation, and reducing bacterial virulence, these essential oils have the potential to revolutionize food safety practices and promote cleaner, more sustainable food preservation methods [84, 85].

Further research is needed to optimize the application methods and concentrations of these essential oils to fully harness their potential in combating foodborne pathogens and ensuring the safety of food products [86–88].

Acknowledgements

I would like to express my deepest gratitude to Dr. Mohammed Elbeeh for his invaluable guidance, continuous support, and insightful feedback throughout the course of this research. His expertise and dedication have significantly contributed to the success of this project. I am truly grateful for his mentorship and for always encouraging me to pursue excellence in my work. The author acknowledges the use of QuillBot for language polishing of the manuscript.

Conflict of interest

The author declares no conflict of interest.

Abbreviations

QS	quorum sensing
MIC	minimum inhibitory concentration
EPS	extracellular polymeric substances
EO	essential oils
S. typhimurium	*Salmonella typhimurium*

Author details

Alaa T. Qumsani
Biology Department, Al-Jamoum University College, Umm al-Qura University, Makkah, Saudi Arabia

*Address all correspondence to: atqumsani@uqu.edu.sa

References

[1] Javanmard Z, Pourhajibagher M, Bahador A. Advancing anti-biofilm strategies: Innovations to combat biofilm-related challenges and enhance efficacy. Journal of Basic Microbiology [Internet]. 2024;**64**(12). DOI: 10.1002/jobm.202400271

[2] Iaconis A, De Plano LM, Caccamo A, Franco D, Conoci S. Anti-biofilm strategies: A focused review on innovative approaches. Microorganisms [Internet]. 2024;**12**(4):639. DOI: 10.3390/microorganisms12040639

[3] Subramani R, Jayaprakashvel M. Bacterial quorum sensing: Biofilm formation, survival behaviour and antibiotic resistance. In: Implication of Quorum Sensing and Biofilm Formation in Medicine, Agriculture and Food Industry [Internet]. 2019. pp. 21-37. DOI: 10.1007/978-981-32-9409-7_3

[4] Crain SL, Coffey RT. Occurrence of ethyl carbamate in foods and beverages: Review of the formation mechanisms, advances in analytical methods, and mitigation strategies. A Comment on: Journal of Food Protection. 84(12):2195-2212 (2021). Journal of Food Protection. 2022;**85**(8):1104-1106. DOI: 10.4315/0362-028x.85.8.1104

[5] Roy MP, Adhikari MD, Tiwary BK. Phytocompound-mediated inhibition of quorum-sensing cascade in pathogenic bacteria. Natural Products [Internet]. 2023:79-101. DOI: 10.1201/9781003300557-5

[6] Cáceres M, Hidalgo W, Stashenko E, Torres R, Ortiz C. Essential oils of aromatic plants with antibacterial, anti-biofilm and anti-quorum sensing activities against pathogenic bacteria. Antibiotics [Internet]. 2020;**9**(4):147. DOI: 10.3390/antibiotics9040147

[7] Brown LG et al. Correction to: Restaurant date-marking practices concerning ready-to-eat food requiring time and temperature control for safety. Foodborne Pathogens and Disease [Internet]. 2022;**19**(1):80-80. DOI: 10.1089/fpd.2021.0003.correx

[8] Popova TP, Bankova R. Antimicrobial activity *in vitro* of essential oils from oregano (*Origanum compactum* L.) and thyme (*Thymus vulgaris* L.). International Journal of Current Microbiology and Applied Sciences [Internet]. 2016;**5**(10):57-68. DOI: 10.20546/ijcmas.2016.510.008

[9] Paudyal N, Pan H, Li X, Fang W, Yue M. Retraction of: Antibiotic resistance in *Salmonella Enteritidis* isolates recovered from chicken, chicken breast, and humans through national antimicrobial resistance monitoring system between 1996 and 2014. Foodborne Pathogens and Disease [Epub ahead of print]. DOI: 10.1089/fpd.2017.2402. Foodborne Pathogens and Disease [Internet]. 2018;15(10):669-669. DOI:10.1089/fpd.2017.2402.retract

[10] Türkmenoğlu A, Özmen D. Allergenic components, biocides, and analysis techniques of some essential oils used in food products. Journal of Food Science [Internet]. 2021;**86**(6):2225-2241. DOI: 10.1111/1750-3841.15753

[11] Li YX, Erhunmwunsee F, Liu M, Yang K, Zheng W, Tian J. Antimicrobial mechanisms of spice essential oils and application in food industry. Food Chemistry [Internet]. 2022;**382**:132312. DOI: 10.1016/j.foodchem.2022.132312

[12] Mahomoodally MF, Gurib-Fakim A, Subratty AH. Screening for alternative antibiotics: An investigation into the

antimicrobial activities of medicinal food plants of Mauritius. Journal of Food Science[Internet]. 2010;**75**(3). DOI: 10.1111/j.1750-3841.2010.01555.x

[13] Ji J, Shankar S, Royon F, Salmieri S, Lacroix M. Essential oils as natural antimicrobials applied in meat and meat products—A review. Critical Reviews in Food Science and Nutrition[Internet]. 2021;**63**(8):993-1009. DOI: 10.1080/10408398.2021.1957766

[14] Broadway PR et al. Correction to: Prevalence and antimicrobial susceptibility of *Salmonella* serovars isolated from U.S. retail ground pork. Foodborne Pathogens and Disease [Internet]. 2021;**18**(5):364-365. DOI: 10.1089/fpd.2020.2853.correx

[15] Ríos JL. Essential oils. In: Essential Oils in Food Preservation, Flavor and Safety [Internet]. 2016. pp. 3-10. DOI: 10.1016/b978-0-12-416641-7.00001-8

[16] Liu J, Huang Y, Lu X, Yu W, Yu K, Peng S, et al. Solidification of plant essential oils by electrostatic adsorption and Ca^{2+} crosslinking for pot-stewed duck neck preservation. Food Control [Internet]. 2025;**174**:111214. DOI: 10.1016/j.foodcont.2025.111214

[17] Glass-Kaastra et al. Correction to: Estimated reduction in the burden of nontyphoidal *Salmonella* illness in Canada circa 2019. Foodborne Pathogens and Disease [Internet]. 2023;**20**(7):313-314. DOI: 10.1089/fpd.2022.0045.correx

[18] Hu et al. Correction to: Probiotic and safety evaluation of twelve lactic acid bacteria as future probiotics. Foodborne Pathogens and Disease [Internet]. 2024. DOI: 10.1089/fpd.2023.0039.correx

[19] Ojha S, Pandey AK, Singh P. *Citrus aurantifolia* essential oil composition, bioactivity, and antibacterial mode of action on *Salmonella enterica*, a foodborne pathogen. Food Science and Engineering [Internet]. 2023:75-88. DOI: 10.37256/fse.4120231615

[20] Gamaryani A, Mukhtar MF, Rahman KU, Ullah I, Dur-e-Nayab AAM, et al. Antimicrobial activity of curcumin against drug-resistant Gram-negative pathogens in skin infections. Indus Journal of Bioscience Research [Internet]. 2025;**3**(1):307-313. DOI: 10.70749/ijbr.v3i1.508

[21] Ait Mammar W, Wilson A, Miche A, Kuntzel T, Salmain M, Boujday S. Smartphone-assisted plasmonic biosensors for rapid on-site detection of foodborne pathogens and allergens. Talanta [Internet]. 2025;**291**:127864. DOI: 10.1016/j.talanta.2025.127864

[22] Ramallo IA, Gago G, Gramajo H, Furlan RLE. Bioautographic method for detecting natural preservatives against *Mycobacterium* in edible essential oils. Food Control [Internet]. 2025;**174**:111224. DOI: 10.1016/j.foodcont.2025.111224

[23] Zare-Zardini H. Antimicrobial peptides with spermicidal activity as new contraceptive agents: Killing two birds with one stone. Current Women`s Health Reviews [Internet]. 2025;**21**(5). DOI: 10.2174/0115734048307970240902095704

[24] Gamaryani A, Mukhtar MF, Rahman KU, Ullah I, Dur-e-Nayab AAM, et al. Antimicrobial activity of curcumin against drug-resistant Gram-negative pathogens in skin infections. Indus Journal of Bioscience Research [Internet]. 2025;**3**(1):307-313. DOI: 10.70749/ijbr.v3i1.508

[25] Ju J. Essential oils in vapor phase as antimicrobial agents. In: Essential Oils as Antimicrobial Agents in Food

Preservation [Internet]. 2023. pp. 69-85. DOI: 10.1201/9781003329268-4

[26] Najeeb LM, Abdul Jalil AA, Koodi MK. Expression of *flmA* and *csgA* genes in uropathogenic *Escherichia coli* treated with supernatant of *Lactobacillus plantarum* plus gentamicin. International Journal of Bioinformatics Research and Applications [Internet]. 2026;**22**(1). DOI: 10.1504/ijbra.2026.10067789

[27] Khan J, Ali S, Usman M, Asif H, Ahmad M, Waheed SF, et al. Role of microbiology in tackling antimicrobial resistance: Implications for food safety and public health. Indus Journal of Bioscience Research [Internet]. 2025;**3**(1):223-235. DOI: 10.70749/ijbr.v3i1.473

[28] Singh S. Can essential oils be a potent alternative to synthetic antioxidants? Advances in Clinical Toxicology [Internet]. 2022;**7**(1). DOI: 10.23880/act-16000229

[29] Moshaverinia M, Sahmeddini S, Lavaee F, Zareshahrabadi Z, Zomorodian K. Antimicrobial and anti-biofilm activities of *Thymus fallax* essential oil against oral pathogens. BioMed Research International [Internet]. 2022;**2022**(1). DOI: 10.1155/2022/9744153

[30] Cáceres M, Hidalgo W, Stashenko E, Torres R, Ortiz C. Essential oils of aromatic plants with antibacterial, anti-biofilm and anti-quorum sensing activities against pathogenic bacteria. Antibiotics [Internet]. 2020;**9**(4):147. DOI: 10.3390/antibiotics9040147

[31] Aparicio-García N, Martínez-Villaluenga C, Frias J, Peñas E. Sprouted oat as a potential gluten-free ingredient with enhanced nutritional and bioactive properties. Food Chemistry [Internet]. 2021;**338**:127972. DOI: 10.1016/j.foodchem.2020.127972

[32] Unusan N. Essential oils and microbiota: Implications for diet and weight control. Trends in Food Science and Technology [Internet]. 2020;**104**:60-71. DOI: 10.1016/j.tifs.2020.07.014

[33] Ju J. The inhibitory activity and mechanism of essential oils on foodborne fungi. In: Essential Oils as Antimicrobial Agents in Food Preservation [Internet]. 2023. pp. 39-68. DOI: 10.1201/9781003329268-3

[34] Wurihan W, Weber AM, Gong Z, Lou Z, Sun S, Zhou J, et al. *GrgA* overexpression inhibits *Chlamydia trachomatis* growth through sigma66- and sigma28-dependent mechanisms. Microbial Pathogenesis [Internet]. 2021;**156**:104917. DOI: 10.1016/j.micpath.2021.104917

[35] Jannat B, Mirza Alizadeh A, Farshi P, Dadgarnejad M, Hosseini H, Hashempour-Baltork F, et al. Anti-biofilm activity of essential oils in fruit and vegetable: A systematic review. Food Control [Internet]. 2023;**152**:109875. DOI: 10.1016/j.foodcont.2023.109875

[36] Ju J. Application of plant essential oils in different fields. In: Essential Oils as Antimicrobial Agents in Food Preservation [Internet]. 2023. pp. 1-11. DOI: 10.1201/9781003329268-1

[37] Sadekuzzaman M, Mizan MFR, Kim HS, Yang S, Ha SD. Activity of thyme and tea tree essential oils against selected foodborne pathogens in biofilms on abiotic surfaces. LWT [Internet]. 2018;**89**:134-139. DOI: 10.1016/j.lwt.2017.10.042

[38] Stapled hairpin antimicrobial peptides with improved stability and activity against drug-resistant Gram-negative bacteria. Journal of Medicinal Chemistry [Internet]. DOI: 10.1021/acs.jmedchem.3c00140.s001

[39] Sallam K, Raslan MT, Sabala RF, Abd-Elghany S, Mahros MA, Elshebrawy H. Antimicrobial effect of garlic against foodborne pathogens in ground mutton. SSRN [Internet]. 2023. DOI: 10.2139/ssrn.4332276

[40] Golcuk Y. From ICU to emergency department: Integrating sustainability for a greener healthcare future – Letter on Bartoli et al. Intensive and Critical Care Nursing [Internet]. 2025;**89**:104006. DOI: 10.1016/j.iccn.2025.104006

[41] Cervantes-Huamán BRH, Vega-Sánchez A, Rolón-Verdún P, Gervilla-Cantero G, Rodríguez-Jerez JJ, Ripolles-Avila C. Effect of *Cinnamomum cassia* essential oil combined with enzymes on the elimination and regrowth potential of *Listeria monocytogenes* and *Salmonella enterica* biofilms formed on stainless steel surfaces. Food Control[Internet]. 2025;**172**:111120. DOI: 10.1016/j.foodcont.2024.111120

[42] A synthetic cyclized antimicrobial peptide with potent effects against drug-resistant skin pathogens. ACS Infectious Diseases [Internet]. DOI: 10.1021/acsinfecdis.2c00598.s001

[43] Meenu M, Padhan B, Patel M, Patel R, Xu B. Antibacterial activity of essential oils from different parts of plants against *Salmonella* and *Listeria* spp. Food Chemistry [Internet]. 2023;**404**:134723. DOI: 10.1016/j.foodchem.2022.134723

[44] Xia Y, Xiao X, Adade SYS, Xi Q, Wu J, Xu Y, et al. Physicochemical properties and gel quality monitoring of surimi during thermal processing using hyperspectral imaging combined with deep learning. Food Control [Internet]. 2025;**175**:111258. DOI: 10.1016/j.foodcont.2025.111258

[45] Ramallo IA, Gago G, Gramajo H, Furlan RLE. Bioautographic method for detecting natural preservatives against *Mycobacterium* in edible essential oils. Food Control [Internet]. 2025;**174**:111224. DOI: 10.1016/j.foodcont.2025.111224

[46] Hofmeisterová L, Bajer T, Walczak M, Šilha D. Chemical composition and antibacterial effect of clove and thyme essential oils on growth inhibition and biofilm formation of *Arcobacter* spp. and other bacteria. Antibiotics [Internet]. 2024;**13**(12):1232. DOI: 10.3390/antibiotics13121232

[47] Kowalska A, Clapham L, Manning L. The role of technology in monitoring and verifying safety, quality and sustainability in agri-food supply chains. In: Improving Standards and Certification in Agri-Food Supply Chains: Ensuring Safety, Sustainability and Social Responsibility [Internet]. 2025. pp. 309-318. DOI: 10.19103/as.2024.0133.06

[48] Broadway PR et al. Correction to: Prevalence and antimicrobial susceptibility of *Salmonella* serovars isolated from U.S. retail ground pork. Foodborne Pathogens and Disease [Internet]. 2021;**18**(5):364-365. DOI: 10.1089/fpd.2020.2853.correx

[49] Oh SY, Yun W, Lee JH, Lee CH, Kwak WK, Cho JH. Effects of essential oil (blended and single essential oils) on anti-biofilm formation of *Salmonella* and *Escherichia coli*. Journal of Animal Science and Technology [Internet]. 2017;**59**(1). DOI: 10.1186/s40781-017-0127-7

[50] He S, Shi X. Microbial food safety in China: Past, present, and future. Foodborne Pathogens and Disease [Internet]. 2021;**18**(8):510-518. DOI: 10.1089/fpd.2021.0009

[51] Granata G, Stracquadanio S, Leonardi M, Napoli E, Malandrino G, Cafiso V, et al. Oregano and thyme essential oils encapsulated in chitosan nanoparticles as effective antimicrobial agents against foodborne pathogens. Molecules [Internet]. 2021;**26**(13):4055. DOI: 10.3390/molecules26134055

[52] Granata G, Stracquadanio S, Leonardi M, Napoli E, Malandrino G, Cafiso V, et al. Oregano and thyme essential oils encapsulated in chitosan nanoparticles as effective antimicrobial agents against foodborne pathogens. Molecules [Internet]. 2021;**26**(13):4055. DOI: 10.3390/molecules26134055

[53] Shaltout FA. Use of essential oils as potential antimicrobial agents in meat preservation. Nutrition and Food Processing [Internet]. 2024;7(8):01-07. DOI: 10.31579/2637-8914/218

[54] Hofmeisterová L, Bajer T, Walczak M, Šilha D. Chemical composition and antibacterial effect of clove and thyme essential oils on growth inhibition and biofilm formation of *Arcobacter* spp. and other bacteria. Antibiotics [Internet]. 2024;**13**(12):1232. DOI: 10.3390/antibiotics13121232

[55] Friedman M. Antimicrobial activities of plant essential oils and their components against antibiotic-susceptible and antibiotic-resistant foodborne pathogens. In: Essential Oils and Nanotechnology for Treatment of Microbial Diseases [Internet]. 2017. pp. 14-38. DOI: 10.1201/9781315209241-2

[56] Song L, Yang H, Meng X, Su R, Cheng S, Wang H, et al. Inhibitory effects of trans-cinnamaldehyde against *Pseudomonas aeruginosa* biofilm formation. Foodborne Pathogens and Disease [Internet]. 2023;**20**(2):47-58. DOI: 10.1089/fpd.2022.0073

[57] Rajkowska K, Nowicka-Krawczyk P, Kunicka-Styczyńska A. Effect of clove and thyme essential oils on *Candida* biofilm formation and the oil distribution in yeast cells. Molecules[Internet]. 2019;**24**(10):1954. DOI: 10.3390/molecules24101954

[58] Ju J. In vivo experiment, stability, and safety of essential oils. In: Essential Oils as Antimicrobial Agents in Food Preservation [Internet]. 2023. pp. 263-284. DOI: 10.1201/9781003329268-14

[59] Friedman M. Antimicrobial activities of plant essential oils and their components against antibiotic-susceptible and antibiotic-resistant foodborne pathogens. In: Essential Oils and Nanotechnology for Treatment of Microbial Diseases [Internet]. 2017. pp. 14-38. DOI: 10.1201/9781315209241-2

[60] Rajkowska K, Nowicka-Krawczyk P, Kunicka-Styczyńska A. Effect of clove and thyme essential oils on *Candida* biofilm formation and the oil distribution in yeast cells. Molecules [Internet]. 2019;**24**(10):1954. DOI: 10.3390/molecules24101954

[61] Arroyave F. Antimicrobial activity of essential oils harvested from Bogota, Colombia, against six pathogenic multiresistant bacterial strains. Morressier [Internet]. 2016. DOI: 10.26226/morressier.56d6be78d462b80296c97a73

[62] Granata G, Stracquadanio S, Leonardi M, Napoli E, Malandrino G, Cafiso V, et al. Oregano and thyme essential oils encapsulated in chitosan nanoparticles as effective antimicrobial agents against foodborne pathogens. Molecules [Internet]. 2021;**26**(13):4055. DOI: 10.3390/molecules26134055

[63] Hofmeisterová L, Bajer T, Walczak M, Šilha D. Chemical

composition and antibacterial effect of clove and thyme essential oils on growth inhibition and biofilm formation of *Arcobacter* spp. and other bacteria. Antibiotics [Internet]. 2024;**13**(12):1232. DOI: 10.3390/antibiotics13121232

[64] Becerril R, Nerín C, Gómez-Lus R. Evaluation of bacterial resistance to essential oils and antibiotics after exposure to oregano and cinnamon essential oils. Foodborne Pathogens and Disease [Internet]. 2012;**9**(8):699-705. DOI: 10.1089/fpd.2011.1097

[65] Sadekuzzaman M, Mizan MFR, Kim HS, Yang S, Ha SD. Activity of thyme and tea tree essential oils against selected foodborne pathogens in biofilms on abiotic surfaces. LWT [Internet]. 2018;**89**:134-139. DOI: 10.1016/j.lwt.2017.10.042

[66] Inhibitory effect on biofilm formation of pathogenic bacteria induced by rubrolide lactam analogues. ACS Omega [Internet]. DOI: 10.1021/acsomega.8b02334.s001

[67] Serag MS, Elfayoumy RA, Mohesien MT. Essential oils as antimicrobial and food preservatives. In: Essential Oils - Advances in Extractions and Biological Applications [Internet]. 2022. DOI: 10.5772/intechopen.103000

[68] Ju J. Essential oils in vapor phase as antimicrobial agents. In: Essential Oils as Antimicrobial Agents in Food Preservation [Internet]. 2023. pp. 69-85. DOI: 10.1201/9781003329268-4

[69] Somrani M, Huertas JP, Iguaz A, Debbabi H, Palop A. Antimicrobial activity of cinnamon, garlic, and onion essential oils against foodborne *Salmonella enteritidis* biofilms. SSRN [Internet]. 2023. DOI: 10.2139/ssrn.4552975

[70] Ju J. Synergistic antibacterial effect of essential oils and antibacterial agent. In: Essential Oils as Antimicrobial Agents in Food Preservation [Internet]. 2023. pp. 87-101. DOI: 10.1201/9781003329268-5

[71] Cui H, Zhao C, Li C, Lin L. Essential oils-based antibacterial agent against *Escherichia coli* O157:H7 biofilm on cucumber. Journal of Food Processing and Preservation [Internet]. 2016;**41**(5):e13140. DOI: 10.1111/jfpp.13140

[72] Schilcher H. Effects and side-effects of essential oils. Essential Oils and Aromatic Plants [Internet]. 1985:217-231. DOI: 10.1007/978-94-009-5137-2_26

[73] Liu J, Gu Y, Xu Z. Biofilm formation of food-borne pathogens. In: Stress Responses of Foodborne Pathogens [Internet]. 2022. pp. 461-497. DOI: 10.1007/978-3-030-90578-1_16

[74] Turgis M, Vu KD, Dupont C, Lacroix M. Combined antimicrobial effect of essential oils and bacteriocins against foodborne pathogens and food spoilage bacteria. Food Research International [Internet]. 2012;**48**(2):696-702. DOI: 10.1016/j.foodres.2012.06.016

[75] Zhou C, Yin L, Zhang Z, Wang Z, Wang L, Li D, et al. Synergistic antimicrobial effect of cinnamon and thyme essential oils on Rhizopus microsporus and its preservation application in berries. SSRN [Internet]. 2024. DOI: 10.2139/ssrn.5022184

[76] Quendera AP, Barreto AS, Semedo-Lemsaddek T. Antimicrobial activity of essential oils against foodborne multidrug-resistant enterococci and aeromonads in planktonic and biofilm state. Food Science and Technology International [Internet]. 2018;**25**(2):101-108. DOI: 10.1177/1082013218799027

[77] Meenu M, Padhan B, Patel M, Patel R, Xu B. Antibacterial activity of

essential oils from different parts of plants against *Salmonella* and *Listeria* spp. Food Chemistry [Internet]. 2023;**404**:134723. DOI: 10.1016/j.foodchem.2022.134723

[78] Evaluation of the antimicrobial activity of essential oils against veterinary pathogens, multidrug-resistant bacteria, and dermatophytes. The Pakistan Veterinary Journal [Internet]. 2024. DOI: 10.29261/pakvetj/2024.165

[79] Sallam K, Raslan MT, Sabala RF, Abd-Elghany S, Mahros MA, Elshebrawy H. Antimicrobial effect of garlic against foodborne pathogens in ground mutton. SSRN [Internet]. 2023. DOI: 10.2139/ssrn.4332276

[80] PEGylation of polyethylenimine lowers acute toxicity while retaining anti-biofilm and lactam potentiation properties against antibiotic-resistant pathogens. ACS Omega [Internet]. DOI: 10.1021/acsomega.0c04111.s001

[81] Ju J. Essential oils in vapor phase as antimicrobial agents. In: Essential Oils as Antimicrobial Agents in Food Preservation [Internet]. 2023. pp. 69-85. DOI: 10.1201/9781003329268-4

[82] Sadekuzzaman M, Mizan MFR, Kim HS, Yang S, Ha SD. Activity of thyme and tea tree essential oils against selected foodborne pathogens in biofilms on abiotic surfaces. LWT [Internet]. 2018;**89**:134-139. DOI: 10.1016/j.lwt.2017.10.042

[83] Atia TS, Moustafa EA, Ibrahim SI. Improving bacterial, oxidative, and sensory quality of meat steaks using cumin, garlic, and thyme essential oils. World's Veterinary Journal[Internet]. 2022:274-283. DOI: 10.54203/scil.2022.wvj34

[84] Meenu M, Padhan B, Patel M, Patel R, Xu B. Antibacterial activity of essential oils from different parts of plants against *Salmonella* and *Listeria* spp. Food Chemistry [Internet]. 2023;**404**:134723. DOI: 10.1016/j.foodchem.2022.134723

[85] Quendera AP, Barreto AS, Semedo-Lemsaddek T. Antimicrobial activity of essential oils against foodborne multidrug-resistant *Enterococci* and *Aeromonads* in planktonic and biofilm state. Food Science and Technology International [Internet]. 2018;**25**(2):101-108. DOI: 10.1177/1082013218799027

[86] Zhou C, Yin L, Zhang Z, Wang Z, Wang L, Li D, et al. Synergistic antimicrobial effect of cinnamon and thyme essential oils on *Rhizopus microsporus* and its preservation application in berries. SSRN [Internet]. 2024. DOI: 10.2139/ssrn.5022184

[87] Ju J. The inhibitory activity and mechanism of essential oils on foodborne fungi. In: Essential Oils as Antimicrobial Agents in Food Preservation [Internet]. 2023. pp. 39-68. DOI: 10.1201/9781003329268-3

[88] Wurihan W, Weber AM, Gong Z, Lou Z, Sun S, Zhou J, et al. GrgA overexpression inhibits Chlamydia trachomatis growth through sigma66- and sigma28-dependent mechanisms. Microbial Pathogenesis [Internet]. 2021;**156**:104917. DOI: 10.1016/j.micpath.2021.104917

Chapter 9

Phytochemicals: A Promising Strategy to Combat Biofilm-Associated Antimicrobial Resistance

Jiddu Joseph, Sanya Boby and Muhammed Shafeekh Muyyarikkandy

Abstract

The impact of antimicrobial resistance (AMR) on global health and the economy is gradually increasing over time. This issue is further exacerbated by biofilms due to their inherent mechanisms that worsen the conditions. Furthermore, biofilms can limit the effectiveness of antibiotics and hinder changes in physiology and gene expression that contribute to AMR. There are several ways biofilms promote the development of AMR among various biofilm-associated bacteria. These include mechanisms that obstruct antibiotic penetration to the matrix, the role of quorum sensing, and the horizontal transfer of AMR genes. It is essential to prevent bacterial biofilms using safer alternatives that can both prevent biofilms and control AMR. Recently, phytochemicals have gained attention as natural products with antibiotic-potentiating effects. Various studies have shown that phytochemicals play different roles in disturbing biofilms, from affecting the extracellular matrix to targeting quorum sensing and DNA replication. Additionally, challenges such as standardizing the mechanisms of action could facilitate approval for therapeutic uses, thus helping to demonstrate the potential use of phytochemicals against biofilms.

Keywords: biofilms, phytochemicals, antimicrobial resistance, antibiotic potentiation, quorum sensing

1. Introduction

Biofilms exhibit distinct physiological properties compared to their planktonic counterparts. Their study is critical for advancing our understanding of microbial survival and pathogenicity to tackle various challenges caused by them including diseases and antimicrobial resistance [1, 2]. Various intricate features of bacterial cells were widely studied. However, the complex community structures of bacteria forming a biofilm are intriguing as they are unexpected, orderly-arranged planktonic cells coordinated to create a population that has more stability against variations in the surrounding environment. They can be established either on a living or non-living surface. These characteristics and community features make the biofilms formed by different pathogenic bacteria problematic [1, 3, 4]. Biofilms account for an economic loss of US $4000 billion a year, and a significant part is due to various health hazards, including food-borne infections and antimicrobial resistance [5, 6]. Additionally, the National Institute of Health (NIH) reports reveal that most biofilms resist standard antimicrobial treatment. Biofilms play a crucial role in increasing antimicrobial resistance (AMR), as their structure makes bacteria less accessible to antibiotics. Therefore, understanding the patterns of AMR is essential to tackling the effects caused by these biofilms [6, 7].

The discovery of penicillin was a milestone in medical history that paved the way to save millions of lives in the twentieth century [8]. Following that, newer antibiotics were used against various pathogens, and subsequently, the resistance of these pathogens towards the antibiotics became stronger, causing more morbidity and mortality associated with infectious diseases [9, 10]. Currently, the World Health Organization (WHO), Centers for Disease Control and Prevention (CDC), and researchers across the globe are giving priority to overcoming AMR by relying on antibiotic alternatives and ways to use the available effectively [11–13]. This even includes biofilms, as they can regulate diseases from periodontitis and food infections to cystic fibrosis [14–16]. Strategies include developing antibiotic alternatives or potentiating the currently available antibiotics. Among the latter, phytochemicals have shown a significant role in recent research [17, 18].

Phytochemicals are bioactive compounds obtained from plants that have shown significant antibacterial effects on the planktonic cells and biofilms. They control biofilms on various surfaces by taking advantage of antibiotics and regulating mechanisms associated with structural formation rather than causing a direct antibacterial effect [19]. There are multiple strategies for phytochemicals targeting biofilms that can be further influenced using antibiotics. One crucial strategy among them includes influencing the cell-to-cell interactions within biofilms [20, 21]. These cell-to-cell communication are called quorum sensing, which is essential for the robustness of biofilms' structural and functional integrity. However, phytochemicals disrupt quorum sensing, which will not develop resistance against them but help disrupt the biofilm structure, enabling the antibiotics to act effectively [19, 21, 22]. They can also alter the motility of bacteria by making structural changes in bacterial pili and fimbriae [22, 23]. In addition, these phytochemicals can influence planktonic cells by inhibiting peptidoglycan synthesis, disrupting the membrane, efflux pump inhibition, suppressing toxins and virulence factors, which makes the antibiotics more effective against multidrug-resistant bacteria [20, 22]. Apart from this, phytochemicals are promising antibiotic potentiators. Various phenolic compounds, phytoestrogens, limonoids, terpenoids, carotenoid alkaloids, organosulfur compounds, and phytosterols have shown promising antioxidant effects against bacteria that can also be used against biofilms [23–25]. Phytochemicals are essential not only because of the mechanism mentioned earlier but also due to their cost-effectiveness, minimal side effects, and capacity for antibiotic potentiation, which is a possible solution against antibiotic resistance [22]. However, the challenges and limitations of phytochemicals as antibiotic potentiators against biofilms also need to be considered.

Even though there are promising effects for phytochemicals against biofilms, their mechanism of action is multifaceted, which means each molecule has multiple targets, making the process complex. Moreover, identifying their mechanism of action is a time-consuming process, especially regarding antibiotic potentiation, in which we need more knowledge about how each antibiotic reacts with a phytochemical molecule on a specific surface [26–28]. This is further complicated by the long screening time of the bioassays, along with the lack of information about the toxicity at cellular levels for phytochemical plus antibiotic combinations [26, 29]. However, this can be resolved through high-throughput screening, multivariate data analysis, and metabolomics. Additionally, newer therapeutic drug delivery strategies, such as nanoparticle-based ones, might be another critical area of improvement that can make more bioavailability of the phytochemicals at various biotic and abiotic surfaces [30, 31]. Addressing this would help develop strategies that can control biofilms and antimicrobial resistance and achieve a global impact in terms of human, animal, and environmental health. This book chapter provides a detailed overview of biofilm-associated antimicrobial resistance and the use of phytochemicals as antibiotic potentiators to overcome the hurdles caused by biofilms.

2. Antimicrobial resistance and biofilms

In bacterial biofilms, cells are reversibly attached to biotic or abiotic surfaces, which are intercalated with a matrix formed by the extracellular polymeric substances (EPS), determining the biofilm architecture and phenotypic function. The matrix is composed of various polysaccharides, proteins, lipids, extracellular DNA (eDNA), cellulose, amyloids, pili, fimbriae, flagella, and water (97%) [32]. The bacteria attach to biotic or abiotic surfaces when there is signal perception for biofilm formation, which is followed by attachment enhancement with the help of extracellular appendages along with the use of adhesins and gene upregulation. This is followed by microcolony formation along with EPS gene upregulation, which results in the maturation of biofilm via quorum-sensing molecules, polysaccharides, and eDNA, as demonstrated in **Figure 1**. However, when there is nutrient limitation or toxic product accumulation, they will disperse to other locations with favorable environments for further proliferation [33]. Along with this, the matrix also helps to provide tolerance towards desiccation by forming hydrogel with the EPS components. Moreover, other inorganic, organic, and metal ions will be sequestrated from the surface to give more stability to the bacterial community [32].

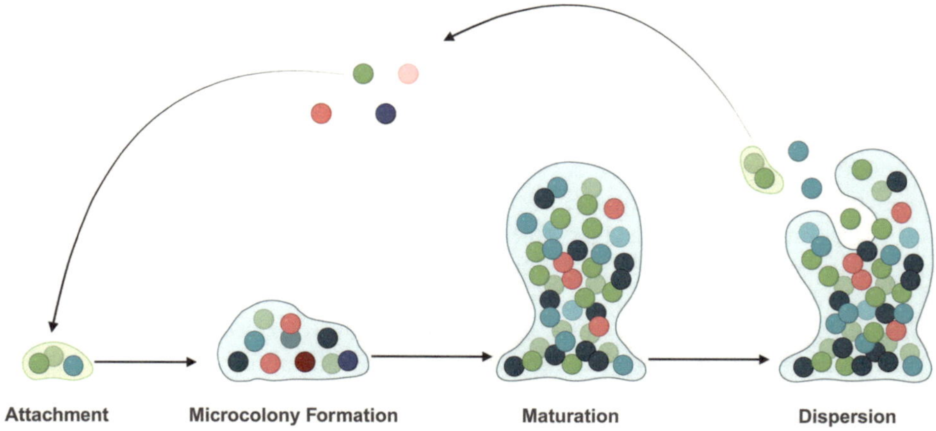

Figure 1.
Steps in biofilm formation.

Microorganisms develop resistance to antibiotics over time. This might be due to various mutations or transfers of genetic elements that have been undergone over time, depending on the environmental and genetic conditions. Biofilms can impact this antimicrobial resistance by not only through a mechanism that prevents antibiotic penetration but also due to various other mechanisms [34, 35]. For a particular antimicrobial to be effective against planktonic cells associated with biofilms, it should overcome high cell density, efflux pumps, antibiotic-modifying enzymes, heterogeneity, hypoxia, reduced growth rates, persistent cells, and resistant mutants. Moreover, the matrix plays a key role in determining which molecules to go inside and interact with planktonic cells. However, the decreased penetration confers an increased resistance that needs further validation [28]. The chemical reactions of the antibiotics with various biofilm molecules might be a possible explanation of what hinders the penetration of the bioactive antibiotic molecules deeper. Apart from that, the role of exopolysaccharides in providing antibiotic resistance was also detected. For example, *Staphylococcus epidermidis* strains, which produce exopolysaccharides, were resistant to multiple antibiotics [36]. The extracellular matrix can be explained as a warehouse for the antimicrobial resistance genes (ARGs), which can help confer resistance to other bacteria and might aggravate the resistance and make the treatments ineffective against various medical conditions [37]. Another possible contributor is the eDNA, which is important in regulating antibiotic resistance by underlying mechanisms affecting the chelation of magnesium ions and triggering pathways responsible for the development of antimicrobial resistance [33, 37]. Additionally, the level of oxygen in the biofilm community and host immunity was also found to contribute to the resistance mechanisms involved with the biofilms, which are discussed in detail in the following section.

2.1 Involvement of biofilm exopolysaccharide

The formation of a thick biofilm matrix is correlated with the community's survival, and exopolysaccharides play an essential role in maintaining the thickness and acting as physical and chemical diffusion barriers. Penetration of the antibiotic into the matrix helps provide either antibiotic efficacy or tolerance [38]. Depleting the antimicrobial agents due to the difficulty in penetration may lead to tolerance. For example, with less penetration, antibiotic-modifying enzyme β- Lactamases can degrade aminoglycosides. The EPS types differ among the bacterial species, which may provide different specific functions [39]. The *Pseudomonas aeruginosa* EPS have Pel, Psl, and alginate, which play a critical role in antimicrobial resistance in their biofilms. Psl is very important for the initial attachment of the colonies and has been shown to provide resistance against various antibiotics such as gentamycin, colistin, polymyxin B, ciprofloxacin, and ceftazidime. Additionally, alginate primarily contributes to mucoid colony formation. It protects the community from various antibiotics, host immune systems, ROS, and antimicrobial peptides, while Pel provides tolerance and resistance antibiotics including aminoglycosides and fluoroquinolones [40]. Apart from this, *S. epidermidis* has PNAG or PIA in the EPS, contributing to various biofilm characteristics, from colonization to antimicrobial resistance [41]. Moreover, some biofilm EPS, such as galactan and glucofuranose shown to be involved in blocking complement components that are important in immunity associated with infections on the biotic surfaces. Overproduction of EPSs is another vital aspect that would contribute to the development of antimicrobial resistance. The expression of *ica* in *S. epidermidis* shows a relationship with antimicrobial resistance towards several antibiotics when given at sub-MIC concentration [36]. Another example would be the sub-MIC use of imipenem against *P. aeruginosa* biofilms, which develops overexpression of the EPS component alginate, which confers an increased antimicrobial resistance. This can be explained as the increased expression of the EPS, which can be attributed to the pressure provided by antibiotics as it may increase the expression of polysaccharides in the matrix, contributing to antimicrobial resistance [35].

The level of heterogeneity of the biofilm structure can also influence the exopolysaccharide types. β-1,3- glucan is an EPS component produced by *Candida albicans* biofilms, which provide ofloxacin resistance. When *Candida* is associated with other bacteria, such as *E. coli* or *Salmonella*, these biofilms also become resistant to ofloxacin, which can be explained by the heterogeneous nature of the biofilms' EPS [42]. There are additional antibacterial effects from the EPS-associated polysaccharides as they can be acetylated to become polycationic, increasing the antimicrobial resistance property through different mechanisms, such as electrostatic repulsion from charged antibiotics. Moreover, the other negatively charged components in the biofilm's matrix can interact with these cationic polysaccharides to develop delayed penetration, contributing to antibiotic tolerance and resistance [39]. Exopolysaccharides of the biofilms were found to influence quorum sensing in the case of antibiotic resistance. *S. aureus* uses auto-inducing proteins (AIPs) to take part in the quorum sensing of the biofilm structure and have a key role in antimicrobial resistance by regulating various sensor kinases and preventing the biofilms from resensitizing against antibiotics [41]. Apart from this, the efflux pumps, such as the RND superfamily in *Pseudomonas*, have mechanisms that influence the antimicrobial resistance in the coming sections. However, most of the mechanisms of resistance are associated with the exopolysaccharide, and it is important to note its significance so that mitigation methods can be targeted based on the EPS.

2.2 Involvement of biofilm eDNA

Genomic DNA (gDNA) is the structure associated with a cell that is packaged inside to coordinate various cellular activities. In biofilms, DNA is present outside the cell in the matrix to coordinate the function of the community, which is called the eDNA. The eDNA coordinates various functions such as maintaining the matrix integrity, participating in host defense responses, maintaining the distribution of charges in the matrix, antibiotic resistance and horizontal gene transfer [43]. Quorum sensing is important to the survival of the biofilms as they impact the cell lysis, which results in the formation of eDNA. Additionally, they are released in the matrix by various other mechanisms such as prophage-mediated release, vesicle-mediated release and various other unknown mechanisms. As mentioned, antibiotics such as aminoglycosides are positively charged and can interact with the negatively charged eDNA molecules to hinder penetration. Moreover, it can participate in forming a physical shield with the host extracellular DNA against antibiotics such as tobramycin to increase resistance [44]. The significant aspect related to the biofilm eDNA is its role in horizontal gene transfer (HGT), which helps distribute AMR genes among large bacterial populations. Extended-spectrum β-lactamase resistance genes such as $bla_{\text{CTX-M}}$ and $bla_{\text{NDM-1}}$ were found to be transferred through HGT associated with biofilms. Among the three mechanisms associated with HGT, conjugation of the AMR gene is reported as the most common mechanism. Interestingly, HGT is reported more frequently in biofilms compared to its planktonic counterparts. The reasons are the wide availability of the AMR genes and eDNA in the community along with its heterogeneous nature. For example, *pbp2x* which is an important penicillin resistance gene, has shown to be transferred between different species of *Streptococcus* in oral biofilms conferring resistance [45]. Besides this, eDNA takes part in antimicrobial resistance through indirect mechanisms involving sequestration of divalent cations such as Mn^{2+}, Ca^{2+}, Mg^{2+}, and Zn^{2} to influence the function of various AMR genes in biofilms. For example, the PhoQ is a sensor in various gram-negative bacteria that detects the $Mg^{2+,}$ and it helps activate various virulence factors. However, in the case of biofilms, cation chelation by DNA is shown to trigger the expression of antibiotic-resistance genes [46]. Moreover, the involvement of eDNA in neutrophil extracellular traps and pattern recognition would make it an excellent component to target antibiofilm activity.

2.3 Involvement of efflux pumps

Bacterial efflux pumps are critical components that help to reduce the influence of endogenous substances that hinder the growth of bacteria. They are of six superfamilies including, ATP-binding cassette (ABC), Major Facilitator (MFS), resistance nodular division (RND), small multidrug resistance (SMR), multidrug and toxic compound extrusion (MATE) and drug metabolite transporter (DMT). They help the bacteria to pump the foreign substances including antibiotics, out of the cell. In biofilms, the over-expression of the efflux pumps in coordination with quorum sensing promotes antimicrobial resistance and even causes multi-drug resistance [34]. There are various efflux pumps involved with emerging multidrug resistance. For example, the efflux pump family TetR acts as a transcriptional repressor, which regulates the function of *tet* genes for tetracycline resistance. The RND type genes, such as *adeB, adeG* and *adeI* could influence the quorum sensing and resistance towards antibiotics such as colistin in *Acinetobacter baumannii*. In *E. coli,* the *AcrAB-TolC*, an RND family gene, was shown to confer resistance against rifampicin, tetracycline, chloramphenicol and fusidic acid. Similarly, MarR- type repressors inactivate a MepA protein, which in turn provides resistance towards antibiotics such as fluoroquinolones and tigecycline [47]. Moreover, efflux pumps can be targeted to determine the presence of antibiotic resistance in biofilms or the level of antibiotics associated. Still, the challenges are due to biofilms' heterogeneous nature, making this more complex. These efflux pumps might be seen as operons in the genome responsible for various other functions that coordinate the overall fitness of the biofilms. This is further influenced by the complex involvement of quorum sensing. Current developments against biofilms and antibiotic resistance focus on efflux pump inhibitors [38]. They are targeted in such a manner to change the level of expression of the genes associated with the pumps, alter the structure of the pump by affecting the assembly, altering the outer membrane in a way that affects the energy efflux which all would ultimately hinder the biofilm formation. The new antibiotic alternatives, including phytochemicals, can be used against these efflux pumps since they play a key role in the multi-drug resistance associated with biofilms.

2.4 Involvement of other factors and limitations

Regarding biofilm-associated antimicrobial resistance, certain other factors also help in the process. The slow growth rate of the biofilms, which resulted from limited nutrient availability, might be one of the reasons. The biofilm cells of *E. coli* and *Staphylococcus*, which had the same level of antibiotic resistance as planktonic cells were found to be showing increased antimicrobial resistance towards ciprofloxacin and the reason was found to be the slow growth rate of the biofilm [35]. In addition, the level of physiological activity and position of the cells in a biofilm structure have effects on the AMR. The cells close to the surface are more vulnerable to antimicrobials than those at a deeper location. Moreover, their level of physiological activity, metabolism, and their level of stress response are also dependent on their location, which is influenced by the phenotype [48]. This is further influenced by the level of *rpoS* regulation in biofilms. Cooperation and competition of cells within the biofilms may develop new interactions, which results in a multifaceted combination of AMR genes that develop emerging combinations of phenotypic resistance, and it is a significant challenge. Furthermore, oxygen availability can be a major determinant of antibiotic resistance in bacteria, including *P. aeruginosa.* Anaerobic conditions prevented *P. aeruginosa* biofilms from antibiotics such as tobramycin, ciprofloxacin, carbenicillin, and ceftazidime when compared to aerobic conditions [49]. Overall, all these factors explain how biofilms develop antimicrobial resistance, which adds to the global burden.

The various methods of antibiotic resistance associated with biofilms will ultimately result in treatment failures of various biofilm-associated foodborne and nosocomial infections. For example, catheter-associated biofilms constitute a significant concern in which hospitalized patients die due to ineffective treatment. Moreover, more than 60% of nosocomial infections are due to biofilms, according to reports from the CDC and NIH, which necessitates the importance of prevention [50]. Various alternatives to antibiotics have been tested against biofilms. These include natural and synthetic antimicrobial peptides, bacteriophages, phage-derived enzymes, combined phage therapy, enzymes, molecules (LP 3134, mannosides), polysaccharides, and phytochemicals. Among these, phytochemicals are promising because of the fewer side effects in the living systems and their ability to potentiate the effect of currently available antibiotics [51].

3. Phytochemicals in controlling biofilms

The increase in drug-resistant pathogens is a concern around the globe since there are rising incidences of treatment failure in humans and animals. Therefore, alternative strategies of treatments against these pathogens are at the highest priority. Among the alternatives, phytochemicals are one of the promising picks due to their efficiency and safety. Phytochemicals are natural metabolites derived from plants that have shown significant roles in various therapeutic applications that are also used as dietary supplements and flavor enhancers in the food industry. The primary classification of the compounds includes phenolic compounds, polyacetylenes, stilbenes, lectins, polypeptides, terpenoids, and alkaloids [51]. Most of these compounds show antibiofilm activities by various mechanisms, including efflux pump inhibition, inhibiting membrane function, interfering with quorum sensing, EPS, adhesion, and synergistic interaction with antimicrobials. These synergistic interactions with antimicrobial agents are relevant as there is increased AMR globally associated with biofilms, and there are fewer efforts to develop newer antibiotics [51]. **Figure 2** shows major mechanisms of action associated with biofilm control by phytochemicals.

Phenolics are a major class of phytochemicals, which includes gallic acid, carvacrol, catechin, coumarin, quercetin, eugenol, and many more which have shown significant roles in infectious and metabolic disease treatments, including

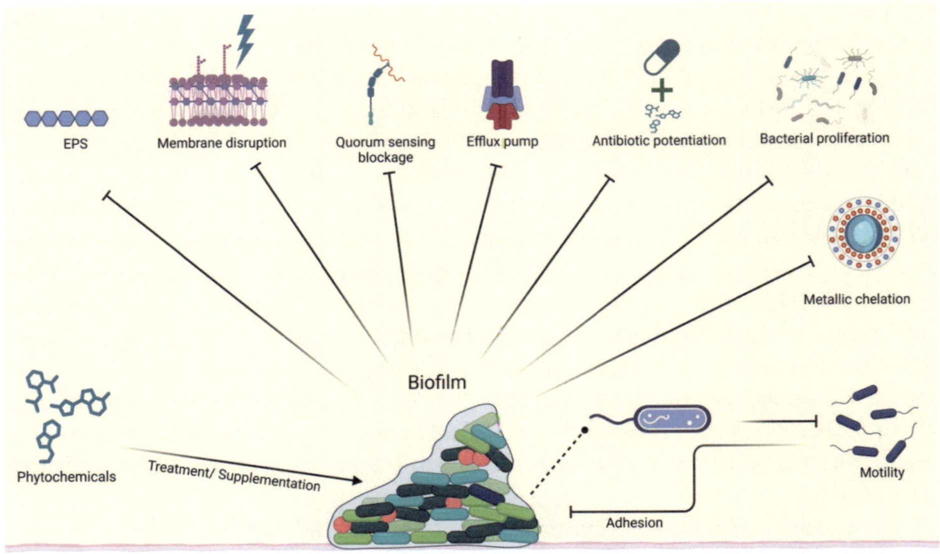

Figure 2.
Mechanisms in which phytochemicals hinder biofilms.

cancer. Alkaloids are another major group comprising compounds such as piperine, reserpine, sanguinarine while carnosic acid, farnesol, and oleanolic acid are some terpenoids [52]. These are beneficial since they are naturally available from plants with fewer side effects and have shown impacts on various bacteria and biofilms. Moreover, synergistic interactions of the currently available antibiotic with phytochemicals have a significant impact since they have been shown to increase the bioavailability and penetration of the antibiotics. Reports are demonstrating the ability of plants to produce inhibitors for drug resistance for their survival. For example, a compound called rhein from rhubarb has been shown to inhibit the multi-drug resistance receptors and potentiate around 2000-fold against various bacteria [53]. As mentioned before, the mechanisms by which the phytochemicals act on biofilms are critical to understanding effective intervention strategies discussed in detail below.

3.1 Inhibition of extracellular polymeric substance synthesis

Extracellular polymeric substances are key matrix components that are synthesized during biofilm formation, stabilizing the biofilm structure in harsh environments required for survival. Therefore, interfering with the synthesis of the elements of the EPS, such as polysaccharides, eDNA, and polypeptides, would significantly impact the stability of the biofilm structure [54]. Some phytochemicals significantly alter the level or production of these matrix components and destroy the integrity of the biofilm matrix. Luteolin, a phenolic flavone, reduces the synthesis of polysaccharides, eDNA, and extracellular proteins in the case of *E. coli* and *Enterobacter cloacae* biofilms, resulting in reduced biofilm biomass and integrity. Furthermore, quercetin reduces the extracellular polysaccharide abundance in *P. aeruginosa* biofilms by interfering with transcription activator, rhl family genes. This significantly affects the matrix structure and functions including quorum sensing, which ultimately leads to the destruction of the biofilm structure [55]. Other examples would be the blocking of the expression of genes such as *gtfB*, *gtfC* and *gtfD* which regulate the synthesis of EPS by an extract from *Cedrus deodara,* a tree in the pine family which is also known as the Monrovia plant. In *S. aureus* biofilms, a phytochemical called sesquiterpenoid or nootkatone was shown to inhibit EPS synthesis, reducing biomass [26]. All the above examples showed the effects of various phytochemicals on the EPS, which destroys the biofilm integrity. However, the exact molecular mechanisms around most of them are still unclear, and they need to be identified with precise evidence so that they can be used therapeutically to target the EPS.

3.2 Membrane disruption

One of the main mechanisms by which antibacterial agents attack bacterial cells is by altering the bacterial membrane. In the case of biofilms, the presence of other matrix components further complicates the process of preventing them from penetrating. This results in increased antibiotic tolerance in addition to antibiotic resistance [48]. Phytochemicals are an excellent choice to potentiate and promote the membrane penetration and killing of the planktonic cells associated with biofilms. This killing might be aided by directly impairing the membrane's structure, which changes the membrane characteristics and physiological function that ultimately leads to death [52]. Essential oils are hydrocarbons and oxygenated derivatives of phytochemicals that are produced by two isoprenoid pathways. They are the plant secondary metabolites that are hydrophobic or lipophilic, mainly consisting of monoterpenes and sesquiterpenes. They have been shown to have a promising membrane-disrupting effect among the phytochemicals against both gram-positive and gram-negative bacteria. The primary reason for the increased penetration is its lipophilic nature, which allows it to interact with the peptidoglycan layer in the cell wall. Moreover, the gram-positive bacteria that have a thick peptidoglycan layer will be more prone to the effects of the essential oils [26]. Furthermore, they can influence cellular functions, starting from altering the morphology, impacting the ion exchange and thereby influencing the membrane potential, influencing metabolic pathways, ATP production, and cell lysis, which leads to leakage and ultimately leading to death of the bacterial cell. For example, terpenes have been shown to have altered the membrane polarization that leads to changes in membrane potential, resulting in damage and leakage of the cellular components, including proteins and nucleic acids of the biofilms associated with *Shigella flexneri* [56]. Additionally, other bacteria such as *S. aureus,* have also been shown to impact the essential oils disrupting the bacterial membrane and ultimately leading to the dissolution of the biofilm.

Apart from essential oil, phenolic compounds are one of the other types of phytochemicals showing promising effects in disrupting the membrane. They also act mainly by membrane depolarization, metabolic pathway alterations, impact on gene expression, altering ATP synthesis, influencing homeostasis, and membrane damage. Carvacrol is one of the phenolic compounds that has shown a membrane-disrupting effect by controlling the ATP synthesis and membrane potential mainly due to its hydrophobic nature. Apart from this, various alkaloids and flavonoids show membrane-disrupting effects primarily by interacting with the lipid bilayer membrane and altering the membrane potential, leading to membrane damage and the biofilm structure's dissolution [52]. Furthermore, membrane disruption would be a good strategy to overcome the AMR when these phytochemicals are used in combination with the currently available phytochemicals.

3.3 Inhibition of quorum-sensing

Quorum-sensing (QS) is an essential property associated with both the planktonic bacteria and a community, which is inevitable for the survival controlling various factors starting from adhesion to virulence. In a bacterial community, intercellular communication is significant for its survival, and considering biofilms, it plays a significant role in its formation and differentiation. In terms of quorum sensing, the cells were not under selective pressure by blocking the sensing pathways when compared to antimicrobials, and hence, the chances of developing resistance might be meager [57]. This strategy makes quorum sensing inhibition an interesting topic for investigating new mechanisms to treat bacterial infections without developing any resistance. The quorum sensing inhibitors show effects on the structural integrity of biofilms by interfering with various pathways, including extracellular polysaccharide production, formation of the microcolonies, and adhesion to surfaces. Phytochemicals have demonstrated significant effects on quorum sensing, thereby interfering with biofilm survival.

Quorum-sensing molecules in gram-positive bacteria are autoinducing peptides (AIPs), while in gram negatives, they use *N*-acyl-homoserine lactones (AHLs). Various classes of phytochemicals have shown QS inhibition on different types of bacterial biofilms. A tannin called hamamelitannin was shown to down-regulate the genes involved with QS and motility of *S. aureus.* More specifically, the phytochemical inhibited the RNAIII in the bacteria primarily involved with the regulation of QS, which is confirmed by graft infection models in rats. Moreover, there were reports of increased susceptibility to vancomycin *in vitro* and *in vivo* models [58]. Naringenin, which is a flavanone, reduced the level of 3-oxo-C12-HSL and C4-HSL, which are molecules helping in quorum sensing for virulence-associated mechanisms in *P. aeruginosa.* Various genes in the *las* and *rhl* family in the QS regulation are down-regulated by this flavanone. Flavonoids extracted from *Glycyrrhiza glabra* or liquorice when interacted with the *A. baumannii* biofilms to down-regulate the gene expression of *abaI,* which is an autoinducer synthase gene to impact the quorum sensing to prevent the structural integrity of biofilms which ultimately leads to dispersion [59]. Terpenoids are another major class of phytochemicals that have shown significant effects on QS. For instance, a monoterpene called thymol inhibited the QS molecules in biofilms of *Listeria monocytogenes*, *P. aeruginosa,* and *S. aureus*. Saponins from the plant *Panax ginseng* reduced the production of *lasA,* which is staphylolysin, and *lasB*, which is an elastase. Both are part of the QS along with the downregulation of other AHLs in *P. aeruginosa*-infected animal models. Even though the phytochemicals affected the different aspects of the quorum sensing pathways, all these biofilms ultimately led to their instability [60]. Apart from this, various other phytochemicals such as benzoic acid derivatives, stilbenes, coumarins, quinones, and alkaloids showed inhibiting effects on the AIPs and AHLs, resulting in biofilm destruction. Additionally, several studies focused on the effects of phytochemicals as quorum-sensing inhibitors; however, most of them failed to explain the exact molecular mechanism behind the disruption of the biofilms. Besides that, more cytotoxicity studies need to be done to analyze the effects of the phytochemicals which support the hypothesis of low or zero side effects and development of inherent resistance.

3.4 Efflux pump inhibition

Bacterial efflux pumps contribute significantly to the development of multidrug resistance globally, which is further complicated by the biofilms associated with various infections. They have been identified as one of the universal targets for AMR, along with various other properties, including virulence and nutrient transport [48]. Moreover, they are one of the key regulators in biofilms associated with the above-mentioned quorum sensing mechanisms, which help communities survive in a coordinated way during extreme stress conditions. Phytochemicals influence the efflux pumps through various mechanisms or targets, which help limit the development of new AMR phenotypes and control bacterial biofilms via quorum sensing inhibition. The possibilities of phytochemicals targeting efflux pumps show a wide possibility for AMR research in which many promising combinations exist for various bacteria. Moreover, modern techniques such as molecular dynamics simulations to screen these combinations with predicted hypotheses based on efflux pump binding sites show a significant breakthrough [61]. However, the efflux pumps can affect the QS both positively and negatively. Hence, identification of the levels of phytochemicals is critical. Reversing the efflux pumps is one of the strategies by which the phytochemicals modify the effectiveness of antibiotics against biofilms [58]. More specifically, the phytochemicals may interact with the EPS and outer membrane to access the efflux pump and its components. This can result in the blockage of their function and increase the drug diffusion inside the cytoplasm. Furthermore, the increase in cytoplasmic concentration of the phytochemicals can influence the ATPase activity, thereby altering the functioning of efflux pumps and downregulating their gene expressions. AcrAB-TolC is an efflux pump in a multi-drug-resistant strain of *Enterobacter*. The chloramphenicol resistance in these bacteria is altered by a phytochemical called geraniol. The genes in *emr*, *acr* and *mdt* families were involved with efflux pump functions in the *E. coli*. Downregulation of these genes resulted in altered biofilm formation due to the effect of phytochemicals [60]. The *NorA* efflux pumps are very important in providing antibiotic resistance in *S. aureus.* Various phytochemicals have shown significant effects blocking these pumps and making antibiotics susceptible. For example, a flavonoid called quercetin was shown to inhibit the *NorA* and reverse the methicillin resistance. Furthermore, reserpine, baicalein, and piperine reversed the ciprofloxacin resistance in *S. aureus* [26]. Additionally, there are many additional examples of phytochemicals, such as isoflavones and coumarins, in blocking the efflux pumps and reversing antibiotic resistance in various bacterial biofilms. This signifies the importance of using phytochemicals by focusing on the efflux pump inhibition. This closely aligns with the concept of antibiotic potentiation, in which currently available antibiotics are more effectively acting against biofilms, overcoming the issues of antimicrobial resistance.

3.5 Antibiotic potentiation

Overcoming antibiotic resistance and treating biofilms with conventional antibiotics were a challenge, as mentioned before, mainly due to their structural and physiological characteristics as a community. Antibiotic potentiation can be mentioned as an outcome of various mechanisms that we have discussed so far, making antibiotics more accessible or effective against biofilms that even contain multidrug-resistant heterogenous communities [14]. Moreover, combining the phytochemicals with antibiotics would help expected outcomes at critically lower doses to overcome the fear of antimicrobial resistance. The most important mechanisms of action resulting in the potentiation of antibiotics are the efflux pump inactivation, membrane permeability changes for antibiotics, inactivation of enzymes inhibiting antibiotics, quorum sensing, and nucleic acid synthesis inhibition [51].

A Flavonoid, quercetin showed antibiotic potentiation for amoxicillin, ampicillin, ceftriaxone, and tetracycline against multi-drug-resistant *S. aureus* and *E. coli* by developing damage in the bacterial membrane by providing more penetration through the biofilm matrix. Furthermore, compounds such as daidzein, myricetin, and genistein provide antibiofilm activity by efflux pump inhibition and potentiate antibiotics such as gentamycin, ciprofloxacin, tetracycline, and vancomycin against *Pseudomonas, Staphylococcus* and *E. coli* [51]. Ellagic acid which is a phytochemical showed potentiation effects against *Propionibacterium* biofilms with tetracycline. Additionally, compounds such as thymol, cinnamaldehyde, and eugenol provided antibiotic potentiation effects with streptomycin against biofilm structures of *Listeria* and *Salmonella*, mainly due to the change in stability to the biofilm architecture. Apart from this, the fact that there might be some antagonistic effects for these phytochemicals in terms of antibiotic resistance could not be neglected in identifying possible combinations. The challenging part of the synergistic interaction between phytochemicals and antibiotics is the identification of the exact combinations or dose levels of the two in providing a synergistic interaction and delivery of the combination to the biofilm site. The former issue can be resolved by various predictive models as mentioned previously however, for solving the latter, new technologies focused on nano drug delivery systems are showing promising results [62]. A good example would be silver and copper nanoparticles loaded with phytochemicals and antibiotics, which provide antibiofilm effects against bacterial species such as methicillin-resistant *S. aureus* [62]. Furthermore, chitosan nanoparticles are one among the drug delivery methods that are widely studied against biofilms involving various pathogens such as *Staphylococcus, Listeria, and E. coli* using various phytochemicals such as essential oils, quercetin, cinnamaldehyde [63]. These aspects highlight the importance of phytochemical synergistic interactions with antibiotics in preventing biofilm-associated infections. Moreover, these applications can be implemented at an industrial level if the exact molecular mechanisms behind the synergism are identified on scientific grounds. This would make a significant breakthrough as naturally available molecules would conceptually have lower side effects in living systems compared to various synthetic derivatives [53, 63].

3.6 Additional mechanisms of action

There are various other mechanisms in which phytochemicals can exert effects on the biofilms in addition to the aspects mentioned above. One of the major mechanisms includes the effects on the metal chelation of the biofilms. Various metal ions, such as calcium, magnesium, copper, manganese, iron and zinc, play a crucial role in all living systems. This is not different in the case of biofilms as they help maintain their structure, signaling, and other virulence-associated mechanisms [64]. When considering the architecture, ions such as calcium and iron are very important in cross-linking the biofilm matrix. Additionally, the metal ions have shown roles in initial bacterial adhesion. Magnesium has been shown to have a role in bacterial multiplication, an association of iron with the release of DNA of *Pseudomonas* biofilms, effects of cation preconditioning with calcium and magnesium induces increased biofilm thickness [26]. All of the abovementioned conclude the importance of metal ions in the survival of bacterial biofilms. Therefore, altering or sequestering the metal ions associated with the biofilms may affect their integrity. Phytochemicals could be one of the many promising alternative strategies to chelate the metal ions associated with the biofilm. Iron chelation is one of the most common effects seen by phytochemicals, mainly because their structure makes them chelate with iron. For example, in flavonoids, the structure contains a dihydroxy chelation site for iron, which helps sequestration. Additionally, PGG, a gallotannin, was found to produce antibiofilm activity in *E. coli* due to iron chelation. Calcium chelation is shown by a phytochemical, alizarin, which is an anthraquinone mainly found in staphylococcal biofilms due to the hydroxyl units associated with its structure [65]. All these results ultimately affected the survivability of the biofilm structure. Division of cells and proliferation is required for the maintenance and survival of the biofilm community. Disruption of these proliferative mechanisms could impair this growth. Phytochemicals can influence growth by interfering with various mechanisms such as DNA and RNA synthesis, inhibiting cell division, growth inhibition, and inhibition of growth regulatory enzymes [66]. Trans cinnamaldehyde, a phytochemical shown to influence the structure of Z-ring by affecting a cell division protein called FtsZ which results in reduced growth of *Enterococcus faecalis*. Another phytochemical that influenced the FtsZ is the sanguinarine [67]. Trans cinnamaldehyde acts in a dose-dependent manner to inhibit cell proliferation in the biofilms and planktonic cells of Methicillin-Resistant *S. aureus* (MRSA). Moreover, this type of dose-dependent inhibition of cell proliferation is seen in MRSA by various other phytochemicals, such as carnosic acid and cineole [67]. Blocking enzymes involved with nucleic acid function is another prominent mechanism in which phytochemicals act. Some targets are topo isomerases I & II, DNA gyrase, and RNA polymerase which are shown by phytochemicals such as quercetin, genistein, berbine, and luteolin against various bacterial pathogens [26]. Most of the mechanism results in reduced biofilm mass and stability, which can be further addressed by alternative measures such as antibiotic potentiation, which would help control biofilm-associated infections.

Motility is a classical feature associated with planktonic cells that helps to establish the biofilm structure initially to a surface. Phytochemicals have shown mechanisms that disrupt the motility and thereby hinder the initial attachment. Antimotility action is mainly explained by the inactivation of the flagella components and the downregulation of genes associated with flagellar function such as families of *fla, fli* and *mot* genes. This is shown by phytochemicals such as eugenol, carvacrol, thymol and many essential oils against pathogens including *Listeria, Staphylococcus, Clostridium* and *E. coli* [68]. Interestingly, carvacrol showed flagellin synthesis inhibition by inducing a heat shock protein GroEL, which made the cells sessile. Further, the motility can impact the establishment of the biofilm architecture. However, the planktonic cells will still be virulent enough to cause diseases. Therefore, a more detailed mechanism of action needs to be uncovered to make it practical [24]. Along with motility, adhesion is another important mechanism required for the attachment of the cells to the surface. Bacterial surface characteristics are an important determinant in the adhesion. For example, the polarity and hydrophobicity are important aspects in determining the interaction with the surface to which they attach. Saponins and coumarins were found to influence the hydrophobicity of the membrane thereby disrupting the attachment. Moreover, phytochemicals such as carvacrol have been shown to affect the length and size of cells, further impacting the adhesive properties [28, 69]. All these mechanisms show the importance of phytochemicals in controlling the biofilms effectively.

Among the various methods discussed above, some promising ones are studied in depth to uncover the underlying mechanism of action. However, a deep understanding is required for others to elucidate their effectiveness. Phytochemicals would be a great choice to control biofilms and associated infections despite the increased burden of global antimicrobial resistance.

4. Challenges and limitations

Among the various mitigation strategies for tackling antimicrobial resistance associated with biofilms, phytochemicals showed a promising outcome. They are more reliable in terms of safety than synthetic compounds. However, some aspects need to be addressed to use them effectively [60].

Most of the research is focused on specific bacterial biofilms and the interactions of phytochemicals. This is different when we observe the actual living systems where multiple species are involved providing a complex heterogenous environment. In that case, the mechanism of action of the phytochemical starting from the penetration to biofilm the structure may differ due to this heterogeneity [32]. Phytochemicals can interact with the host tissue in the same way as the biofilm structure if it is in a living system. There can be metabolism and degradation of this phytochemical by the host system, which might reduce its bioavailability. Furthermore, the solubility and stability of different phytochemicals might be influenced by many factors that need to be studied. Bacteria have inherent mechanisms to fight the antimicrobial agents, which results in increased antimicrobial resistance. Therefore, there is a chance that bacteria will develop resistance against phytochemicals through various mechanisms, including efflux pumps and QS. Still, it might be a slow process compared to the traditional synthetic antimicrobial. For example, quercetin and resveratrol have been shown to selectively enhance resistance in certain bacteria, such as *S. aureus,* when used in sub-optimal concentration, leading to AMR. Understanding the mechanisms of action and composition of the phytochemicals at a cellular level is important. They can interact with various cellular components and act in a toxic way detrimental to the host cells in addition to the biofilm components. Further, it may influence beneficial organisms associated with the host cells. Therefore, it is imperative to determine the cellular effects of each phytochemical to understand and use them at their full potential. Standardization and quality control is another major challenge involved with phytochemicals. Each phytochemical might have different extraction mechanisms, depending on various factors involving extraction methods, plant characteristics, and environmental conditions. Variations in the same phytochemical product might influence the efficiency and mechanism of action. Standardization of the products is a key technique to reduce this variation, but the cost of the purification involving large-scale production might be a major challenge in addition to providing a sustainable supply of phytochemicals [52]. Another major challenge would be the absence of clinical trials involving biofilms and phytochemicals. The exact mechanism by which most phytochemicals interact with biofilms has yet to be understood. Moreover, most of the studies are pre-clinical, involving animal models, and lack human trials. Additionally, the regulatory approval of these products is quite challenging. The main issue is the confusion regarding various regulatory agencies' consideration of phytochemicals as therapeutics or dietary supplements [70]. The complexity of the phytochemicals is another challenge; for example, various essential oils have multiple active components, which makes the demonstration of individual effects very difficult. There can be challenges with intellectual property protections as they are naturally occurring compounds compared to synthetic ones, which is an independent discovery. Apart from these facts, some of the phytochemicals have shown hepatotoxicity, nephrotoxicity and antagonistic activities, making the regulations and approval process much more difficult compared to synthetic therapeutic molecules [70].

Considering these factors, priority should be given to the standardization of the phytochemicals to maintain the reproducibility of the experiments and approvals by introducing advanced analytical methods. This is followed by legitimate clinical trials, which can pave ways to streamline more convenient regulatory processes considering the promising efficiency of phytochemicals as antibiofilm agents or antibiotic potentiating agents.

5. Future directions

Phytochemicals have shown exceptional activity against biofilms by interfering with various mechanisms, starting from attachment to quorum sensing. Addressing the limitations would make them a good source for overcoming antimicrobial resistance, which is aggravated by the biofilms [16]. Identification of the synergistic combinations for antibiotic potentiation is a time-consuming process. The application of next-generation computing for this process has been shown to produce significant results in a short amount of time [71]. Moreover, predictive models based on machine learning would be a good approach since they can even predict the mechanisms of action behind the synergistic combinations, which clinical research can further validate. Advanced drug delivery systems are another avenue of research that would benefit the use of phytochemicals against biofilms. Various types of nanoparticles, such as gold, silver, and chitosan particles, have successfully delivered various biomolecules with increasing stability, solubility, and release profile. Hence, if the research can be focused on delivering standardized phytochemicals into biofilm structures by these nanoparticles, it would help to provide the expected mechanisms of action [72]. Furthermore, for biofilms associated with hospitalized infections, coating the susceptible medical devices such as catheters and implants with successful antibiofilm phytochemicals would be a possible strategy. Epigallocatechin gallate has been studied for its anti-biofilm properties in medical devices by surface coating [73]. However, the tissue-specific or site-specific mechanisms or drug delivery, such as in the case of chronic wounds, should be investigated further to create new avenues for phytochemical applications against biofilms.

Another important mechanism that needs further exploration might be the mechanism that phytochemicals can elicit in the host against the biofilms. This could be understood based on the antibiotic tolerance and immune regulations in the host that can be addressed by antibiotic potentiation with phytochemicals. Moreover, many phytochemicals have traditionally shown anti-inflammatory effects, which can be useful along with antibiotics against biofilms [74]. Advancements in therapeutic strategies also need much attention. For example, phytochemical profiling for personalized therapies would be one of the possible strategies to influence the effectiveness of treatment with phytochemicals. It is widely practiced in other avenues of research, such as cancer. Additionally, more comprehensive and promising pharmacodynamics studies should be conducted to validate the antibiotics' effectiveness. These future directions represent a multifaceted approach to combating biofilm-associated infections and enhancing the effectiveness of antibiotics using phytochemicals. The combination of molecular insights, advanced delivery systems, and clinical validation will be key to realizing the full potential of phytochemicals in this area.

6. Conclusion

In conclusion, the increasing global prevalence of antimicrobial resistance (AMR), particularly in biofilm-associated infections, presents a significant challenge to public health and clinical treatments. Biofilms, which consist of extracellular polymeric substances (EPS) and display altered metabolic states, contribute to the enhanced resistance of microorganisms to conventional antibiotics. Furthermore, the mechanisms of horizontal gene transfer and biofilm-mediated protection complicate treatment strategies, particularly in nosocomial and foodborne infections. Phytochemicals, with their diverse categories including alkaloids, terpenoids, flavonoids, and phenolic acids, offer promising alternatives in combating biofilms and AMR. These compounds demonstrate potent biofilm inhibition, quorum sensing disruption, and EPS degradation, contributing to antibiotic potentiation. Several *in vitro* and *in vivo* studies have demonstrated successful synergistic effects when combining phytochemicals with antibiotics, highlighting their potential for enhancing the efficacy of existing antimicrobial therapies.

However, challenges still need to be addressed in the widespread application of phytochemicals, primarily due to issues related to bioavailability, stability, and the complexities of regulatory approval. Moreover, potential bacterial resistance to these compounds requires further investigation. Emerging solutions, such as the use of nanotechnology for drug delivery and personalized treatment strategies, hold promise in overcoming these limitations. The future of phytochemical research in AMR will likely focus on developing novel delivery systems and combination therapies and exploring new phytochemical sources, aiming to provide a sustainable solution to the growing threat of biofilm-related infections and antibiotic resistance.

Conflict of interest

The authors declare no conflict of interest.

Author details

Jiddu Joseph, Sanya Boby and Muhammed Shafeekh Muyyarikkandy*
Department of Animal and Food Sciences, University of Delaware, Newark, DE, USA

*Address all correspondence to: msm@udel.edu

References

[1] Flemming H, Wuertz S. Bacteria and archaea on earth and their abundance in biofilms. Nature Reviews Microbiology. 2019;**17**:247-260. DOI: 10.1038/s41579-019-0158-9

[2] Squyres GR, Newman DK. Biofilms as more than the sum of their parts: Lessons from developmental biology. Current Opinion in Microbiology. 2024;**82**:102537. DOI: 10.1016/j.mib.2024.102537

[3] Crabbe A, Jensen PO, Bjarnsholt T, Coenye T. Antimicrobial tolerance and metabolic adaptations in microbial biofilms. Trends Microbiology. 2019;**27**:850-863. DOI: 10.1016/j.tim.2019.05.003

[4] Shapiro JA. Bacteria as multicellular organisms. Scientific American. 1988;**258**:82-89. Available from: https://www.jstor.org/stable/24989125

[5] Hofer U. The cost of biofilms. Nature Reviews Microbiology. 2022;**20**:445. DOI: 10.1038/s41579-022-00758-1

[6] Camara M, Green W, MacPhee CE, Rakowska PD, Raval R, Richardson MC, et al. Economic significance of biofilms: A multidisciplinary and cross-sectoral challenge. npj Biofilms and Microbiomes. 2022;**8**:42. DOI: 10.1038/s41522-022-00306-y

[7] Metcalf DG, Bowler PG. Biofilm delays wound healing: A review of the evidence. Burns and Trauma. 2013;**1**:2321-3868. DOI: 10.4103/2321-3868.113329

[8] Fleming A. On the antibacterial action of cultures of a penicillium, with special reference to their use in the isolation of *B. Influenzae*. British Journal of Experimental Pathology. 1929;**10**:226

[9] Dhingra S, Rahman NAA, Peile E, Rahman M, Sartelli M, Hassali MA, et al. Microbial resistance movements: An overview of global public health threats posed by antimicrobial resistance, and how best to counter. Frontiers in Public Health. 2020;**8**:535668. DOI: 10.3389/fpubh.2020.535668

[10] Antimicrobial resistance in the environment and the food supply: Causes and how it spreads [Internet]. 2024. Available from: https://www.cdc.gov/antimicrobial-resistance/causes/environmental-food [Accessed: September 13, 2024]

[11] Tang KW, Millar BC, Moore JE. Antimicrobial resistance (AMR). British Journal of Biomedical Science. 2023;**80**:11387. DOI: 10.3389/bjbs.2023.11387

[12] Tetz G, Tetz V. Overcoming antibiotic resistance with novel paradigms of antibiotic selection. Microorganisms. 2022;**10**:2383. DOI: 10.3390/microorganisms10122383

[13] Hauser AR, Mecsas J, Moir DT. Beyond antibiotics: New therapeutic approaches for bacterial infections. Clinical Infectious Diseases. 2016;**63**:89-95. DOI: 10.1093/cid/ciw200

[14] Krukiewicz K, Kazek-Kęsik A, Brzychczy-Wloch M, Los MJ, Ateba CN, Mehrbod P, et al. Recent advances in the control of clinically important biofilms. International Journal of Molecular Sciences. 2022;**23**:9526. DOI: 10.3390/ijms23179526

[15] Balducci E, Papi F, Capialbi DE, Del BL. Polysaccharides' structures and functions in biofilm architecture of antimicrobial-resistant (AMR)

pathogens. International Journal of Molecular Sciences. 2023;**24**:4030. DOI: 10.3390/ijms24044030

[16] Nadar S, Khan T, Patching SG, Omri A. Development of antibiofilm therapeutics strategies to overcome antimicrobial drug resistance. Microorganisms. 2022;**10**:303. DOI: 10.3390/microorganisms10020303

[17] Gangwar B, Kumar S, Darokar M. Antioxidants Phytochemicals as Novel Therapeutic Strategies against Drug-Resistant Bacteria [Internet]. London, United Kingdom: IntechOpen; 2023. DOI: 10.5772/intechopen.108220 [Accessed: January 27, 2025]

[18] Cheema HS, Maurya A, Kumar S, Pandey VK, Singh RM. Antibiotic potentiation through phytochemical-based efflux pump inhibitors to combat multidrug resistance bacteria. Medicinal Chemistry. 2024;**20**:557-575. DOI: 10.2174/0115734064263586231022135644

[19] Simoes M, Bennett RN, Rosa EA. Understanding antimicrobial activities of phytochemicals against multidrug-resistant bacteria and biofilms. Natural Product Reports. 2009;**26**:746-757. DOI: 10.1039/b821648g

[20] Kumar A, Khan IA, Koul S, Koul JL, Taneja SC, Ali I, et al. Novel structural analogs of piperine as inhibitors of the NorA efflux pump of Staphylococcus aureus. Journal of Antimicrobial Chemotherapy. 2008;**61**:1270-1276. DOI: 10.1093/jac/dkn088

[21] Davies DG, Parsek MR, Pearson JP, Iglewski BH, Costerton JW, Greenberg EP. The involvement of cell-to-cell signals in the development of a bacterial biofilm. Science. 1998;**280**:295-298. DOI: 10.1126/science.280.5361.295

[22] Kungwani NA, Panda J, Mishra AK, Chavda N, Shukla S, Vikhe K, et al. Combating bacterial biofilms and related drug resistance: Role of Phyto-derived adjuvant and nanomaterials. Microbial Pathogens. 2024;**195**:106874. DOI: 10.1016/j.micpath.2024.106874

[23] Thakur M, Singh K, Khedkar R. Phytochemicals: Extraction process, safety assessment, toxicological evaluations, and regulatory issues. Functional and preservative properties of phytochemicals. In: Prakash B, editor. Functional and Preservative Properties of Phytochemicals. London, United Kingdom: Academic Press; 2020. pp. 341-361. DOI: 10.1016/B978-0-12-818593-3.00011-7

[24] Andrade M, Malheiro J, Borges F, Saavedra MJ, Simões M. The potential of phytochemical products in biofilm control. In: Simoes M, Borges A, Simoes LC, editors. Recent Trends in Biofilm Science and Technology. Amsterdam, Netherlands: Elsevier; 2020. pp. 273-293. DOI: 10.1016/B978-0-12-819497-3.00012-X

[25] Huang Y, Xiao D, Burton-Freeman BM, Edirisinghe I. Chemical changes of bioactive phytochemicals during thermal processing. Food Science. 2016;**9**:1-9. DOI: 10.1016/B978-0-08-100596-5.03055-9

[26] Borges AJ, Saavedra M, Simoes M. Insights on antimicrobial resistance, biofilms and the use of phytochemicals as new antimicrobial agents. Current Medicinal Chemistry. 2015;**22**:2590-2614. DOI: 10.2174/0929867322666150530210522

[27] Taraszkiewicz A, Fila G, Grinholc M, Nakonieczna J. Innovative strategies to overcome biofilm resistance. Biomed Research International. 2013;**2013**(1):150653. DOI: 10.1155/2013/150653

[28] Bjarnsholt T, Ciofu O, Molin S, Givskov M, Høiby N. Applying insights from biofilm biology to drug development can a new approach be developed. Nature Reviews Drug Discovery. 2013;**12**:791-808. DOI: 10.1038/nrd4000

[29] Borges A, Abreu AC, Dias C, Saavedra MJ, Borges F, Simões M. New perspectives on the use of phytochemicals as an emergent strategy to control bacterial infections including biofilms. Molecules. 2016;**21**:877. DOI: 10.3390/molecules21070877

[30] Martin C, Low WL, Gupta A, Amin MC, Radecka I, Britland S, et al. Strategies for antimicrobial drug delivery to biofilm. Current Pharmaceutical Design. 2015;**21**:43-66. DOI: 10.2174/1381612820666140905123529

[31] Birk SE, Boisen A, Nielsen LH. Polymeric nano and microparticulate drug delivery systems for treatment of biofilms. Advanced Drug Delivery Reviews. 2021;**174**:30-52. DOI: 10.1016/j.addr.2021.04.005

[32] Flemming H, Wingender J, Szewzyk U, Steinberg P, Rice SA, Kjelleberg S. Biofilms: An emergent form of bacterial life. Nature Reviews Microbiology. 2016;**14**:563-575. DOI: 10.1038/nrmicro.2016.94

[33] Armbruster CR, Parsek MR. New insight into the early stages of biofilm formation. Proceedings of the National Academy of Sciences. 2018;**115**:4317-4319. DOI: 10.1073/pnas.1804084115

[34] de Brito FA, de Freitas AP, Nascimento MS. Multidrug-resistant biofilms (MDR): Main mechanisms of tolerance and resistance in the food supply chain. Pathogens. 2022;**11**:1416. DOI: 10.3390/pathogens11121416

[35] Jorge P, Magalhaes AP, Grainha T, Alves D, Sousa AM, Lopes SP, et al. Antimicrobial resistance three ways: Healthcare crisis, major concepts and the relevance of biofilms. FEMS Microbiology Ecology. 2019;**95**:fiz115. DOI: 10.1093/femsec/fiz115

[36] Arciola CR, Campoccia D, Gamberini S, Donati ME, Pirini V, Visai L, et al. Antibiotic resistance in exopolysaccharide-forming *Staphylococcus epidermidis* clinical isolates from orthopedic implant infections. Biomaterials. 2005;**26**:6530-6535. DOI: 10.1016/j.biomaterials.2005.04.031

[37] Rasamiravaka T, Labtani Q, Duez P, El JM. The formation of biofilms by *Pseudomonas aeruginosa*: A review of the natural and synthetic compounds interfering with control mechanisms. Biomed Research International. 2015;**15**:759348. DOI: 10.1155/2015/759348

[38] Liu J, Zhang J, Guo L, Zhao W, Hu X, Wei X. Inactivation of a putative efflux pump (LmrB) in *Streptococcus mutans* results in altered biofilm structure and increased exopolysaccharide synthesis: Implications for biofilm resistance. Biofouling. 2017;**33**:481-493. DOI: 10.1080/08927014.2017.1323206

[39] Gupta P, Pruthi PA, Pruthi V. Role of exopolysaccharides in biofilm formation. In: Introduction to Biofilm Engineering ACS. Washington DC, USA: ACS publications; 2019. pp. 17-57. DOI: 10.1021/bk-2019-1323.ch002

[40] Emami S, Nikokar I, Ghasemi Y, Ebrahimpour M, Ebrahim-Saraie HS, Araghian A, et al. Antibiotic resistance pattern and distribution of pslA gene among biofilm producing *Pseudomonas aeruginosa* isolated from wastewater of a burn center. Jundishapur Journal of Microbiology. 2015;**8**(11):e23669. DOI: 10.5812/jjm.23669

[41] Begun J, Gaiani JM, Rohde H, Mack D, Calderwood SB, Ausubel FM, et al. Staphylococcal biofilm exopolysaccharide protects against Caenorhabditis elegans immune defenses. PLoS Pathogens. 2007;**3**:e57. DOI: 10.1371/journal.ppat.0030057

[42] Yasir M, Willcox MDP, Dutta D. Action of antimicrobial peptides against bacterial biofilms. Materials. 2018;**11**:2468. DOI: 0.3390/ma11122468

[43] Carrolo M, Frias MJ, Pinto FR, Melo-Cristino J, Ramirez M. Prophage spontaneous activation promotes DNA release enhancing biofilm formation in *Streptococcus pneumoniae*. PLoS One. 2010;**5**:e15678. DOI: 10.1371/journal.pone.0015678

[44] Alhede M, Alhede M, Qvortrup K, Kragh KN, Jensen PO, Stewart PS, et al. The origin of extracellular DNA in bacterial biofilm infections *in vivo*. Pathogens and Disease. 2020;**78**:ftaa018. DOI: 10.1093/femspd/ftaa018

[45] Chi F, Nolte O, Bergmann C, Ip M, Hakenbec R. Crossing the barrier: Evolution and spread of a major class of mosaic pbp2x in *Streptococcus pneumoniae*, *S. Mitis* and *S. Oralis*. International Journal of Medical Microbiology. 2007;**297**:503-512. DOI: 10.1016/j.ijmm.2007.02.009

[46] Johnson L, Mulcahy H, Kanevets U, Shi Y, Lewenza S. Surface-localized spermidine protects the *Pseudomonas aeruginosa* outer membrane from antibiotic treatment and oxidative stress. Journal Bacteriology. 2012;**194**:813-826. DOI: 10.1128/jb.05230-11

[47] Dabul ANG, Avaca-Crusca JS, Van TD, Gilmore MS, Camargo ILBC. Resistance in *in vitro* selected tigecycline-resistant methicillin-resistant *Staphylococcus aureus* sequence type 5 is driven by mutations in mepR and mepA genes. Microbial Drug Resistance. 2018;**24**:519-526. DOI: 10.1089/mdr.2017.0279

[48] Mah TC, O'Toole GA. Mechanisms of biofilm resistance to antimicrobial agents. Trends in Microbiology. 2001;**9**:34-39. DOI: 10.1016/S0966-842X(00)01913-2

[49] Borriello G, Werner E, Roe F, Kim AM, Ehrlich GD, Stewart PS. Oxygen limitation contributes to antibiotic tolerance of *Pseudomonas aeruginosa* in biofilms. Antimicrobial Agents and Chemotherapy. 2004;**48**:2659-2664. DOI: 10.1128/aac.48.7.2659-2664.2004

[50] Soto GMJ, Rodriguez RLM, Luo C, Elk M, Ryu H, Hoelle J, et al. Biofilms on hospital shower hoses: Characterization and implications for nosocomial infections. Applied and Environmental Microbiology. 2016;**82**:2872-2883. DOI: 10.1128/AEM.03529-15

[51] Paul D, Chawla M, Ahrodia T, Narendrakumar L, Das B. Antibiotic potentiation as a promising strategy to combat macrolide resistance in bacterial pathogens. Antibiotics. Bazel, Switzerland: Multidisciplinary Digital Publishing Institute; 2023;12:1715. DOI: 10.3390/antibiotics12121715

[52] Cragg GM, Newman DJ. Natural products: A continuing source of novel drug leads. Biochimica et Biophysica Acta (BBA)-General Subjects. Amsterdam, Netherlands: Elsevier; 2013;1830:3670-3695. DOI: 10.1016/j.bbagen.2013.02.008

[53] Kalan L, Wright GD. Antibiotic adjuvants: Multicomponent anti-infective strategies. Expert Reviews in Molecular Medicine. 2011;**13**:e5. DOI: 10.1017/s1462399410001766

[54] Miao J, Lin S, Soteyome T, Peters BM, Li Y, Chen H, et al. Biofilm formation

of *Staphylococcus aureus* under food heat processing conditions: First report on CML production within biofilm. Scientific Reports. 2019;**9**:1312. DOI: 10.1038/s41598-018-35558-2

[55] Qian W, Fu Y, Liu M, Zhang J, Wang W, Li J, et al. Mechanisms of action of luteolin against single-and dual-species of *Escherichia coli* and *Enterobacter cloacae* and its antibiofilm activities. Applied Biochemistry and Biotechnology. 2021;**193**:1397-1414. DOI: 10.1007/s12010-020-03330-w

[56] Huang J, Yang L, Zou Y, Luo S, Wang X, Liang Y, et al. Antibacterial activity and mechanism of three isomeric terpineols of Cinnamomum longepaniculatum leaf oil. Folia Microbiologica. 2021;**66**:59-67. DOI: 10.1007/s12223-020-00818-0

[57] Gohil N, Ramírez-García R, Panchasara H, Patel S, Bhattacharjee G, Singh V. Quorum sensing vs. quorum quenching: A battle with no end in sight. Frontiers in Cellular Infectious Microbiology. 2018;**8**:106. DOI: 10.3389/fcimb.2018.00106

[58] Kiran MD, Adikesavan NV, Cirioni O, Giacometti A, Silvestri C, Scalise G, et al. Discovery of a quorum-sensing inhibitor of drug-resistant staphylococcal infections by structure-based virtual screening. Molecular Pharmacology. 2008;**73**:1578-1586. DOI: 10.1124/mol.107.044164.Epub 2008 Feb 26

[59] Bhargava N, Singh SP, Sharma A, Sharma P, Capalash N. Attenuation of quorum sensing-mediated virulence of *Acinetobacter baumannii* by Glycyrrhiza glabra flavonoids. Future Microbiology. 2015;**10**:1953-1968. DOI: 10.2217/fmb.15.107

[60] Ta CAK, Arnason JT. Mini review of phytochemicals and plant taxa with activity as microbial biofilm and quorum sensing inhibitors. Molecules. 2015;**21**:29. DOI: 10.3390/molecules21010029

[61] Verma P, Tiwari M, Tiwari V. In silico high-throughput virtual screening and molecular dynamics simulation study to identify inhibitor for AdeABC efflux pump of *Acinetobacter baumannii*. Journal of Biomolecular Structure and Dynamics. 2018;**36**:1182-1194. DOI: 10.1080/07391102.2017.1317025

[62] Shamprasad BR, Lotha R, Nagarajan S, Sivasubramanian A. Metal nanoparticles functionalized with nutraceutical kaempferitrin from edible Crotalaria juncea, exert potent antimicrobial and antibiofilm effects against methicillin-resistant *Staphylococcus aureus*. Scientific Reports. 2022;**12**:7061. DOI: 10.1038/s41598-022-11004-2

[63] Guidotti TM, Ribeiro LNM, Santos FAL, Rossi DA, Lucia FD, de Melo RT. Essential oil-based nanoparticles as antimicrobial agents in the food industry. Microorganisms. 2022;**10**:1504. DOI: 10.3390/microorganisms10081504

[64] Porcheron G, Garenaux A, Proulx J, Sabri M, Dozois CM. Iron, copper, zinc, and manganese transport and regulation in pathogenic Enterobacteria: Correlations between strains, site of infection and the relative importance of the different metal transport systems for virulence. Frontiers in Cellular and Infection Microbiology. 2013;**3**:90. DOI: 10.3389/fcimb.2013.00090

[65] Lee J, Kim Y, Yong RS, Lee J. Calcium-chelating alizarin and other anthraquinones inhibit biofilm formation and the hemolytic activity of Staphylococcus aureus. Scientific Reports. 2016;**6**:19267. DOI: 10.1038/srep19267

[66] Nowicki D, Maciąg DM , Bogucka K, Szalewska PA, Herman AA. Various modes of action of dietary phytochemicals, sulforaphane, and phenethyl isothiocyanate, on pathogenic bacteria. Scientific Reports. 2019;**9**:13677. DOI: 10.1038/s41598-019-50216-x

[67] Ali IAA, Matinlinna JP, Levesque CM, Neelakantan P. Trans-cinnamaldehyde attenuates *enterococcus faecalis* virulence and inhibits biofilm formation. Antibiotics. 2021;**10**:702. DOI: 10.3390/antibiotics10060702

[68] Upadhyay A, Arsi K, Wagle BR, Upadhyaya I, Shrestha S, Donoghue AM, et al. Trans-cinnamaldehyde, carvacrol, and eugenol reduce *campylobacter jejuni* colonization factors and expression of virulence genes *in vitro*. Frontiers in Microbiology. 2017;**8**:713. DOI: 10.3389/fmicb.2017.00713

[69] Madsen JS, Burmolle M, Hansen LH, Sorensen SJ. The interconnection between biofilm formation and horizontal gene transfer. FEMS Immunology & Medical Microbiology. 2012;**65**:183-195. DOI: 10.1111/j.1574-695X.2012.00960. x

[70] Panossian A. Challenges in phytotherapy research. Frontiers in Pharmacology. 2023;**14**:1199516. DOI: 10.3389/fphar.2023.1199516

[71] Moshawih S, Goh HP, Kifli N, Idris AC, Yassin H, Kotra V, et al. Synergy between machine learning and natural products cheminformatics: Application to the lead discovery of anthraquinone derivatives. Chemical Biology and Drug Design. 2022;**100**:185-217. DOI: 10.1111/cbdd.14062

[72] Wang S, Su R, Nie S, Sun M, Zhang J, Wu D, et al. Application of nanotechnology in improving bioavailability and bioactivity of diet-derived phytochemicals. Journal of Nutritional Biochemistry. 2014;**25**:363-376. DOI: 10.1016/j.jnutbio.2013.10.002

[73] Meesaragandla B, Hayet S, Fine T, Janke U, Chai L, Delcea M. Inhibitory effect of epigallocatechin Gallate-silver nanoparticles and their lysozyme bioconjugates on biofilm formation and cytotoxicity. ACS Applied Bio Materials. 2022;**5**:4213-4221. DOI: 10.1021/acsabm.2c00409

[74] Wang T, Cui X, Cai S, Zou X, Zheng S, Li Y, et al. Multifunctional phytochemical nano platform for comprehensive treatment of all-stage MRSA biofilm-associated infection and its accompanying inflammation. Chemical Engineering Journal. 2024;**480**:147951. DOI: 10.1016/j.cej.2023.147951

Section 3

Biofilm-Mediated Risks from Industrial to Clinic Applications

Chapter 10

Biofilms and Their Multidimensional Impacts: From Combating Industrial and Clinical Risks to Unlocking Opportunities in Sustainable Agriculture

Atiye Karadoğan, Fatma Azgin, Esra Sündüz Yiğittekin and Sadik Dinçer

Abstract

Biofilms are microbial communities embedded in a matrix of extracellular polymeric substances (EPS) that irreversibly adhere to surfaces in natural, industrial, and clinical environments. Their formation involves a dynamic, multi-step process influenced by microbial interactions, EPS production, and surface properties. Biofilms provide microorganisms with protection against environmental stresses and antimicrobial agents, creating significant challenges in healthcare and industry. In industrial settings, Microbial Induced Corrosion (MIC) is a major issue, with biofilms contributing to the degradation of metallic and nonmetallic surfaces through mechanisms like electrochemical cell formation and the production of corrosive metabolites. Sulfate-reducing bacteria (SRB) and other microbes accelerate this process, impacting the lifespan of pipelines, marine structures, and industrial equipment. Clinically, biofilm-associated infections constitute 70% of all infections, resisting antibiotics and immune responses. These infections complicate treatment, impair medical implants, and are linked to chronic conditions like cystic fibrosis and diabetic foot ulcers. Emerging diagnostic tools, such as biosensors, and treatments like nanoparticles, conjugated antimicrobials, and phage therapy, offer promising solutions. In agriculture, biofilms enhance the virulence of pathogens but also support beneficial effects. Plant Growth Promoting Bacteria (PGPB) within biofilms help plants combat biotic and abiotic stresses while promoting growth through beneficial metabolite production.

Keywords: extracellular polymeric substance (EPS), exopolysaccharide, microbial induced corrosion (MIC), quorum sensing (QS), antibiotic resistance, ESKAPE, plant growth promoting Bacteria (PGPB)

1. Introduction

A biofilm is a community of cells organized in microcolonies, irreversibly attached to a surface and embedded in an organic polymer matrix of microbial origin formed at the interface between a liquid medium and a surface [1, 2]. Bacteria form biofilms in natural and industrial environments as a defense mechanism against antibacterial chemicals, environmental bacteriophages, and phagocytes. Biofilms are capable of developing on various surfaces, including living tissues, medical devices, pipelines in industrial or drinking water systems, and natural water sources. The solid-liquid interface provides an ideal environment for microorganisms to adhere and multiply [3].

The formation of biofilms is a complex and dynamic process that begins with the following steps: Planktonic bacteria are delivered to solid surfaces through hydrodynamic forces and mechanisms of physical or chemical adsorption. Extracellular structures such as flagella, folds, fimbriae or pili, and outer membrane proteins facilitate bacterial recognition and interaction with surfaces. These interactions are crucial for biofilm development as they allow bacterial cells to overcome long-range repulsive forces near the surface. Additionally, these processes are modulated by the physicochemical properties of the substrate surface, including factors such as charge and hydrophobicity. At this stage, bacteria typically show Brownian motion and can be easily removed from the surface by shear forces. Once initial attachment occurs, flagellar movement is restricted, and attached cells begin to produce extracellular polymeric substances (EPS) (**Figure 1**). EPS production shifts bacterial attachment from a reversible to an irreversible state. Due to the EPS matrix, these attached cells become increasingly difficult to detach from the surface. The composition of EPS varies depending on the bacterial species and growth conditions. As cells proliferate and accumulate more EPS, these micron-scale aggregates grow into mature biofilms, forming three-dimensional structures [4].

The extracellular polymeric substances (EPS) play a critical role in biofilm architecture by anchoring biofilm cells and maintaining them in proximity. This close spatial arrangement promotes intense interactions, including intercellular communication and the establishment of synergistic micro-consortia [5]. The composition of EPS includes polysaccharides, proteins, extracellular DNA (eDNA),

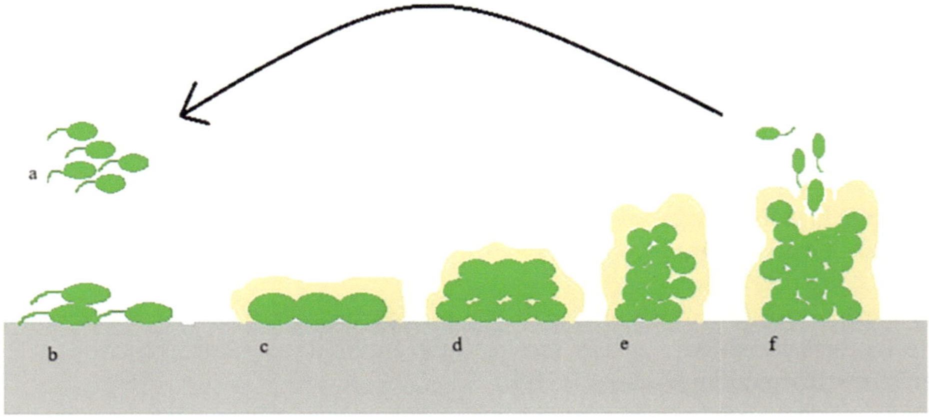

Figure 1.
Development of a biofilm and microstructures. (a) Planktonic organisms, (b) reversible attachment, (c) irreversible attachment and bacterial colonization, (d) adhesion and production of exopolymeric substances (EPS), (e) formation of mature biofilm, and (f) dispersion stage.

and lipids. The structural integrity of the biofilm matrix is preserved through non-covalent interactions, which are mediated by weak physicochemical forces between the components of the EPS [1].

2. Biofilms in industry

Impacts corrosion is a harmful process that occurs when metals undergo chemical or electrochemical reactions with their environment. This electrochemical phenomenon involves the release of electrons from the metal at anodic sites and their acquisition at cathodic sites [6, 7].

$$M \rightarrow M^{2+} + 2e^{-} \text{ Anodic reaction} \quad (1)$$

$$1/2O_2 + H_2O + 2e^{-} \rightarrow 2OH^{-} \text{ Cathodic reaction } \textit{at} \text{ neutral or alkaline pH} \quad (2)$$

Microbial Induced Corrosion (MIC) is a type of corrosion caused by the presence and activities of microorganisms, leading to the deterioration of both metallic and nonmetallic materials [7]. MIC is considered the direct cause of severe corrosion failures and leads to damage costs reaching billions of U.S. dollars annually. Microorganisms such as bacteria, fungi, archaea, and microalgae can directly or indirectly influence corrosion, depending on specific interactions between the microorganism, the material, and the electrolyte [8].

Biofilms actively contribute to corrosion through various mechanisms such as accumulation of cells at different concentrations, production of corrosive substances, changes in anion ratios, and inactivation of corrosion inhibitors [7].

When a metal surface is covered by a biofilm, the portion of the metal outside the biofilm remains exposed to oxygen, while the metal beneath the biofilm is shielded from oxygen exposure. This disparity in oxygen availability results in the formation of a corrosion cell within the anodic zone under the biofilm, where metal ions are generated, leading to localized pitting corrosion. Electrons migrate to the metal surface outside the biofilm to facilitate oxygen reduction (cathodic reaction), during which hydroxyl ions are produced (**Figure 2**). These systems are referred to as oxygen concentration cells and are frequently linked to microbially influenced

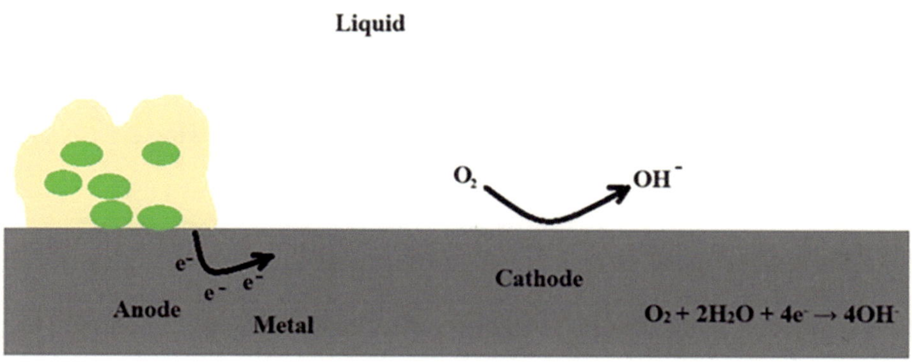

Figure 2.
MIC mechanism.

corrosion. Liu et al. [9] demonstrated that the adhesion of *Vibrio natriegens* to a surface enhances the anodic reaction rate, thereby accelerating the dissolution of aluminum.

Biofilms diminish the efficacy of corrosion inhibitors by establishing a diffusion barrier that obstructs direct interaction between the metal surface and the inhibitors present in the environment. Additionally, microorganisms are capable of degrading specific corrosion inhibitors, such as aliphatic amines and nitrites. This microbial degradation not only compromises the performance of the inhibitors but also facilitates the proliferation of microbial populations, thereby accelerating the corrosion process [10].

Microorganisms produce both inorganic and organic acids that can have corrosive effects on metals. The primary inorganic acid involved in metal corrosion is sulfuric acid, which is produced by acidophilic and sulfur-oxidizing bacteria. These bacteria thrive in environments where sulfur compounds are reduced and can produce very low pH levels (pH 2–5) when oxygen is present. Important microorganisms include *Thiobacillus thiooxidans* and *Thiobacillus ferrooxidans*; the latter is often associated with acidic mine drainage [11].

Sulfate-reducing bacteria (SRB) are the microorganisms most strongly linked to microbial-induced corrosion (MIC). These bacteria utilize sulfate as a terminal electron acceptor in their metabolic processes, resulting in the production of hydrogen sulfide (H_2S). They belong to a diverse group of anaerobic microorganisms that inhabit a wide range of environments. The metabolic activities of SRB contribute to the accumulation of sulfur compounds near metal surfaces, significantly accelerating the corrosion process. SRBs are a critical area of focus in MIC research, with several corrosion mechanisms attributed to their activity, including:

- Cathodic depolarization via dehydrogenase enzymes
- Anodic depolarization processes
- Secretion of exopolysaccharides that bind metal ions
- Sulfur-induced stress corrosion cracking
- Hydrogen-induced cracking and bubbling
- Formation of metal sulfides

These effects of SRB play an important role in the degradation of metal surfaces [10].

von Wolzogen Kuhr and van der Vlugt [12] proposed the following electrochemical reactions related to the MIC performed by SRB:

$$4Fe \rightarrow 4Fe^{2+} + 8e^{-}\ (\text{anodic reaction}) \tag{3}$$

$$8H_2O \rightarrow 8H^{+} + 8OH^{-}\ (\text{water dissociation}) \tag{4}$$

$$8H^{+} + 8e^{-} \rightarrow 8H\ (\text{cathodic reaction}) \tag{5}$$

$$SO_4^{2-} + 8\mathrm{H} \rightarrow \mathrm{S}^{2-} + 4\mathrm{H_2O}\,(\text{bacterial consumption}) \tag{6}$$

$$Fe^{2+} + \mathrm{S}^{2-} \rightarrow FeS\,(\text{corrosion products}) \tag{7}$$

$$4\mathrm{Fe} + SO_4^{2-} + 4\mathrm{H_2O_3} \rightarrow Fe(OH)_2 + FeS + 2\mathrm{OH}^- \tag{8}$$

Ilhan-Sungur et al. [13] showed that sulfate-reducing bacteria (*Desulfovibrio* sp.) are responsible for corrosion of galvanized steel.

Cetin and Aksu conducted a study demonstrating that the corrosion rate of steel samples significantly increased when exposed to *Desulfotomaculum* sp. bacteria. Scanning Electron Microscopy (SEM) and Energy Dispersive X-ray Spectroscopy (EDS) analyses revealed that these bacteria caused severe corrosion on the steel surface [14].

Misoni and Ihejirika investigated the microbiologically influenced corrosion of mild steel and aluminum in seawater caused by the sulfate-reducing bacterium *Desulfotomaculum* sp. Their findings revealed that in the presence of SRB, the average corrosion rate of mild steel and aluminum coupons was four times higher compared to those in environments without *Desulfotomaculum* sp. [15].

Anandkumar et al. investigated the presence of the sulfate-reducing bacterium *Desulfobulbus propionicus* in the cooling towers of a petroleum refinery and analyzed its corrosion behavior on steel. Electrochemical and weight loss analyses revealed that *D. propionicus* significantly increased pitting corrosion in cooling towers. Their findings also demonstrated that the presence of this bacterium accelerated the corrosion rate through the production of corrosive H_2S [16].

While SRB are among the most extensively studied microorganisms in MIC, other bacterial groups have also been implicated in metal deterioration.

Aruliah and Ting conducted a study aimed at characterizing the corrosive bacterial communities present in water samples collected from a cooling tower. They identified seven aerobic bacterial species: *Pseudomonas putida*, *Pseudomonas aeruginosa*, *Massilia timonae*, *Massilia albidiflava*, *Pseudomonas mosselii*, *Massilia* sp., and *Pseudomonas* sp. Notably, the *Massilia* genus was detected for the first time in cooling tower water, and it was observed to form a thin bacterial biofilm and cause pitting corrosion on copper metal surfaces [17].

MIC is common in a variety of environments such as soil, freshwater and seawater, and in numerous industries, including petroleum, power generation and marine sectors. Systems with high microbial populations that are not effectively controlled, systems operating in stagnant or low flow conditions, and environments with temperatures that support microbial life are more susceptible to MIC. This susceptibility is often seen in industries such as power plants, refineries, petrochemical plants, steel mills, paper and pulp mills, and marine infrastructure [8, 18].

Given all these problems caused by MIC, it is necessary to develop an effective prevention strategy. Appropriate treatment methods should be selected to prevent biofilm formation or eliminate existing biofilm. Microbial Influenced Corrosion (MIC) is estimated to be responsible for approximately 20% of corrosion-related damage. In the UK, 10% of corrosion incidents are believed to be caused by biocorrosion. In addition, the lifespan of flowlines in Western Australia has been reduced from the intended 20+ years to less than 3 years due to MIC. Microbial corrosion is also considered one of the main causes of corrosion problems in underground pipelines [18].

Various methods are used to reduce biofilm accumulation on engineering surfaces. These methods include adding oxidizing or nonoxidizing biocides to water to eliminate microorganisms from entering the system or slow their growth within the biofilm, mechanically removing biofilms from surfaces using tools such as sponge balls or brushes, and treating water by aeration or deaeration to reduce the number and types of microorganisms [10].

The most common method used in industries to prevent biofilm formation and thus microbial corrosion is the use of biocides that inhibit the growth of microorganisms or kill them.

Biocides used in industrial water treatment are inevitably released into the environment over time. Ideally, a biocide should only target the specific microorganisms for which it is intended. However, all chemicals have different degrees of impact on plant and animal life depending on their concentration. It is generally assumed that dilution and natural degradation will neutralize biocides. Laboratory studies have shown that commercially available biocides are biodegradable. However, these findings do not necessarily mean that such degradation will readily occur in the natural environment [19].

Considering all these factors, the use of environmentally friendly products should be encouraged. Prevention of biofilm formation using plant extracts and coating metal surfaces with metabolites of lactic acid bacteria with biosurfactant properties can be preferred as an alternative to the use of biocides.

3. Biofilms as a health concern

It is estimated that approximately 70% of clinically significant infections are biofilm-associated. Compared to their planktonic forms, bacteria within biofilms exhibit higher resistance to physical and chemical factors, complicating treatment, prolonging hospital stays, increasing healthcare costs, and ultimately categorizing them as an economic and social issue [20].

Current diagnostic methods still primarily focus on isolating bacteria, which can lead to the oversight of infections that develop on a biofilm basis. Bacteria in biofilm form can tolerate antibiotics up to 1000 times more effectively, rendering antibiotic treatment insufficient and increasing the likelihood of resistance development. When infections are identified as biofilm-based, a change in therapeutic direction becomes necessary. The global spread of antibiotic resistance and the insufficiency of antibiotics in combating biofilm-associated infections have laid the groundwork for the development of novel therapeutic approaches and antimicrobial/anti-biofilm agents. The development of materials to prevent biofilm formation for medical device manufacturing is considered a preventive measure. The development of electrochemical biosensors, particularly Electrochemical Impedance Spectroscopy (EIS), has shown promising results. This method is projected to support significant research, especially in detecting biofilms without causing tissue damage, developing anti-biofilm agents, and monitoring treatment progress [21].

The three-dimensional structure of biofilms includes a region deep within the biofilm containing dormant bacteria known as “persister” cells. These cells constitute approximately 1% of the biofilm. In the event of chemical or physical damage to the biofilm, persister cells can restore the biofilm structure once conditions return to normal. Due to their slowed metabolism, these cells are unaffected by antimicrobials [22].

Exopolysaccharides form a matrix structure that retains water, facilitating the transport of nutrients, gene transfer, and the distribution of signaling molecules within the biofilm. Data indicate that *Pseudomonas aeruginosa* polysaccharides are associated with virulence [23]. The extracellular DNA (eDNA) within biofilms was once thought to be a gene pool enabling horizontal gene transfer or merely remnants of dead bacteria. However, it has been shown that eDNA molecules are part of supramolecular structures, such as stable filamentous networks, common to both environmental and pathogenic biofilms. These molecules contribute to escaping immune responses, neutralizing antimicrobials, and serving as an energy source during starvation. However, the mechanisms of eDNA release and regulation within biofilms remain unknown. The discovery of programmed cell lysis within biofilms suggests it may contribute to the biofilm's polymeric structure [24]. The use of DNase has been shown to inhibit biofilms of *P. aeruginosa* and *Staphylococcus aureus* [25], as well as to enhance the penetration of antibiotics into biofilms, making it effective in immature biofilm structures [26].

Lipids within the matrix contribute to biofilm formation by reducing surface tension, allowing biofilms to adhere to challenging surfaces.

The insufficiency of biofilm detection underlying infections, coupled with increasing research data on biofilm structure and function, inspires the development of new methodologies. The development of electrochemical biosensors, particularly EIS, has shown promising results. The identification of biofilm-based infection foci in clinical settings will facilitate accurate diagnosis and treatment decisions.

In biofilm formation, both Gram-negative and Gram-positive bacteria produce "biofilm-associated proteins" (bap) that exhibit structural and functional similarities. Bap, a bacterial surface protein of high molecular weight, plays a role in maintaining cell surface hydrophobicity, a key factor in biofilm formation. It promotes strong intercellular adhesion by forming amyloid structures under environmental conditions [27].

Quorum Sensing (QS) is a chemical communication system through which bacteria within biofilms coordinate gene expression. QS employs signal molecules, known as autoinducers (AIs), which accumulate to a threshold level to facilitate bacterial coordination in response to population density and changes in the host environment. QS enables biofilms to function as multicellular structures. Autoinducers are classified into three main categories: autoinducing peptides (AIPs) found in Gram-positive bacteria, acyl-homoserine lactones (AHLs) present in Gram-negative bacteria, and autoinducer-2 (AI-2), which is common to both types [28].

Divalent cations such as Ca/Mg contribute to the physical stability of the anionic EPS structure, playing significant roles in the maturation phase of biofilms [29].

In 2017, the World Health Organization (WHO) published a list of antibiotic-resistant microorganisms requiring urgent development of new antimicrobial therapies. These bacteria, collectively referred to as ESKAPE, include *Enterococcus faecium*, *Staphylococcus aureus*, *Klebsiella pneumoniae*, *Acinetobacter baumannii*, *Pseudomonas aeruginosa*, and *Enterobacter* spp. The shared characteristic among these bacteria is their ability to develop biofilm-based infections [30].

3.1 Biofilm-associated diseases

Microorganisms can attach to a variety of tissue surfaces in the body, including skin, connective tissues, intestinal mucosa, heart valves, and the oral cavity, where they can form biofilms that persist and spread until an inflammatory response is triggered. These biofilm formations may enter the circulatory system, potentially causing embolism, impacting other organs, and posing severe life-threatening risks to patients.

In the oral cavity, microorganisms adhere to structures such as enamel, dentin, and mucosal epithelial tissues, creating biofilms commonly referred to as dental plaque. In advanced stages, this biofilm can contribute to significant dental issues, including tooth loss [31].

One complication of diabetes mellitus, diabetic foot ulcers (DFUs), occurs in 15–25% of cases. DFUs have been shown to be biofilm-based infections [32]. Studies of diabetic foot microbiota have revealed less diversity and a higher prevalence of opportunistic pathogens compared to healthy individuals [33].

Infective Endocarditis (IE) is a highly fatal biofilm-based infection affecting heart valves, with approximately 25% of patients succumbing to the disease. Implants used in treatment can also cause similar issues, with *S. aureus* being the primary causative agent in nearly all IE cases.

Biofilms forming over the thick mucus layer that acts as a barrier between the intestinal microbiota and tissue have not been associated with any pathogenesis. These biofilms may exhibit commensal behavior, competing for space and nutrients and producing inhibitory metabolites such as acetate or butyrate to limit pathogenic colonization. However, disruption of the mucus layer due to host genetics or dietary factors can lead to bacterial contact with epithelial tissue and the formation of biofilms associated with intestinal dysbiosis, colorectal tumors, and Crohn's disease [34]. *Helicobacter pylori*, a causative agent of peptic ulcers and gastric cancer, has been shown to cover 97% of urease-positive biopsy surfaces in ulcer patients with biofilms, compared to only 1.6% in urease-negative controls [35]. This highlights the potential severity of biofilm-associated pathogenesis.

Cystic fibrosis (CF) is an autosomal recessive genetic disorder resulting from mutations in the gene responsible for encoding the cystic fibrosis transmembrane conductance regulator (CFTR) protein. Dysfunction of CFTR damages epithelial tissues and mucus-covered surfaces, including the lungs, leading to chronic inflammation. CF patients are infected by biofilm-forming pathogens, initially *S. aureus*, followed by *P. aeruginosa*. In CF, biofilm structures display three-dimensional architecture, remaining suspended within lung tissues rather than adhering to surfaces [36]. *P. aeruginosa*'s biofilm strategy involves producing at least three polysaccharides—alginate, Psl, and Pel. These polysaccharides contribute to adhesion, immune evasion, and resistance against antibiotics, demonstrating a close relationship between their ratios and biofilm virulence [23].

Osteomyelitis, involving bone tissue infection, can occur endogenously through hematologic spread or exogenously via implants. While *S. aureus* is commonly implicated in hematologic osteomyelitis, biofilms involving multiple species such as *P. aeruginosa* and *Escherichia coli* can cause chronic osteomyelitis.

3.2 Medical device-associated biofilm infections

Implants such as cochlear devices, dental implants, orthopedic implants (e.g., knee and hip prostheses), heart valves, and vascular stents, particularly in association with surgical interventions, frequently develop biofilm-based infections involving ESKAPE bacteria. Devices used in invasive procedures, such as urinary catheters, central venous catheters, and intrauterine devices, provide a liquid-solid interface conducive to bacterial colonization and biofilm formation. These complications can endanger patients' lives, often necessitating implant removal [37].

3.3 Treatment strategies for biofilm-associated infections

Treatment of biofilm-associated infections has become more effective with the elucidation of biofilm structure and physiology. However, traditional treatment methods are increasingly insufficient, necessitating the urgent development of new antimicrobial agents and anti-biofilm materials.

The biofilm's matrix structure, composed of common components such as polysaccharides, lipids, proteins, and eDNA, forms the primary framework during biofilm's lifecycle, from initial microbial colonization to maturation and virulence expression. Therapeutics targeting the matrix structure can enhance antibiotic efficacy, activate immune responses, and eliminate multispecies biofilms. Mechanical disruption of the matrix structure, as in dental cleaning or wound debridement, can increase treatment effectiveness.

Antimicrobial peptides (AMPs) have gained attention as alternatives to traditional antibiotics. AMPs are synthesized by various organisms, ranging from plants to animals, with molecular weights between 1 and 5 kDa. Their nonspecific mechanisms, targeting multiple sites, reduce the likelihood of resistance development. However, to enhance their effectiveness and resistance to proteases, modifications or synthetic production methods are employed [38].

Methods targeting the QS mechanism, known as quorum quenching (QQ), aim to disrupt biofilm formation and disassemble existing biofilms by inhibiting signal production, degrading signal molecules, or blocking receptors. Compounds like farnesol and triclosan inhibit QS signal molecule production, while enzymes such

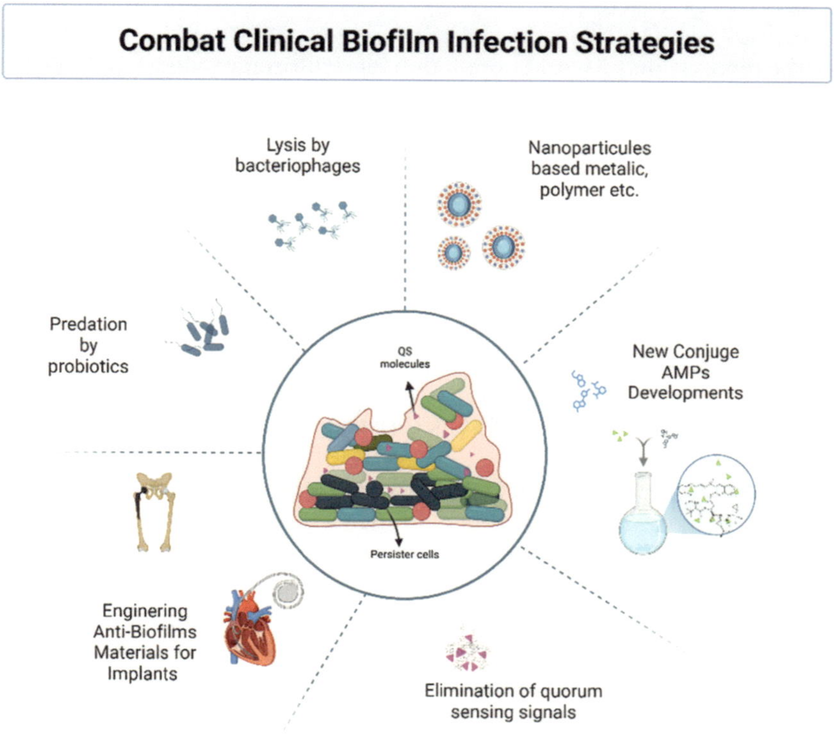

Figure 3.
Innovative strategies need to be developed to combat biofilm in the clinic.

as AHL lactonases degrade signal molecules. Receptor blockers such as furanones and naringenin prevent QS signaling. While promising, challenges such as selectivity, resistance development, and unintended virulence increases necessitate further research (**Figure 3**) [39].

Nanoparticles, with dimensions of 1–100 nm, offer innovative and effective solutions for both antimicrobial and anti-biofilm targets. Nanoparticles can penetrate biofilm matrixes, disrupt extracellular polymeric substances, and neutralize persister cells with reactive oxygen species. They also block efflux pumps, increase bacterial membrane permeability, and interfere with quorum sensing. Despite their advantages, concerns regarding biocompatibility and toxicity, especially at high concentrations, remain. Strategies such as surface modification and green synthesis are being developed to address these issues [30].

Enhancing the anti-biofilm properties of medical implants is a preferred preventive measure. Surface coating techniques, drug delivery systems, antibacterial substances, and nanotechnology-based approaches aim to prevent biofilm formation, reduce microbial adhesion, and decrease antibiotic dependency. Challenges such as improving the mechanical durability and biocompatibility of coatings must still be overcome [27].

Probiotics such as Lactobacillus species and natural compounds like plant extracts have been shown to inhibit biofilms. Phage therapy, due to its specificity and non-toxicity, is another potential approach for combating biofilms. However, challenges such as dosage determination, evaluation of combination therapies, toxicity, and insufficient *in vivo* studies necessitate further development.

4. Biofilms in agriculture

With the increase in the world population, agricultural production needs to increase by approximately 50% by 2050 in order to meet the food demand [40]. However, the intensification of production to achieve this goal leads to excessive use of chemical fertilizers [41]. Farmers intensively use chemical fertilizers and pesticides to increase productivity and meet food demand. The overuse of these chemicals threatens sustainable agriculture by causing environmental degradation, changes in soil pH, and excess fertilizer leaching into groundwater and damaging aquatic ecosystems [42].

A healthy soil is essential for plant growth. Functions of soil microorganisms such as nutrient cycling, organic matter decomposition, plant nutrition and disease resistance contribute to soil health. Soil microorganisms interact both with each other and with plants to improve soil structure and increase plant resistance to harsh environmental conditions [43].

Plant Growth Promoting Bacteria (PGPB) are a group of beneficial bacteria commonly found in the root environment of plants that promote plant growth and the absorption and utilization of mineral nutrients. Playing an important role in soil health and agricultural sustainability, PGPBs include well-characterized species such as *Pseudomonas fluorescens*, *Bacillus subtilis*, *Azospirillum brasilense*, *Rhizobium leguminosarum*, *Streptomyces lydicus*, and *Burkholderia phytofirmans* [44, 45]. These microorganisms establish either symbiotic relationships with plant roots or thrive as free-living organisms in the rhizosphere.

The mechanisms of action of PGPBs and the molecular mechanism of the symbiotic relationship they form with plants and the development of methods of their use in agricultural fields have become of increasing research interest in recent years.

One of the most desirable characteristics of PGPBs is their ability to effectively colonize plant roots and leaf surfaces. This colonization is possible only if the bacteria form a biofilm structure. In nature, bacteria develop biofilm organizations rather than planktonic forms. A biofilm is a form of colonization in which different species often have synergistic relationships. Biofilms refer to communities of microorganisms organized in extracellular polymeric substance (EPS) that they produce by attaching to a living or nonliving surface. Although the structure of EPS varies according to abiotic conditions and the diversity of microorganisms gathered, it generally contains exopolysaccharides, protein, lipid, and eDNA (**Figure 4**) [46].

It has been shown that QS molecules of PGPB bacteria are active in regulating gene expression of activities such as nitrogen fixation, ACC deaminase activity, and phytohormone synthesis [47]. Furthermore, among these QS molecules, AHLs significantly enhance plant defense responses, thereby increasing resistance against pathogens. These molecules activate the Mitogen-Activated Protein Kinase (MAPK) signaling cascade (particularly MPK3/MPK6), triggering various defense mechanisms, including callose deposition, stomatal closure, and phytoalexin production [48]. Notably, specific AHLs such as 3-oxo-C8-HSL coordinate both salicylic acid (SA) and jasmonic acid/ethylene (JA/ET) pathways, reducing *Pseudomonas syringae* proliferation by up to 70% [49]. These findings demonstrate the potential of AHL-based biostimulants as sustainable alternatives to chemical pesticides in agricultural applications.

Induced Systemic Resistance (ISR) is a natural resistance mechanism of plants against pathogens. Compounds such as lipopolysaccharide, siderophore, and volatile

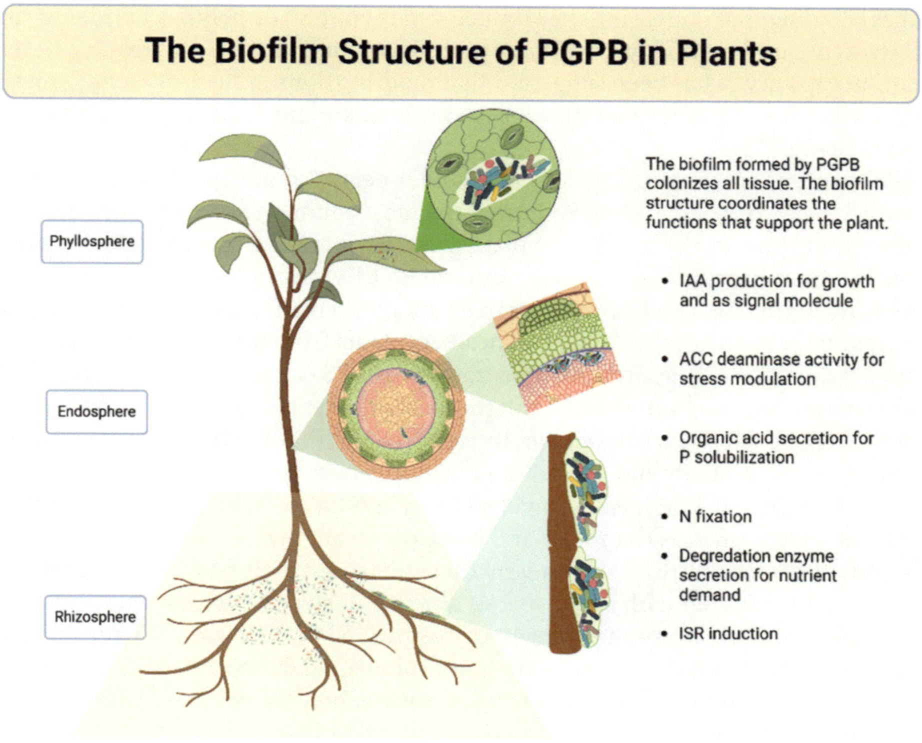

Figure 4.
Biofilm formation of Plant Growth Promoting Bacteria (PGPB) is located in the endosphere, phyllosphere, and rhizosphere.

organic compound (VOC) that enable the plant to generate an ISR response by PGPBs have been characterized. PGPBs regulate the signaling pathways that enable the synthesis of these compounds within the biofilm more strongly compared to mutants with inhibited biofilm formation [50, 51].

The skeleton of the biofilm structure is formed by exopolysaccharides with high water retention capacity. Exopolysaccharides function in biotic and abiotic stress management of PGPB bacteria. Global Climate Change (GCC) is exposing crops to more abiotic stresses and risks from extreme weather events.

As a result of the GCC, surface waters are decreasing with increasing temperatures and excessive evaporation. While this situation causes drought, it leads to increased precipitation and floods in areas where vapors are concentrated. The decrease in surface water and the change in the world water distribution result in drought, which is the abiotic stress that affects agricultural areas the most. Strategies to manage drought include the development of drought-tolerant crops as well as the use of PGPB bacteria that show stress-reducing activities. Drought in the microenvironment of PGPB bacteria causes changes in the composition of the exopolysaccharides they produce. *Azospirillum brasilense* Sp245, a rhizospheric bacterium, with the modification of producing carbohydrate complexes with high molecular weight (lipopolysaccharide-protein and polysaccharide-lipid complexes), forms a biofilm layer with high water retention capacity, increasing the water content of the rhizosphere and thus allowing the plant metabolism to adapt to drought [52].

The soil aggregation formed by the biofilm structures of PGPBs in the rhizospheric area facilitates the uptake of water and minerals from the roots and forms a barrier to prevent the plant from being affected by the lack of water in the bulk soil. There are studies showing that increasing the D-glucuronate content of polysaccharides in the EPS structure under drought conditions promotes plant growth by increasing water retention capacity. It has been suggested that modifications in the functional groups of bacterial exopolysaccharides may trigger antioxidant mechanisms that manage stress in plants [53].

Globally, 20% of irrigated agricultural land is degraded due to salinity, and this is projected to reach 50% by 2050. Sodium is the most common and most harmful agent in soil salinization. In the biofilms of plant growth promoting bacteria (PGPB) present in the rhizospheric zone, exopolysaccharides (EPS) play a critical role by binding cations, including Na^+, and preventing their uptake by plant roots. This mechanism helps maintain the K^+/Na^+ balance and protects plants from the adverse effects of salinity. Numerous studies have demonstrated that EPS can render Na^+ inaccessible to plant roots through sodium chelation in the soil [54]. For instance, EPS produced by *Pseudomonas* sp. AK-1 has been shown to bind free Na^+ in soil, effectively reducing its uptake by soybean plants and promoting normal growth even under saline conditions of up to 200 mM NaCl [55]. Additionally, plants in saline soils increase the exudation of specific sugars, such as rhamnose and trehalose, from their roots, which attract salt-tolerant bacteria to the root zone, further enhancing their resilience to salinity.

Soil is contaminated with heavy metals due to industrial activities, excessive use of pesticides, and nitrogen-phosphorus-potassium (NPK) fertilizers. Heavy metals, which are a permanent threat due to their non-biodegradability, can have toxic effects even in trace amounts on living organisms in nature. Biofilm structure adsorbs heavy metals and acts as a barrier, preventing their bioavailability to plants [56]. Heavy metals can be immobilized and detoxified by biofilms through mechanisms such as biosorption, reduction, oxidation, and precipitation. With these mechanisms, metals can be transformed into less harmful forms, as well as removing metals from soil and water. In addition, it has been shown that bacteria that improve the growth of plants used in phytoremediation have high biofilm formation abilities [57].

The ability of plant pathogens to form biofilms is seen as part of their virulence. Biofilm-forming pathogens are able to neutralize immune responses and antimicrobials synthesized by the plant. The extremely slow metabolism of persister cells within the biofilm makes it almost impossible for biofilms to be completely eradicated in the face of changing conditions such as UV radiation, drought, and insufficient nutrient availability. The advanced survival strategies of biofilm-forming phytopathogens make them more detrimental to crop yield and quality [58].

Rosmarinic acid, one of the plant defense compounds, is effective against planktonic pathogens [59]. The biofilm structure of pathogens makes them resistant to this compound. *Pseudomonas syringae* pv. *Syringae* is the causal agent of brown spot disease on leaves, and biofilms have been shown to play an important role in its virulence [60]. *Xanthomonas campestris* pv. *Campestris* causes black rot disease of cruciferous crops by colonizing the xylem. Biofilm colonization of these bacteria is mediated by virulence factors such as degrading enzymes and xanthan gum, an exopolysaccharide [61]. *Clavibacter michiganensis* subsp. *Sepedonicus* causes bacterial ring rot by forming biofilm on potato plants through exopolysaccharides [62].

5. Conclusion

Biofilms are complex microbial communities with significant impacts in industrial, clinical, and agricultural fields. Their formation processes, driven by microbial interactions and the production of extracellular polymeric substances (EPS), enable microorganisms to acquire resistance to environmental stresses but also pose significant challenges. In industrial systems, biofilms are the primary cause of microbial-induced corrosion (MIC), leading to material degradation and economic losses. The mechanisms of MIC, such as the production of corrosive metabolites, inactivation of inhibitors, and the formation of localized electrochemical cells, highlight the need for effective control strategies. In clinical settings, biofilm-based infections show increasing resistance to antibiotics and immune responses, complicating treatment and increasing healthcare costs. The development of innovative diagnostics, such as biosensors, could enable the identification of biofilm structures without compromising tissue integrity. Nanoparticles that target the biofilm structure and eliminate infections, the development of antimicrobial agents, and effective treatment methods to be conjugated with conventional therapies are being studied. Phage therapies also target the biofilm structure. It is important for medical device developers to develop materials with anti-biofilm properties. The biofilm formation of PGPBs is crucial to improve plant growth and make plants more resistant to biotic and abiotic stresses. However, they increase the virulence of phytopathogens, making biofilms an agricultural problem.

Effective biofilm management requires a multidisciplinary approach that combines environmental sustainability with technological innovation. Environmentally friendly solutions such as plant-derived biocides, biosurfactants, and advanced coatings hold promise as alternatives to conventional chemical treatments. Future research should prioritize the development of cost-effective, environmentally friendly, and scalable strategies to address the diverse challenges presented by biofilms, increase the lifespan and efficiency of industrial systems, improve clinical outcomes, and support sustainable agricultural practices.

Author details

Atiye Karadoğan, Fatma Azgin, Esra Sündüz Yiğittekin and Sadik Dinçer*
Biology Department, Faculty of Art and Science, Çukurova University, Adana, Turkey

*Address all correspondence to: sdincer@cu.edu.tr

References

[1] Martino D, Patrick. Extracellular polymeric substances, a key element in understanding biofilm phenotype. AIMS Microbiology. 2018;**4**(2):274. DOI: 10.3934/microbiol.2018.2.274

[2] Donlan RM. Biofilms: Microbial life on surfaces. Emerging Infectious Diseases. 2002;**8**(9):881. DOI: 10.3201/eid0809.020063

[3] Arampatzi SI, Giannoglou G, Diza E. Biofilm formation: A complicated microbiological process. Aristotle University Medical Journal. 2011;**38**(2):21-29

[4] Chapman J. Microstructures of biofilm. In: Biofilm and Materials Science. Cham: Springer International Publishing; 2015. pp. 35-43. DOI: 10.1007/978-3-319-14565-5_5

[5] Flemming H-C, Wingender J. The biofilm matrix. Nature Reviews Microbiology. 2010;**8**(9):623-633. DOI: 10.1038/nrmicro2415

[6] Uhlig HH, Revie RW. Corrosion and Corrosion Control. 3rd ed. New York: Wiley; 1985. DOI: 10.1002/9780470277270

[7] Zarasvand KA, Rai VR. Microorganisms: Induction and inhibition of corrosion in metals. International Biodeterioration & Biodegradation. 2014;**87**:66-74. DOI: 10.1016/j.ibiod.2013.10.023

[8] Little BJ et al. Microbially influenced corrosion—Any progress? Corrosion Science. 2020;**170**:108641. DOI: 10.1016/j.corsci.2020.108641

[9] Liu T et al. Investigations on reducing microbiologically-influenced corrosion of aluminum by using super-hydrophobic surfaces. Electrochimica Acta. 2010;**55**(18):5281-5285. DOI: 10.1016/j.electacta.2010.04.082

[10] Little BJ, Lee JS. Microbiologically influenced corrosion. In: Kirk-Othmer Encyclopedia of Chemical Technology. Hoboken: Wiley; 2009. DOI: 10.1002/0471238961.micrlitt.a01

[11] Iverson WP. Microbial corrosion of metals. Advances in Applied Microbiology. 1987;**32**:1-36. DOI: 10.1016/S0065-2164(08)70077-7

[12] Von Wolzogen Kühr CAH, Van Der Vlugt LS. Aerobic and anaerobic iron corrosion in water mains. Journal of American Water Works Association. 1953;**45**(1):33-46. Available from: https://www.jstor.org/stable/41253241

[13] Ilhan-Sungur E, Cansever N, Cotuk A. Microbial corrosion of galvanized steel by a freshwater strain of sulphate reducing bacteria (*Desulfovibrio* sp.). Corrosion Science. 2007;**49**(3):1097-1109

[14] Cetin D, Aksu ML. Corrosion behavior of low-alloy steel in the presence of *Desulfotomaculum* sp. Corrosion Science. 2009;**51**(8):1584-1588. DOI: 10.1016/j.corsci.2009.04.001

[15] Misoni PJ, Ihejirika CE. Effects of *Desulfotomaculum* sp on corrosion behaviour of mild steel and aluminium in sea water. Zastita Materijala. 2023;**64**(2):190-197. DOI: 10.5937/zasmat2302190I

[16] Anandkumar B et al. Corrosion behavior of SRB *Desulfobulbus propionicus* isolated from an Indian petroleum refinery on mild steel.

Materials and Corrosion. 2012;**63**(4):355-362. DOI: 10.1002/maco.201005883

[17] Aruliah R, Ting Y-P. Characterization of corrosive bacterial consortia isolated from water in a cooling tower. International Scholarly Research Notices. 2014;**2014**(1):803219. DOI: 10.1155/2014/803219

[18] Javaherdashti R. Microbiologically influenced corrosion (MIC). In: Javaherdashti R, editor. Microbiologically Influenced Corrosion. Engineering Materials and Processes. Cham: Springer; 2017. pp. 61-102. DOI: 10.1007/978-3-319-44306-5_4

[19] Cloete TE. Biofouling control in industrial water systems: What we know and what we need to know. Materials and Corrosion. 2003;**54**(7):520-526. DOI: 10.1002/maco.200390115

[20] Ben-Amram H, Azrad M, Cohen-Assodi J, Sharabi-Nov A, Edelstein S, Agay-Shay K, et al. Biofilm formation by hospital-acquired resistant bacteria isolated from respiratory samples. Journal of Epidemiology and Global Health. 2024;**14**(2):291-297. DOI: 10.1007/s44197-024-00215-7

[21] Ameer S, Ibrahim H, Yaseen MU, Kulsoom F, Cinti S, Sher M. Electrochemical impedance spectroscopy-based sensing of biofilms: A comprehensive review. Biosensors-Basel. 2023;**13**(8):777. DOI: 10.3390/bios13080777

[22] Wood TK, Knabel SJ, Kwan BW. Bacterial persister cell formation and dormancy. Applied and Environmental Microbiology. 2013;**79**(23):7116-7121. DOI: 10.1128/AEM.02636-13

[23] Jennings LK, Dreifus JE, Reichhardt C, Storek KM, Secor PR, Wozniak DJ, et al. Pseudomonas aeruginosa aggregates in cystic fibrosis sputum produce exopolysaccharides that likely impede current therapies. Cell Reports. 2021;**36**(3):108782. DOI: 10.1016/j.celrep.2021.108782

[24] Turnbull L, Toyofuku M, Hynen AL, Kurosawa M, Pessi G, Petty NK, et al. Explosive cell lysis as a mechanism for the biogenesis of bacterial membrane vesicles and biofilms. Nature Communications. 2016;**7**:11220. DOI: 10.1038/ncomms11220

[25] Sharma K, Singh AP. Antibiofilm effect of DNase against single and mixed species biofilm. Food. 2018;**7**(3):42. DOI: 10.3390/foods7030042

[26] Das T, Simone M, Ibugo AI, Witting PK, Manefield M, Manos J. Glutathione enhances antibiotic efficiency and effectiveness of DNase I in disrupting *Pseudomonas aeruginosa* biofilms while also inhibiting pyocyanin activity, thus facilitating restoration of cell enzymatic activity, confluence and viability. Frontiers in Microbiology. 2017;**8**:2429. DOI: 10.3389/fmicb.2017.02429

[27] Negut I, Albu C, Bita B. Advances in antimicrobial coatings for preventing infections of head-related implantable medical devices. Coatings. 2024;**14**(3):256. DOI: 10.3390/coatings14030256

[28] Papenfort K, Bassler BL. Quorum sensing signal–response systems in Gram-negative bacteria. Nature Reviews. Microbiology. 2016;**14**(9):576-588. DOI: 10.1038/nrmicro.2016.89

[29] Wu RX, Zhang Y, Guo ZQ, Zhao B, Guo JS. Role of Ca2+ and Mg2+ in changing biofilm structure and enhancing biofilm formation of *P. stutzeri* strain XL-2. Colloids and Surfaces. B, Biointerfaces. 2022;**220**:112972. DOI: 10.1016/j.colsurfb.2022.112972

[30] Sarkar S, Roy A, Mitra R, Kundu S, Banerjee P, Acharya Chowdhury A, et al. Escaping the ESKAPE pathogens: A review on antibiofilm potential of nanoparticles. Microbial Pathogenesis. 2024;**194**:106842. DOI: 10.1016/j.micpath.2024.106842

[31] Mirzaei R, Mohammadzadeh R, Alikhani MY, Shokri Moghadam M, Karampoor S, Kazemi S, et al. The biofilm-associated bacterial infections unrelated to indwelling devices. IUBMB Life. 2020;**72**(7):1271-1285. DOI: 10.1002/iub.2266

[32] Malik A, Mohammad Z, Ahmad J. The diabetic foot infections: Biofilms and antimicrobial resistance. Diabetes and Metabolic Syndrome: Clinical Research and Reviews. 2013;**7**:101-107. DOI: 10.1016/j.dsx.2013.02.006

[33] Gontcharova V, Youn E, Sun Y, Wolcott RD, Dowd SE. A comparison of bacterial composition in diabetic ulcers and contralateral intact skin. The Open Microbiology Journal. 2010;**4**:8-19. DOI: 10.2174/1874285801004010008

[34] Jandl B, Dighe S, Baumgartner M, Makristathis A, Gasche C, Muttenthaler M. Gastrointestinal biofilms: Endoscopic detection, disease relevance, and therapeutic strategies. Gastroenterology. 2024;**167**(6):1098-1112.e5. DOI: 10.1016/j.gastro.2024.07.023

[35] Coticchia JM, Sugawa C, Tran VR, et al. Presence and density of Helicobacter pylori biofilms in human gastric mucosa in patients with peptic ulcer disease. Journal of Gastrointestinal Surgery. 2006;**10**(6):883-889. DOI: 10.1016/j.gassur.2006.01.003

[36] Cheng T, Torres NS, Chen P, Srinivasan A, Cardona S, Lee GC, et al. A facile high-throughput model of surface-independent Staphyl-ococcus aureus biofilms by spontaneous aggregation. mSphere. 2021;**6**(3):e00186-21. DOI: 10.1128/mSphere.00186-21

[37] Bouhrour N, Nibbering PH, Bendali F. Medical device-associated biofilm infections and multidrug-resistant pathogens. Pathogens. 2024;**13**(5):393. DOI: 10.3390/pathogens13050393

[38] Di Somma A, Moretta A, Canè C, Cirillo A, Duilio A. Antimicrobial and antibiofilm peptides. Biomolecules. 2020;**10**(4):652. DOI: 10.3390/biom10040652

[39] Krzyżek P. Challenges and limitations of anti-quorum sensing therapies. Frontiers in Microbiology. 2019;**10**:2473. DOI: 10.3389/fmicb.2019.02473

[40] Alexandratos N, Bruinsma J. World Agriculture towards 2030/2050: The 2012 Revision. Rome: Food and Agriculture Organization of the United Nations (FAO); 2012. ESA Working Paper No. 12-03. DOI: 10.22004/ag.econ.288998

[41] Canfield DE, Glazer AN, Falkowski PG. Theevolution andfuture of Earth's nitrogen cycle. Science. 2010;**330**:192-196. DOI: 10.1126/science.1186120

[42] Angus AA, Hirsch AM. Biofilm formation in the rhizosphere: Multispecies interactions and implications for plant growth. Molecular Microbial Ecology of the Rhizosphere. 2013;**2**:701-712. DOI: 10.1002/9781118297674.ch66

[43] Chen Q, Song Y, An Y, Lu Y, Zhong G. Soil microorganisms: Their role in enhancing crop nutrition and health. Diversity. 2024;**16**(12):734

[44] Glick BR. Plant growth-promoting bacteria: Mechanisms and applications.

Scientifica. 2012; Article ID 963401. DOI: 10.6064/2012/963401

[45] Sahu PK, Singh DP, Prabha R, Meena KK, Abhilash PC. Connecting microbial capabilities with the soil and plant health: Options for agricultural sustainability. Ecological Indicators. 2019;**105**:601-612. DOI: 10.1016/j.ecolind.2018.05.084

[46] Rafique M, Naveed M, Mumtaz MZ, et al. Unlocking the potential of biofilm-forming plant growth-promoting rhizobacteria for growth and yield enhancement in wheat (*Triticum aestivum* L.). Scientific Reports. 2024;**14**:15546. DOI: 10.1038/s41598-024-66562-4

[47] Jung BK, Ibal JC, Pham HQ, Kim MC, Park GS, Hong SJ, et al. Quorum sensing system affects the plant growth promotion traits of *Serratia fonticola* GS2. Frontiers in Microbiology. 2020;**11**:536865. DOI: 10.3389/fmicb.2020.536865

[48] Lazarus HPS, Easwaran N. Molecular insights into PGPR fluorescent Pseudomonads complex mediated intercellular and interkingdom signal transduction mechanisms in promoting plant's immunity. Research in Microbiology. 2024;**175**:104218. DOI: 10.1016/j.resmic.2024.104218

[49] Shrestha A, Grimm M, Ojiro I, Krumwiede J, Schikora A. Impact of quorum sensing molecules on plant growth and immune system. Frontiers in Microbiology. 2020;**11**:1545. DOI: 10.3389/fmicb.2020.01545

[50] Salwan R, Sharma M, Sharma A, Sharma V. Insights into plant beneficial microorganism-triggered induced systemic resistance. Plant Stress. 2023;**7**:100140. DOI: 10.1016/j.stress.2023.100140

[51] Zhu L, Huang J, Lu X, Zhou C. Development of plant systemic resistance by beneficial rhizobacteria: Recognition, initiation, elicitation, and regulation. Frontiers in Plant Science. 2022;**13**:952397. DOI: 10.3389/fpls.2022.952397. Correction in: Front Plant Sci. 2023; 13:1118073

[52] Fedonenko YP, Zdorovenko EL, Konnova SA, et al. A comparison of the lipopolysaccharides and O-specific polysaccharides of *Azospirillum brasilense* Sp245 and its Omegon-Km mutants KM018 and KM252. Microbiology. 2004;**73**:143-149. DOI: 10.1023/B:MICI.0000023980.08347.ee

[53] Ajijah N, Fiodor A, Pandey AK, Rana A, Pranaw K. Plant growth-promoting bacteria (PGPB) with biofilm-forming ability: A multifaceted agent for sustainable agriculture. Diversity. 2023;**15**(1):112. DOI: 10.3390/d15010112

[54] Li Y, Narayanan M, Shi X, Chen X, Li Z, Ma Y. Biofilms formation in plant growth-promoting bacteria for alleviating agro-environmental stress. Science of The Total Environment. 2024;**907**:167774. DOI: 10.1016/j.scitotenv.2023.167774

[55] Kasotia A, Varma A, Choudhary DK. Pseudomonas-mediated mitigation of salt stress and growth promotion in *Glycine max*. Agricultural Research. 2015;**4**:31-41. DOI: 10.1007/s40003-014-0139-1

[56] Xing Y, Tan S, Liu S, Xu S, Wan W, Huang Q, et al. Effective immobilization of heavy metals via reactive barrier by rhizosphere bacteria and their biofilms. Environmental Research. 2022;**207**:112080. DOI: 10.1016/j.envres.2021.112080

[57] Roy B, Maitra D, Sarkar S, Podder R, Das T, Ghosh J, Mitra AK. Biofilm and

metallothioneins: A dual approach to bioremediate the heavy metal menace. Environmental Quality Management. 2024;**33**(4):659-676. DOI: 10.1002/tqem.22139

[58] Carezzano ME, Paletti Rovey MF, Cappellari LR, Gallarato LA, Bogino P, Oliva MM, et al. Biofilm-forming ability of phytopathogenic bacteria: A review of its involvement in plant stress. Plants. 2023;**12**(11):2207. DOI: 10.3390/plants12112207

[59] Walker TS, Bais HP, Déziel E, Schweizer HP, Rahme LG, Fall R, et al. *Pseudomonas aeruginosa*-plant root interactions. Pathogenicity, biofilm formation, and root exudation. Plant Physiology. 2004;**134**:320-331

[60] Monier J-M, Lindow SE. Frequency, size, and localization of bacterial aggregates on bean leaf surfaces. Applied and Environmental Microbiology. 2004;**70**:346-355. DOI: 10.1128/AEM.70.1.346-355.2004

[61] Dow JM, Crossman L, Findlay K, He Y-Q, Feng J-X, Tang J-L. Biofilm dispersal in Xanthomonas campestris is controlled by cell-cell signaling and is required for full virulence to plants. Proceedings. National Academy of Sciences. United States of America. 2003;**100**:10995-11000

[62] Marques L, De Boer S, Ceri H, Olson M. Evaluation of biofilms formed by *Clavibacter michiganensis* subsp sepedonicus. Phytopathology. 2003;**93**:S57

Chapter 11

Harnessing Biofilms: From Pathogenicity to Industrial Applications

Nimra Irfan and Mirza Imran Shehzad

Abstract

Complex microbial colonies called biofilms significantly impact businesses, healthcare, and natural environments. These problems include nosocomial infections in medical equipment, microbial-induced corrosions, and industrial inefficiencies due to their remarkable resistance to medicines and disinfectants. Biofilm production causes significant losses for industries, including food processing, electricity generation, and oil and gas. Biofilms, however, also have enormous promise for bioremediation, wastewater treatment, and bioleaching, offering environmentally acceptable answers to environmental problems. The management and use of biofilms are being revolutionized by new tactics such as enzymatic interventions, quorum sensing disruption, bacteriophages, and nanoparticles. This chapter examines the dual nature of biofilms, highlighting creative ways to reduce their hazards while maximizing their advantages for long-term environmental and industrial progress.

Keywords: biofilms, quorum sensing, industries, environment, food pathogenicity, corrosion, bioremediation

1. Introduction

Biofilm thus refers to structured microbial cells that are highly resistant to antibiotics and other environmental stresses and are 1000-fold more resistant than planktonic bacteria. Present in the natural environment, biofilms such as those of *Yersinia pestis* can promote pathogen spread. Their structure allows for slow growth and increased competitiveness, as they are attached to surfaces by a solid matrix of polysaccharides, proteins, and nucleic acids (**Figure 1**) [1, 2].

Biofilms, with their ability to enable bacteria to rapidly attach to surfaces such as plastic, glass, or metal, create fully developed structures in a few hours to days. These structures, while assisting microbes in enduring harsh conditions, also compromise food quality, raise energy consumption, and affect equipment reliability. More alarmingly, they can cause diseases, highlighting the potential threat of biofilms [3]. There are known and unknown advantages and disadvantages of biofilms in human life. The harmless bacteria include *Staphylococcus epidermidis.* The actions of harmless bacteria subdue and augment the effects of dangerous bacteria. Nevertheless, there is a correlation between biofilms and severe infections, for example, in cystic fibrosis (CF), when the bacterium

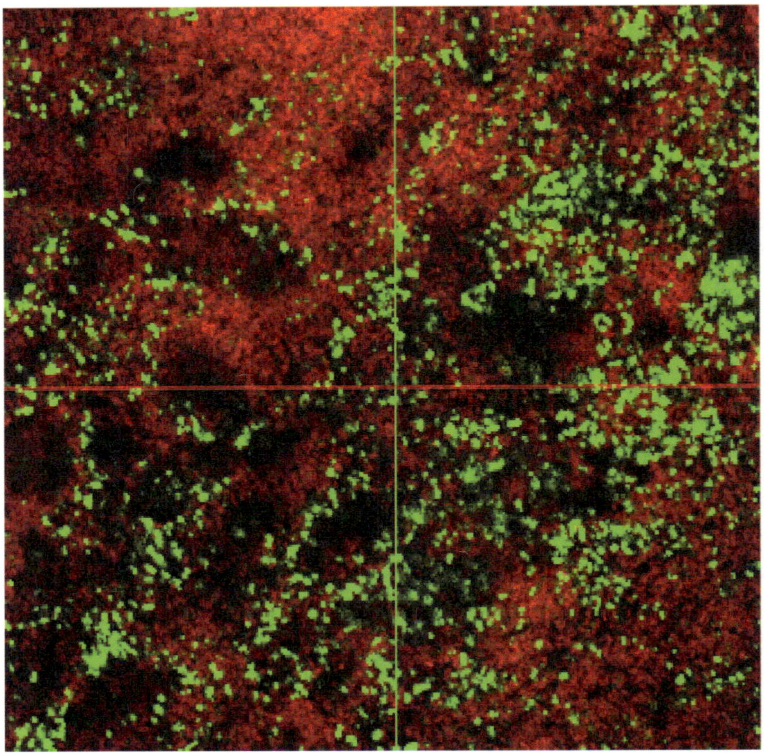

Figure 1.
Polymicrobial biofilm formed by P. aeruginosa *(red) and* S. epidermidis *(green).*

Pseudomonas aeruginosa forms a mucoid biofilm in a chronic phase that is virtually invulnerable to antibiotics and causes recurrent inflammation of the lung tissue (**Figure 2**) [4].

1.1 Biofilm formation

Bacteria form three-dimensional biofilms through a four-phase process. The four significant patterns identified include cohesiveness, clustering, growth, and dispersion. First, the planktonic cells can attach to the surface of host tissues through extracellular matrix molecules such as surface protein and eDNA. The major adhesins are CMSRAMMs, Srf, SdrC, SdrD, SdrE, Fib, ClfA, ClfB, and FnBPs. When nutrients are available, bacteria, once attached, grow. During the aggregation phase, they also alter their response to environmental stimuli to increase biofilm thickness plus the protective layers hitherto produced to fight drugs and the human immune system. If one extrapolates this hypothesis, this increased thickness may result in cell release from graft surfaces [5, 6].

During biofilm maturation, bacteria form colonies that collect detritus and planktonic bacteria, creating a complex structure. extracellular polymeric substances (EPS) facilitate adhesion between cells and surfaces. Quorum sensing (QS) is vital for this process, allowing bacteria to communicate based on density, and it can occur both within and between species. Different bacteria employ varying QS systems; gram-positive bacteria use peptides, while gram-negative bacteria use acylated homo-serine lactones for signaling (**Figure 3**).

The text discusses aspects of bacterial communication systems, mainly how they regulate gene expression by producing and detecting autoinducers. It also describes

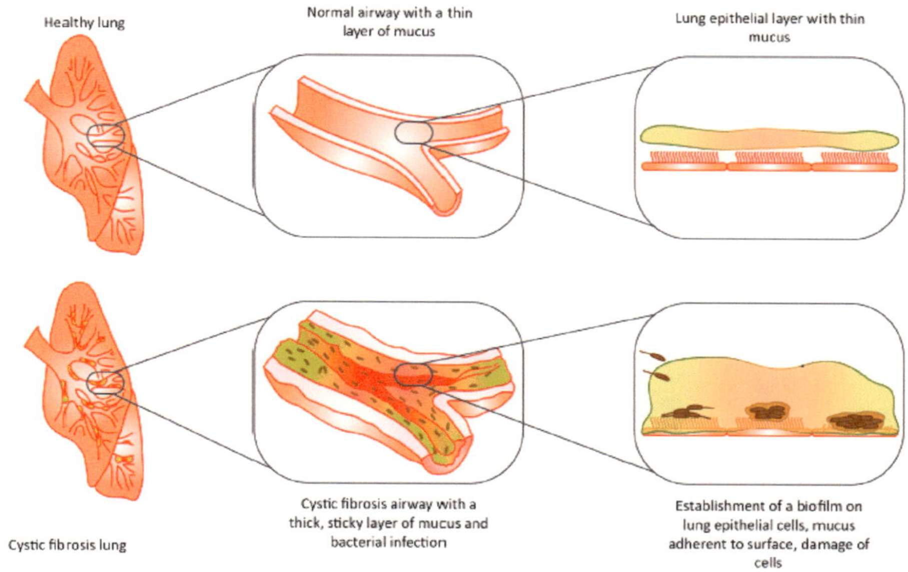

Figure 2.
Role of biofilm in cystic fibrosis.

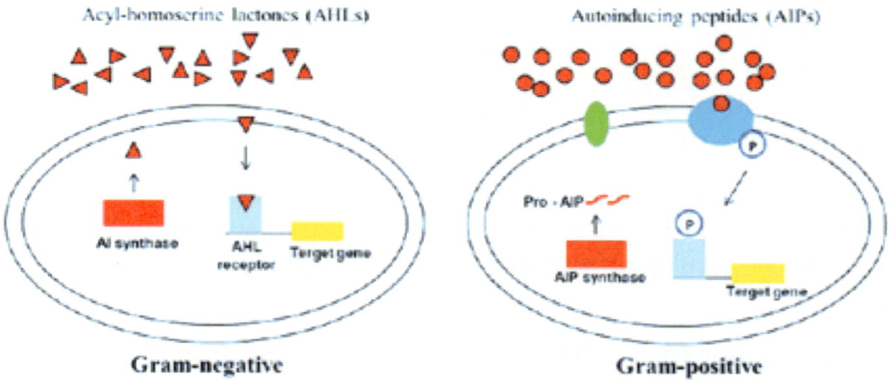

Figure 3.
Quorum sensing systems in bacteria.

the structure of a mature biofilm, which consists of three layers: a basal layer, an interfacial layer, and a surface biofilm where free-growing bacteria can thrive and expand [7].

Biofilms can accumulate toxic substances and spread infections as microbial cells move from an implant surface to seek nutrients. Bacterial dispersion occurs in three steps: individual cells detach from the microcolony, locate a new surface to attach to and start forming a new biofilm. There are two types of dispersion: adherent and non-adherent. Adherent dispersion results from both passive and active mechanisms, including antimicrobial pressure and nutrient scarcity, which increase the detachment force of bacteria from the implant surface (**Figure 4**) [8].

Multi-bacterial species exhibit synthetic values that increase their susceptibility to biofilms in natural environments. Various bacteria can trigger biofilm production

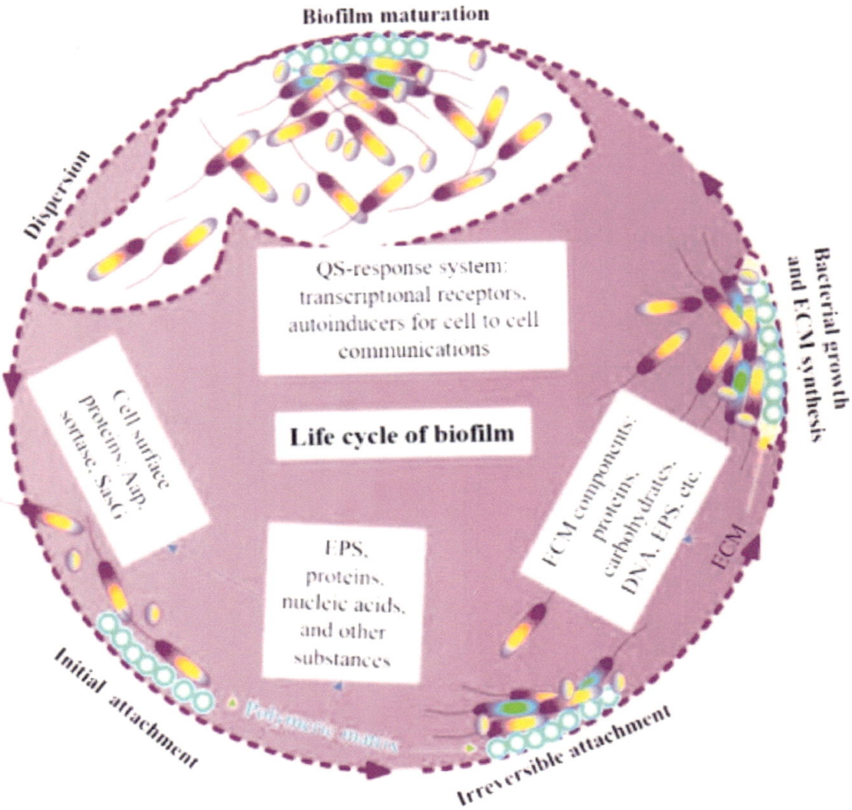

Figure 4.
Life cycle of microbial biofilm.

in specific species, resulting in biofilms that are less diverse and more resistant to multiple biocides than those formed by a single species [9].

2. Biofilms in industry: Impacts, control, and future directions

Microbial biofilms are a significant factor in effluence and human health problems and result in the loss of billions of dollars to the US industry through microbiologically influenced corrosion (MIC). Examples of sectors most impacted are power, textile, chemical, and construction. In textile products, microbial activity results in the development of smell, stain, and fabric deterioration, particularly when the product is exposed to heat and humidity. The construction industry has substantial pecuniary losses from microbial attacks on concrete, particularly the influence of bacterial species such as *Thiobacillus sp.* and *Fusarium sp.,* which erode the concrete structure's strength (**Figure 5**) [10].

The mixture for concrete used Lucky Cement with natural sand (4 mm maximum size) and micro silica amounting to 5% of cement by mass while maintaining a water/binder ratio at 0.80 for high permeability. We prepared test samples with control and fiber-enhanced concrete compositions and added 0.8 kg/m^3 GSF 0520 steel fibers. After curing for 30 days in sterile Milli-Q water, 72 prisms were categorized into four groups based on surface roughness and fiber inclusion. We tested cement samples

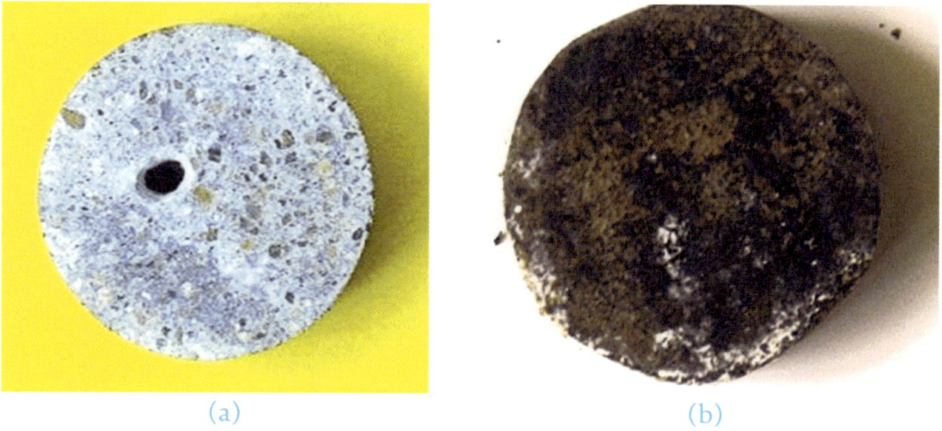

Figure 5.
Fusarium sp. *fungal growth in a year (a) without exposure to a humidity chamber (b) with exposure to a humidity chamber.*

with these four conditions against a smooth fiber-free surface and a rough fiber-free surface [11].

There were four treatments in the experiment, with and without steel fibers and with and without surface roughening treatment (**Table 1**). A thin, slightly viscous layer of biofilm developed on all the concrete surfaces that were tested (**Figure 6**). In all the samples containing steel fibers, there was a formation of yellow deposits. In

Parameter	System A	System B	System C	System D	Seawater
Fiber reinforcement	No fibers	Steel fibers	No fibers	Steel fibers	—
Surface texture type	Smooth	Smooth	Rough	Rough	—
Water pH	8.30 ± 0.09	8.35 ± 0.08	8.34 ± 0.08	8.37 ± 0.08	8.20 ± 0.10
Electrical conductivity	53.05 ± 1.60	52.90 ± 1.30	53.50 ± 1.25	53.80 ± 1.55	50.20 ± 1.10
Bicarbonate alkalinity	128 ± 13	132 ± 5	126 ± 6	138 ± 8	101 ± 16
Dissolved organic carbon	4.10 ± 2.15	5.10 ± 3.15	4.70 ± 2.75	4.20 ± 2.90	2.50 ± 1.20
Total nitrogen content	0.070 ± 0.060	0.095 ± 0.085	0.090 ± 0.080	0.065 ± 0.050	0.065 ± 0.065
Calcium ion concentration	505 ± 98|	515 ± 150	475 ± 110	460 ± 120	455 ± 170
Silica concentration	2.370 ± 1.320|	2.190 ± 1.080	2.230 ± 1.260	2.140 ± 1.200	1.920 ± 1.030
Iron content	0.210 ± 0.020	0.215 ± 0.015	0.200 ± 0.025	0.215 ± 0.030	0.220 ± 0.025

Table 1.
Chemical composition of water in systems and seawater.

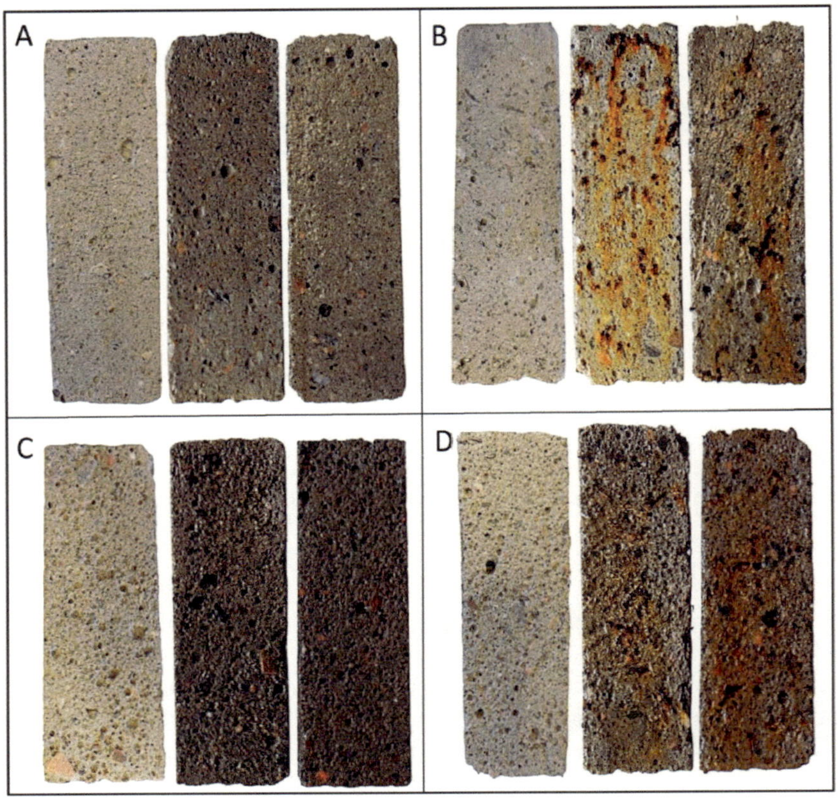

Figure 6.
Blocks of concrete from (A): System 1 (B): System 2 (C): System 3 (D): System 4. Samples are taken from Day 1 to Day 30 of each system's three blocks.

terms of the biofilm formation patterns, there was found to be no significant disparity between the smooth as well as rough surfaces of the concrete structures.

Biofilms in industrial food processing lines can lead to food spoilage and foodborne diseases, as they often harbor pathogens responsible for most bacterial infections in the US. Bacillus cereus is a notable organism that forms resilient biofilms on food-contact surfaces like tanks and conveyor belts. These biofilms produce substances such as surfactants and enzymes that can alter the sensory qualities of food [3].

Biofilm formation is more prevalent on hydrophobic surfaces than hydrophilic ones. Inconsistent cleaning can leave biofilm residues trapped in areas like crevices. Additionally, organisms in free water can harm established biofilms, as extracellular polymeric substances (EPS) help protect biofilms from stressors like sanitizers and disinfectants more effectively than free-floating cells [12].

Microorganisms that form biofilms often colonize surfaces and equipment in the food industry. The extracellular matrix, composed of DNA, proteins, and polysaccharides, facilitates adhesion to various surfaces and enhances biofilm stability by promoting nutrient and oxygen diffusion. It also aids in cell communication and protects cells from harmful substances. In dual- or multiple-species biofilm models, foodborne pathogenic bacteria can interact with resident flora in food processing environments [13].

To speed up microbial growth, the surfaces used to handle food were infected with *Bacillus cereus*, *Escherichia coli*, *Staphylococcus aureus*, and *Pseudomonas* species. Scientists tested for biofilm production with crystal violet tests and specialized media. The research group tested both cooked and raw goods for changes in how they felt. In addition, they checked how well sanitizers fight bacteria that live in clusters [14–16]. **Table 2** shows how bacterial biofilm forms and affects food spoilage, as explained in detail.

Microbiologically influenced corrosion (MIC) is a major concern for the oil and gas industries. MIC affects pipelines, pumps, and de-aeration towers, mainly through bacterial infection from return water injected into oil reservoirs. Some events associated with MIC are pipeline leakage in New Mexico, methane leakage in California, and oil spillage in Alaska. To carbon steel, risks arise from sulfate-reducing bacteria (SRB), especially *Desulfovibrio desulfuricans*, as they increase corrosion rates at the metal/solution interface [17, 18].

The work was done to analyze the approaches of *Desulfovibrio desulfuricans* to affect the Microbiologically Influenced Corrosion (MIC) in the anaerobic environment of the B7 medium. Carbon steel coupons were exposed to B7 medium and exposed to the bacterium *Desulfovibrio desulfuricans* under anaerobic conditions [19]. When *Desulfovibrio desulfuricans* grows, then sulfate decreases and is reduced to sulfide, which reacts with iron to give iron sulfide. During the sampling period of forty-eight days, the samples were subjected to examination of the deposited iron sulfide on the metal surface and its re-dissolution due to the growth of the size of the sulfide crystals and nutrient limitations. Corrosion was observed based on biofilm formation, the amount of iron sulfide, and the extent of corrosion at the metal surface (**Figure 7**, **Table 3**) [24].

Constructed wetlands (CWs) are efficient, low-cost solutions with a 20–50-year lifespan, particularly beneficial in developing countries. However, they can become clogged by biofilms, plant roots, or inorganic particles, with biofilms being the main issue. This clogging can negatively affect industrial applications, increasing prevention and treatment costs. For instance, unintended biofilm growth near wellbores can decrease injectivity and cause formation damage, significantly reducing oil recovery efficiency [25, 26].

Bacterial biofilms developed on medical devices like contact lenses and urinary catheters make healthcare-associated infections more likely. These infections emerge from tough pathogens such as *Pseudomonas aeruginosa* and methicillin-resistant *Staphylococcus aureus*. Health officials across all nations consider these infections major global healthcare problems. Biofilm growth triggers over 80% of microbial diseases in humans, which cause problems like bone infections and damage to implanted medical equipment. CAUTIs from biofilm growth represent the major medical device-related infection problem and affect more than 150 million people globally [27–29].

A flexible multichannel endoscope is a reusable medical instrument that may be exposed to the possibility of developing biofilm when processes are not strictly followed. Once a device is inserted into the body, bacteria can colonize and form biofilms in the wet, nutritional environment of the endoscope's lumen. Bacterial colonization is initiated by placing the EPDM material onto this protein layer. In large numbers, some bacteria can spread into the bloodstream, causing severe infections [30].

Bioremediation is an effective method for removing environmental pollutants, with biofilm-based technology showing particular promise. Unlike traditional pelagic microbes, biofilm-forming bacteria like *Rhodococcus, Alcanivorex, Cycloclasticus, Bacillus,* and *Arthrobacter* are capable of adapting to extreme conditions, making them efficient in degrading hazardous substances in various contaminated environments [31, 32].

Invader	Characteristics	Food contamination	Adverse spoilage repercussions	Results	Ref.
Bacillus cereus	Anaerobic, facultative anaerobic, spore-forming, and gram-positive	Meat, veggies, rice, and dairy goods	Symptoms of vomiting and diarrhea	Utilization of biofilm results in insensitivity to sanitizers; hence, despite cleaning, there may be recurrent contamination and spoilage of foods.	[13, 14]
Escherichia coli	The rod-shaped, gram-negative	Fresh meat, fruits, veggies, and raw milk	Outbreaks of diarrhea and hemolytic uremic syndrome	Despite forming a biofilm, *E. coli* shows increased tolerance to environmental stress factors, including antimicrobial agents, which extend the effective shelf life on food-contact surfaces.	[15]
Staphylococcus aureus	Facultative anaerobic, gram-positive, non-motile, and non-spore-forming	Products made from meat, poultry, eggs, dairy, salads, baked goods, (particularly cakes and pastries with cream filling, and sandwich fillings)	Methicillin resistance may result in diarrhea and vomiting	The *S. aureus* found in a biofilm also has enhanced virulence and might lead to different symptoms than the regular *S. aureus* thus, effects may last longer.	[16, 17]
Pseudomonas spp.	Rod-shaped, psycotrophic, motile and gram- negative	Meat surfaces, fruits, vegetables, and low-acid dairy products	Gives fresh cheese a blue discoloration	Psychrotrophic *Pseudomonas spp.* on dairy products can cause rapid spoilage and discoloration when the bacteria form biofilms on the products, even when stored at low temperatures.	[18]

Table 2.
Pathogenic bacteria that cause the spoilage of food.

DOI: http://dx.doi.org/10.5772/intechopen.1009283

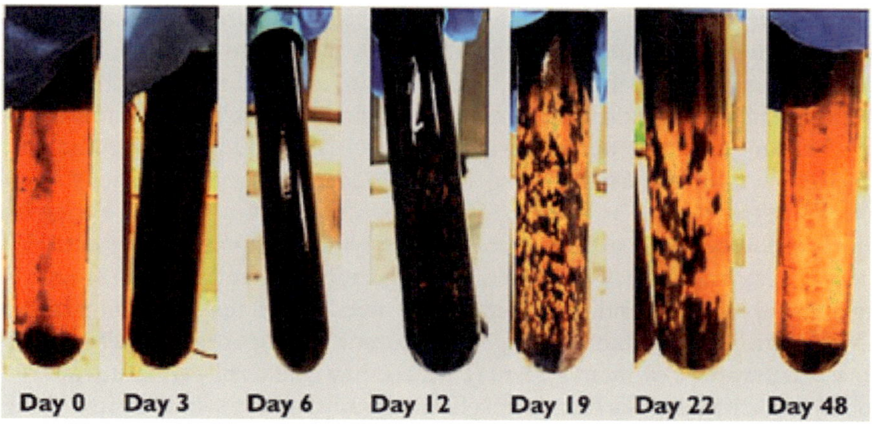

Figure 7.
The growth of Desulfovibrio desulfuricans *in the B7 medium demonstrates the early formation of iron sulfide on the glass wall, followed by the eventual dissolution of this coating as a result of the enlargement of crystal size and nutrient constraints.*

Day	Formation of iron sulfide	Corrosion patterns	Development of biofilms	Ref.
0	Iron sulfide's early development is seen on the metal surface	No apparent corrosion; early growth of biofilms	*Desulfovibrio desulfuricans'* initial infestation on a metal surface	[20, 21]
3	Deposition of iron sulfide on metal has increased	Increased iron sulfide deposition and mild metal surface corrosion	Sulfide production and active biofilm growth	[22, 23]
6	An increase in iron sulfide crystal formation	Early indications of metal surface corrosion; iron sulfide formation persists	As the biofilm develops, its surface area increases	[21, 23]
12	Iron sulfide development on the metal surface is significant	Signs of corrosion worsen, and more iron sulfide is formed	Dense biofilm development was noted	[20, 23]
19	Larger crystals of iron sulfide are developing and coating the metal surface	Increased corrosion activity and some iron sulfide dissolution were noted	A well-developed biofilm with significant amounts of corrosion	[20, 22]
22	On metal surfaces, iron sulfide still forms	Iron sulfide crystals that are seen to corrode and dissolve	Maximum thickness of biofilm	[21, 23]
48	Deposits of black iron sulfide sink to the bottom	Iron sulfide has dissolved, but corrosion has slowed	Biofilm drastically decreased as a result of nutrient loss	[20, 22]

Table 3.
Iron sulfide production and corrosion patterns in B7 medium infected with Desulfovibrio desulfuricans *throughout a 48-day period.*

Microbial communities, commonly known as biofilms, can be used in phytoremediation; these include the removal of heavy metals, petroleum products, herbicides, and insecticides from soil and water. Biofilm formation for bioremediation technique is substituted in several industries to remove contaminated soil and groundwater. Though biofilms can cause numerous health concerns in food processing and hospitals, they are helpful in waste recycling and water management. Advanced bioremediation technologies such as bio-filters, rotary disk contacts, and granular sludge reactors are widely embraced eco-friendly strategies for revitalizing polluted contexts [33].

Bacteria help break down heavy metals lead, cadmium, and copper through their ability to make cell walls and bind metals with metalloproteins. Still, fungi transform metals into harmless substances using hydroxamate siderophores. Bacterial biofilms improve wastewater treatment systems because they shield cells while encouraging microbial growth and make it easier to eliminate contaminants in activated sludge and attached growth systems [34–36]. The natural process of biofilm attachment and enzyme activity helps break antibiotic medications in biofilm-based systems. These systems are also highly effective at degrading lignin, with a specific bacterial consortium showing great potential in cleaning up effluents from agro-processing and pulp mills, removing harmful organic and inorganic pollutants like lignin [37, 38].

Microplastics (MPs) result from the breakdown of large plastic waste exposed to weather and UV light. They harm marine ecosystems by negatively affecting the organs of fish and shrimp, triggering immune responses, and generating reactive oxygen species. Additionally, when microbes colonize MPs, it increases their ability to absorb environmental pollutants, including harmful chemicals and heavy metals [39]. The effectiveness of microplastics biofilm degradation depends upon the type, quality, and amount of biofilm under consideration (**Figure 8**). Temperature, pH, ultraviolet radiation, nutrient availability, and microplastics' characteristics influence biofilm formation. Furthermore, biofilms influence the characteristics of the polymer, such as the material's biodegradation rate (**Figure 9**) [41].

The problem of multidrug resistance in bacteria becomes critical; according to the CDC, around 2.8 million bacterial antibiotic-resistant infections occur in the United States annually, and one in 10 of these patients die. Resistance to antibiotics makes management of standard forms of infections a real issue, let alone the threat of deadly bloodstream infections. The World Health Organization has said that if nothing is done, more than 10 million deaths from bacteria resistant to antibiotics will occur in the next three decades. Since biofilms are dense, there is a significant problem of inaccessibility when administering treatment to affected infections (**Figure 10**). Furthermore, the experts added that antimicrobial drugs are metabolized in the human body to make treatment difficult, and recurrent infections become common [42–45].

Biofouling in piped systems and ship hulls incurs over $250 million annually due to issues like biofilm formation. Traditional mitigation methods, such as repainting and hull cleaning, are not financially sustainable (**Figure 11**). Biofouling negatively impacts marine ecosystems by reducing water flow and increasing disease risk in fish. It also hampers the efficiency of cooling systems in coastal power plants and affects water treatment processes like reverse osmosis by increasing membrane resistance. Environmental and hydrodynamic factors influence the extent of macro fouling, which can further reduce heat transfer and system performance [46].

Biofilms that form on metals increase corrosion of steel and iron products, resulting in substantial financial losses. Researchers have now found two new ways for microorganisms to take electrons from metals and use them for their processes, including sulfate and nitrate reduction. The bacterial type *Desulfovibrio vulgaris*

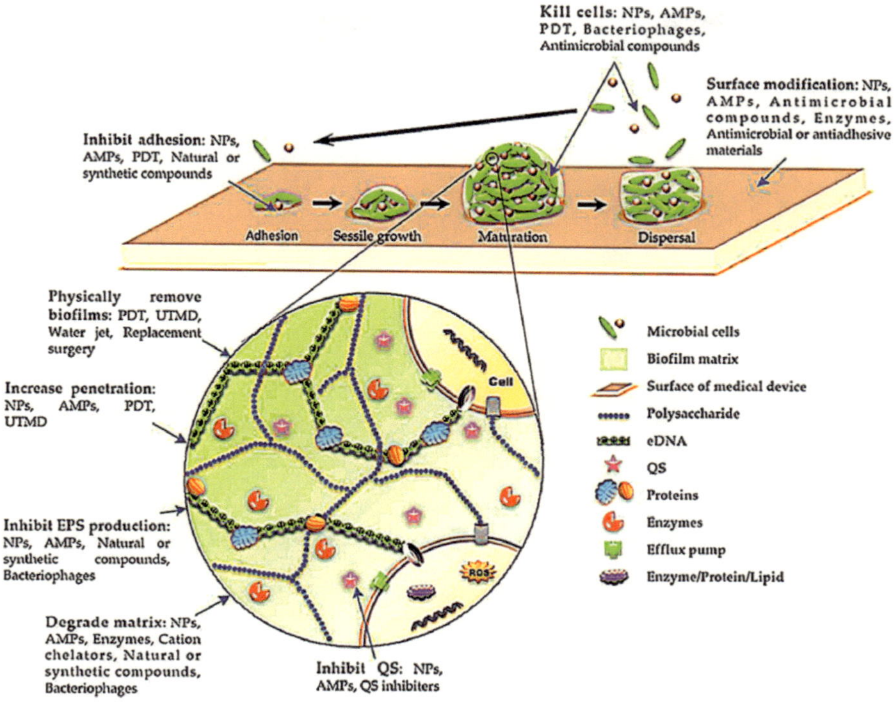

Figure 8.
Phases of biofilm development on the medical equipment's surfaces; Reprinted from MDPI, Basel, Switzerland (copyright © 2021) by the authors and licensee [40].

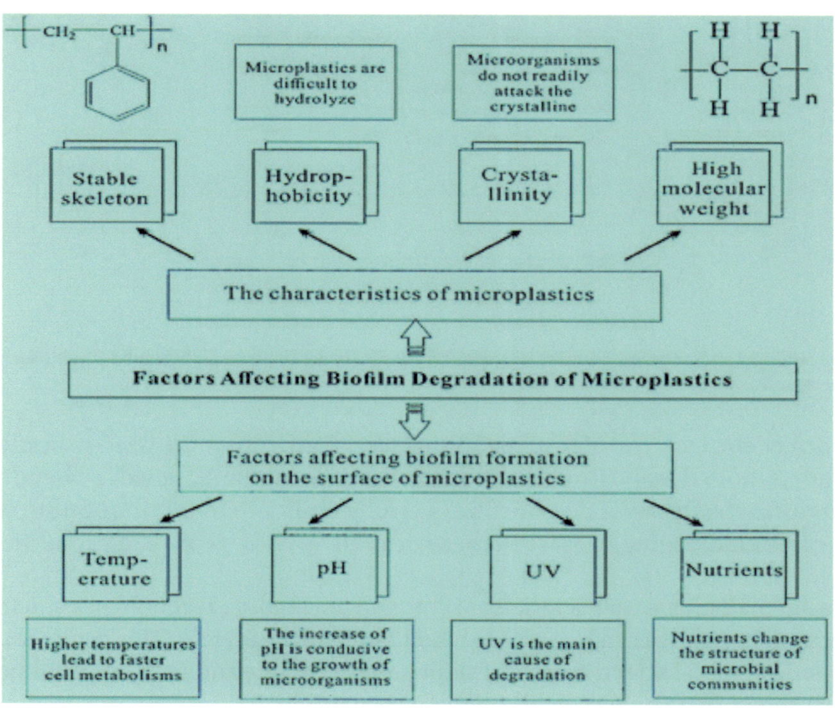

Figure 9.
Factors affecting biofilm degradation of microplastics.

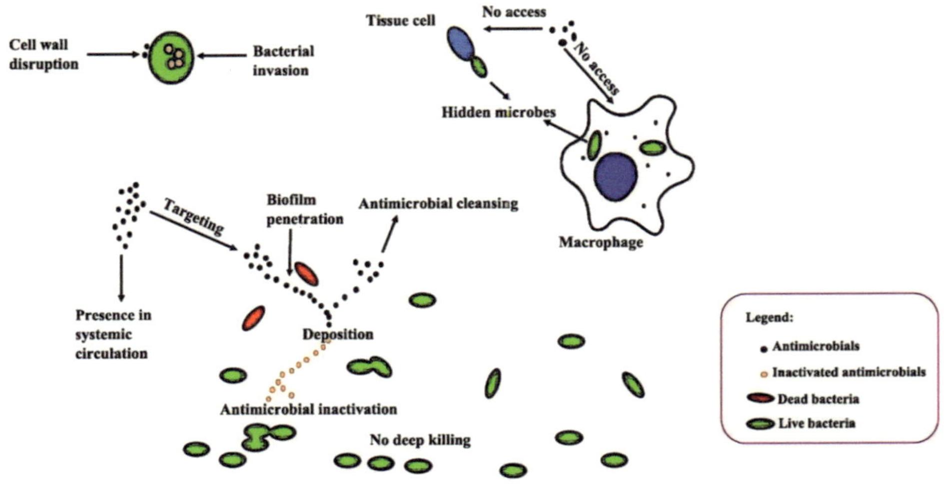

Figure 10.
A summary of the traditional problems that have arisen in the antimicrobial control of pathogenic biofilms.

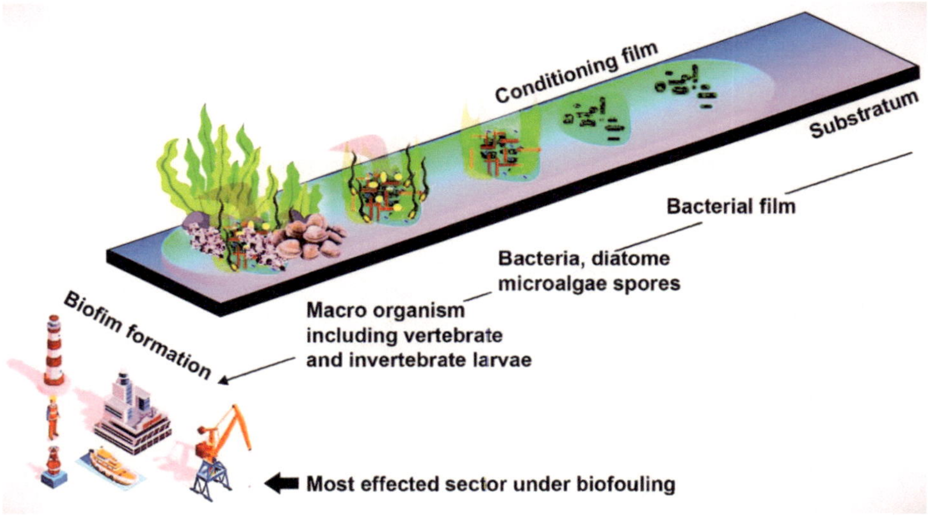

Figure 11.
Biofouling incidents in the marine industry may result from significant stages in biofilm production (Source: Freepik.com; retrieved October 27, 2022).

shows direct electron transfer to metal surfaces, confirming the need to study this process more deeply. Producer-born *Salmonella* and milk powder-friendly *Anoxybacillus flavithermus* demonstrate a strong ability to build films on surfaces that become challenging to erase because of their specific processing conditions [47, 48].

Coating materials with bactericidal films and antifouling technologies enhance antimicrobial properties in biomaterials and biomedical devices. This combination boosts antimicrobial effectiveness through both releasable and non-releasable agents. Research shows that employing lipids and nanoparticles for antibacterial coatings significantly reduces implant-related infections and improves the functionality of biomedical devices (**Figure 12**) [28].

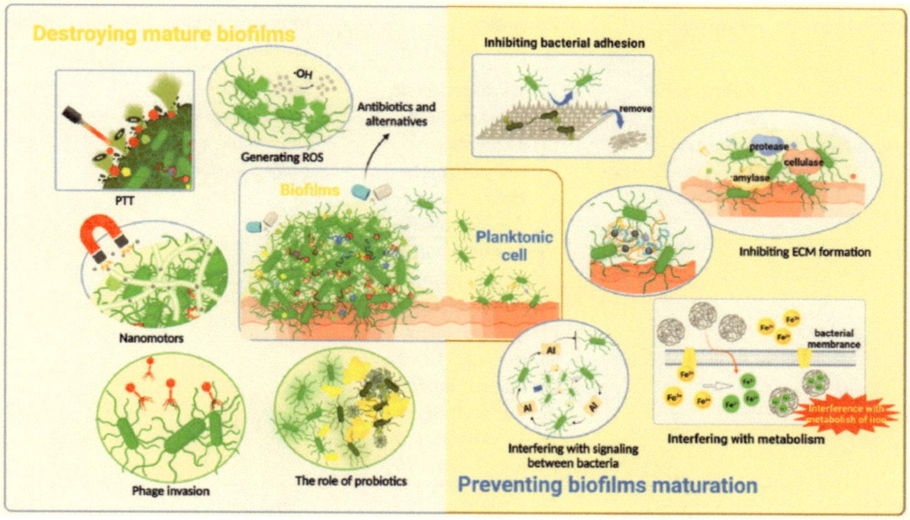

Figure 12.
Controlling the growth of biofilms and removing them using different techniques. Reprinted from Elsevier Ltd. (Amsterdam, The Netherlands) by the authors and licensee under copyright © 2023.

Microorganisms form protective biofilms that block disinfectants from reaching them, which causes food to spoil more often and raises disease danger levels. Successful biofilm control methods impact cell surfaces, manage internal chemistry, and work through physical action. Despite limited sterilization possibilities, regular disinfection with quaternary ammonium compounds, fat-harming peroxides, and chlorine chemicals remains indispensable for preserving food safety (**Table 4**) [55].

Special second-generation anti-biofilm agents like small molecules, DNAse, and proteinase K plus small molecules reduce resistance from bacterial biofilms by dismantling the biofilm protective structure. Biofilms quickly degrade through benzimidazole and N-acetylcysteine treatment, but microbe growth stops when exposed to organophosphates and polyaminocarboxylic acids. Research into nanoparticles helps doctors make more stable and effective treatments with improved medical delivery methods (**Figure 13**) [56].

Nanomaterials inhibit biofilms through several molecular mechanisms, including 1: Breaking down peptidoglycans in gram-negative and gram-positive bacteria, 2: Disrupting cell membrane integrity, 3: Targeting the electron transport chain (ETC), 4: Causing microbial DNA damage, 5: Inactivating microbial enzymes, 6: Disassembling ribosomes, 7: Denaturing intracellular proteins, 8: Inhibiting extracellular DNA, and 9: Suppressing extracellular polymeric substances (EPS) (**Figure 14**) [45].

Because of their huge surface area, metal nanoparticles ranging from 10 to 100 nanometers help create sensors and medical tools in addition to blocking bacterial film growth. When used in small amounts, metals such as gold, silver, iron, zinc, and copper show excellent anti-biofilm activity by crossing bacterial cell walls and destroying the polysaccharide glue layer while blocking essential signaling proteins. They create reactive oxygen species (ROS), which makes oxidative stress break down both the protective layers and genetic material in a film structure [57, 58].

Application of 100 μL of 1.3% nutrient broth, 100 μL of NPs solution, and 20 μL of bacterial cultures to the 96-well microtiter plate, and it was then incubated at 37°C for 24 hours. Samples were washed with phosphate-buffered saline and stained with

Disinfecting agents	Features	Purpose	Microorganism types in action	Citation
QACs, (quaternary ammonium)	Hydrophobic activity, membrane-active agents, and surface-active agents	Causes dispersion in the liquid to aid in the elimination of microorganisms by lowering surface tension and forming micelles. Interact with both the yeast's plasma membrane and the bacterial cytoplasmic membrane. Efficient against viruses that include lipids. Interact with targets inside cells and hind to DNA.	*Bacillus cereus, Pseudomonas spp., Staphylococcus spp.,* and *Listeria monocytogenes.*	[49, 50]
Peroxide of hydrogen (H_2O_2)	High capacity for oxidation	Free radical production has an impact on the biofilm matrix.	*Vibrio spp., Pseudomonas aeruginosa,* and *Staphylococcus aureus*	[50–52]
PAA, (per-acetic acid)	Potent oxidizers	Capable of damaging DNA bases, disrupting membranes, or oxidizing thiol groups in proteins.	*Pseudomonas aeruginosa, Staphylococcus aureus,* and *Listeria monocytogenes.*	[50, 53]
NaClO, (sodium-hypochlorite)	Potent oxidizing agents	Get rid of cells because they can oxidize the sulfhydryl groups of several enzymes involved in the glycolytic cascade and penetrate cell membranes. Able to react with a variety of biological substances, including lipids, proteins, peptides, amino acids, and DNA, at physiological pH levels.	*Fusobacterium nucleatum, Staphylococcus aureus, Prevotella intermedia, Streptococcus intermedius, Pseudomonas, Pepto-streptococcus miros, Listeria monocytogenes,* and *Enterococcus faecalis*	[49, 54]

Table 4.
Lists representative compounds for the most often used disinfectants in food sector sanitary disinfection programs.

crystal violet, fixed, and then demineralized with glacial acetic acid. Od 630 nm was obtained on an ELISA reader, alongside the positive control—ampicillin and the negative control—nutrient broth [59, 60].

Using an anti-biofilm assay, it was revealed that ZnO nanoparticles with *n*-Hex and EtOAc were found highly effective against biofilm formation in all the tested bacteria; in particular, *n*-Hex-ZnO NPs significantly inhibited *Bacillus subtilis,* and EtOAc-ZnO NPs inhibited *Staphylococcus aureus*. DCM-ZnO NPs possessed a moderate level of inhibition, followed by the MetOH-ZnO NPs. Based on these results, ZnO NPs with specific solvents of *n*-Hex and EtOAc intermediate solvents appear to be suitable candidates for biofilm-targeting uses (**Table 5**).

The FAO and World Health Organization (WHO) define probiotics as beneficial live bacteria consumed in sufficient amounts. The most common types are

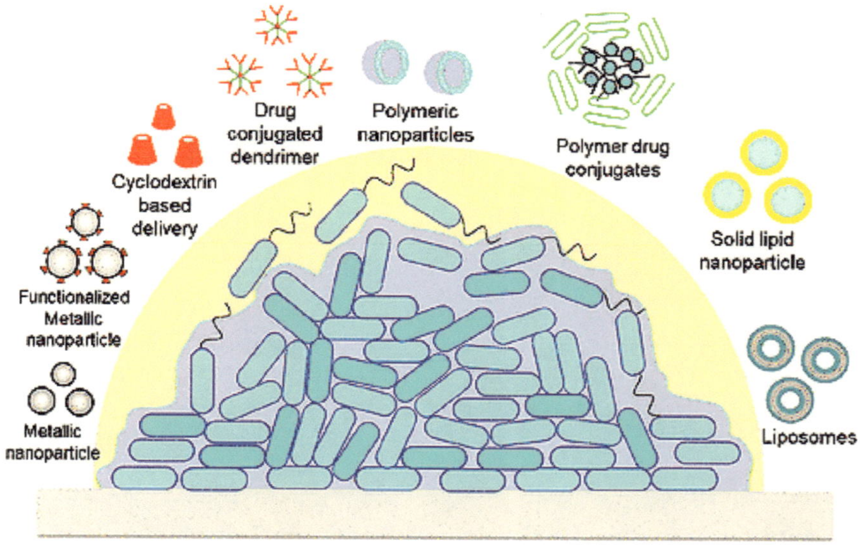

Figure 13.
Sophisticated nanotechnological methods for managing microbial biofilms.

Lactobacillus and *Bifidobacterium,* found in supplements and fermented foods like dairy. Probiotic regulation varies by region, with the European Food Safety Authority (EFSA) implementing the Qualified Presumption of Safety (QPS) process for evaluating the safety of microorganisms, including probiotics [61, 62]. Regulation of probiotic foods and their nutrition and health claims are governed by EU Regulation (EC) No. 1924/2006 and the FDA's GRAS system in the United States of America, which induces interest in their use as preservatives, active packaging to replace chemical preservatives, and biofilm controllers in food processing (**Figure 15**). Using particular bacteria and their antimicrobial compounds helps extend and reduce the spoilage of products. Further, the integration of probiotics with non-thermal technologies to eliminate undesirable microorganisms in the finished foods significantly enhances food safety [63].

Bacterial biofilms can be effectively treated with micro-needles (MNs) that penetrate the biofilm's EPS barrier for direct delivery of antibacterial agents. Research by Yi et al. (2021) demonstrated that chitosan-zinc (CS-Zn [II]) micro-needles effectively eliminated *S. aureus* and *E. coli* biofilms, thanks to their high surface area, acicular design, and favorable cytocompatibility [64].

Chemical techniques for eliminating bacterial biofilms are often ineffective, unstable in warm climates, and costly, with hazardous byproducts. In contrast, newer biological methods like bacteriophage, bacteriocin, enzyme therapy, and novel antimicrobial peptides (AMPs) show greater efficacy in preventing and removing biofilms. AMPs, as cationic agents, can inhibit biofilm formation by targeting genes, preventing bacterial adhesion, and disrupting communication signals among bacteria. They can be used alone or with antibiotics to treat biofilm-related infections effectively [65].

Catabolite control protein A (CcpA) is essential for regulating carbon catabolite repression in bacteria, particularly in *Staphylococcus aureus.* It influences the expression of genes related to virulence, antibiotic resistance, and biofilm formation. Inhibitors of CcpA, such as silver, can impair its DNA-binding capability, leading to

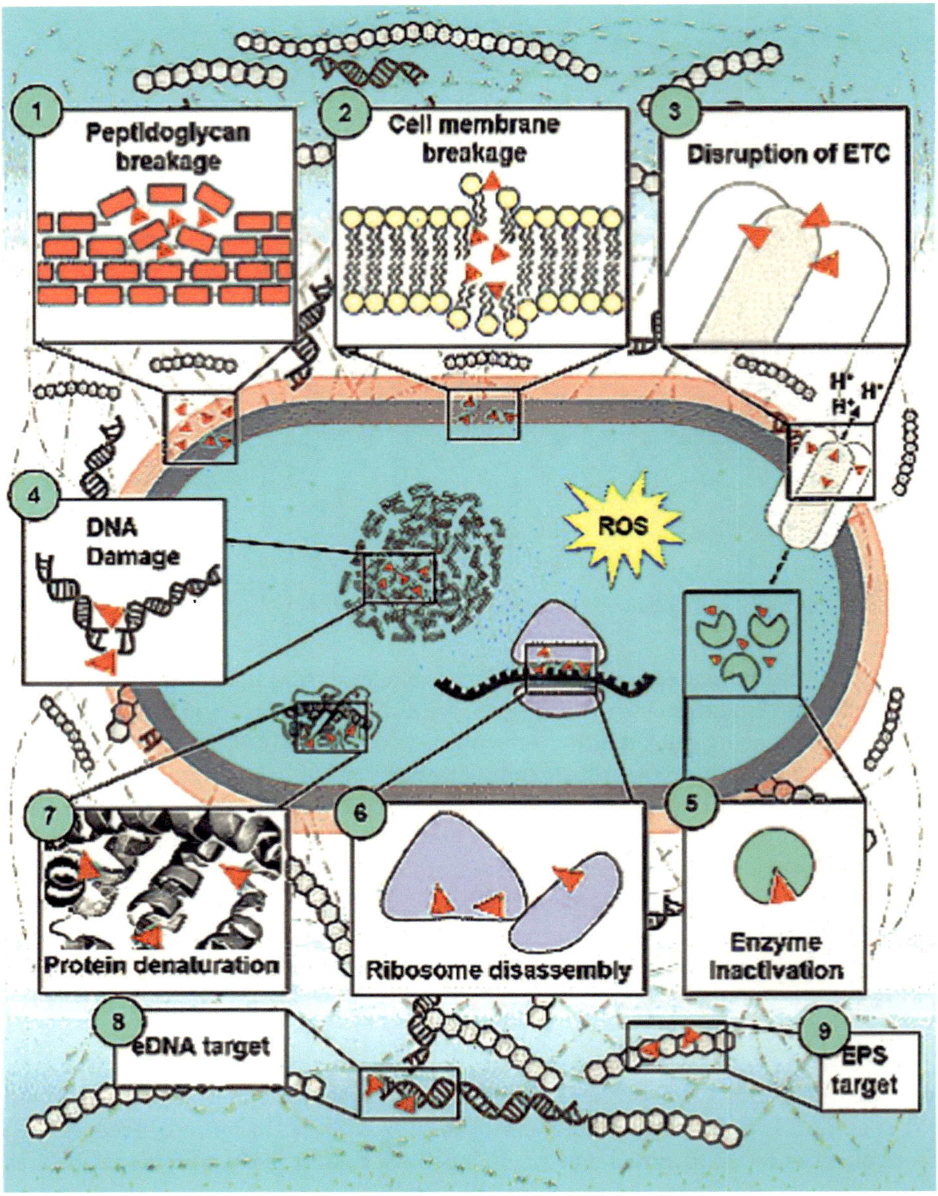

Figure 14.
Nanomaterials' molecular mechanisms and targets for inhibiting biofilms.

reduced expression of pathogenic factors like alpha-hemolysin and lower bacterial pathogenicity [66].

Bacteriophages are becoming popular in replacing conventional antibiotics since they selectively kill bacteria. They have the added advantage of being able to produce targeted actions within bacterial biofilms, thereby increasing their efficiency. Also, it was discovered that a phage-derived enzyme, hemolysinase, can degrade the peptidoglycan layer of bacterial cells, thus also affecting the structural integrity of biofilms (**Figure 16**) [67].

Bacterial strain	NPS	Avg abs	Std. dev	SEM	% Biofilm inhibition (±SEM)
	MtOH	0.410	19.87	14.14	73.26%
	n-Hex	0.275	3.28	2.32	82.01%
Bacillhus subtilis	DCM	1.100	9.84	6.96	28.09%
	EtOAc	0.590	5.77	4.08	61.37%
	-ve control	1.531	0.00	0.00	0%
	Ampicillin	0.575	0.00	0.00	62.44%
	MtOH	0.688	14.86	10.51	52.78%
	n-hex	0.560	32.10	22.70	61.47%
	DCM	0.530	28.82	21.09	63.50%
E. coli	EtOAc	0.450	4.75	6.37	69.40%
	-ve control	1.456	0.00	0.00	0%
	Ampicillin	0.380	0.00	0.00	74.01%
	MtOH	0.512	21.98	15.55	72.33%
	n-hex	1.680	57.06	40.35	51.70%
	DCM	0.390	14.82	10.48	78.94%
K. pneumoniae	EtOAc	0.635	9.39	6.64	65.72%
	-ve control	1.846	0.00	0.00	0%
	Ampicillin	0.365	0.00	0.00	80.20%
	MtOH	0.670	22.30	15.77	61.46%
	n-hex	0.540	14.45	10.22	67.60%
	DCM	0.485	28.16	19.91	73.73%
S.aureus	EtOAc	0.320	8.96	6.34	81.65%
	-ve control	1.753	0.00	0.00	0%
	Ampicillin	0.825	0.00	0.00	52.86%

Table 5.
%I of biofilm by bacterial strains.

The QS (quorum sensing) system regulates the activation of virulence genes at various stages of bacterial biofilm development. Research indicates that inhibiting this mechanism can prevent biofilm formation. Autoinducers facilitate communication among microorganisms by impacting bacterial density and gene expression. The expression levels of specific genes correlate with biofilm production and virulence factors. Key QS signaling molecules include N-acyl-homoserine lactones (AHLs), Auto-inducer peptides (AIPs), and Autoinducer-2 (AI-2) [68].

Enzymes are crucial in forming and managing extracellular polymeric substances (ESPs), intercellular communication, biofilm development, and dispersion. They can inhibit bacterial biofilms by disrupting their extracellular framework and quorum sensing systems. Key anti-biofilm enzymes include polysaccharide-degrading enzymes, oxidase, and proteolytic enzymes, which can hydrolyze components of ESP. Consequently, enzymes are preferred in biological methods for preventing biofilms [69].

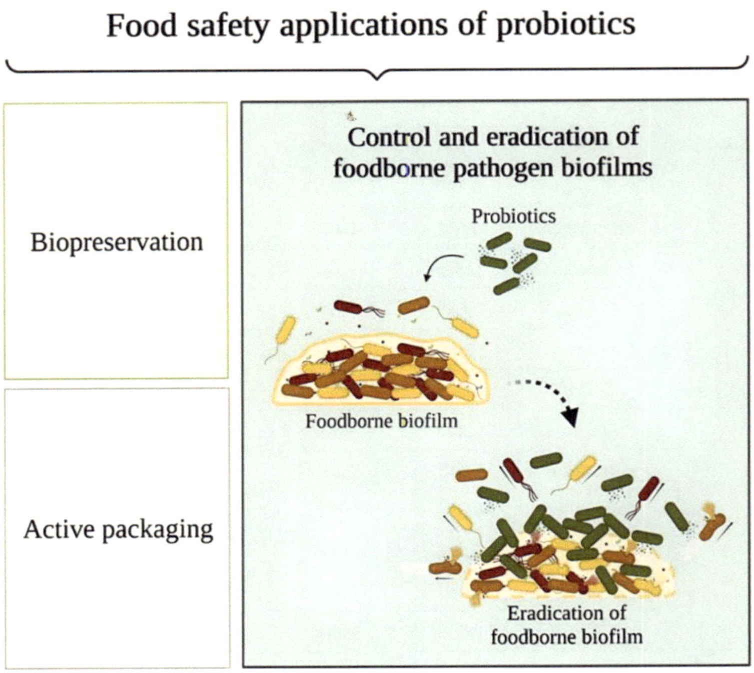

Figure 15.
Probiotics' uses in food safety: Packaging, preservation, and the management and elimination of foodborne pathogen biofilms.

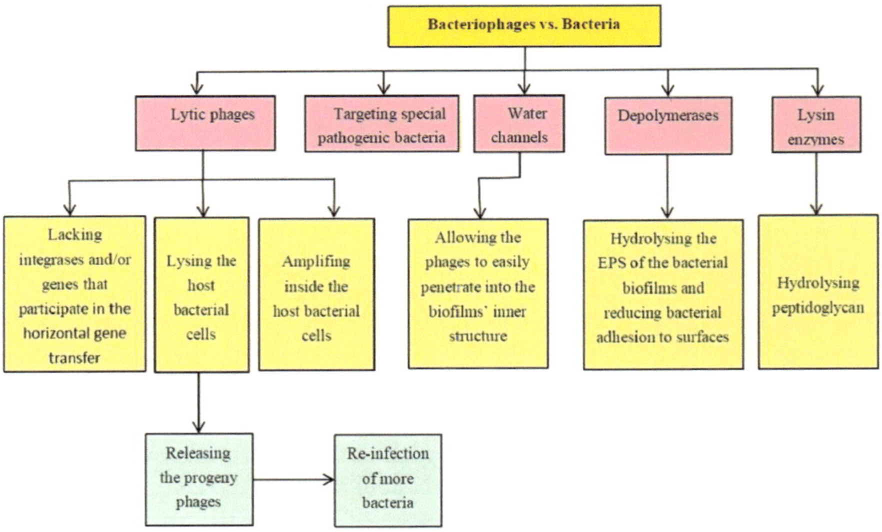

Figure 16.
Role of bacteriophage against bacteria.

Aptamers are one-stranded oligonucleotides or peptides produced in vitro that selectively bind to various molecules, including cells and proteins. Their unique three-dimensional structure allows them to recognize antimicrobial agents and bacterial biofilms specifically. Their antibacterial effects are believed to stem from

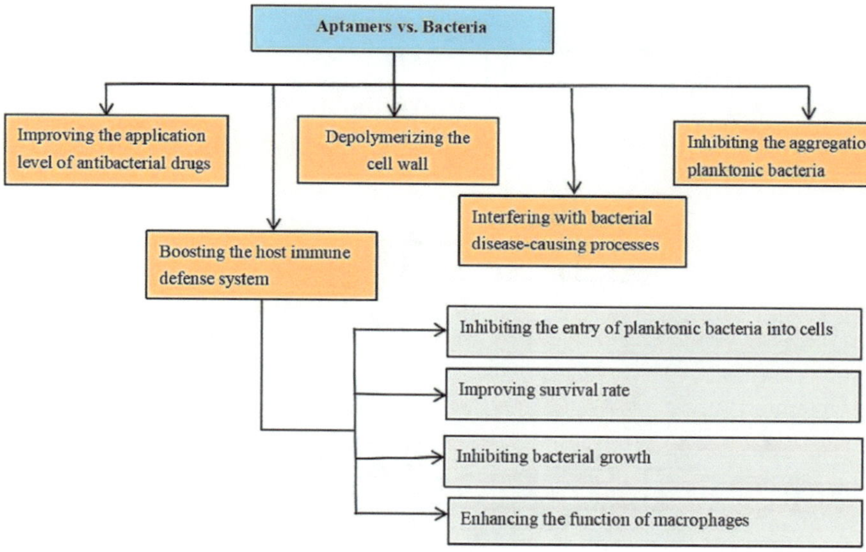

Figure 17.
Role of aptamers against bacteria.

the depolarization of bacterial cell walls, making aptamers potential alternatives for inhibiting biofilm formation (**Figure 17**) [70].

The vaccine potential of infectious disease antigens from biofilm increases when researchers study outer membrane vesicles (OMVs) from these communities. These vesicles protect better than previously studied antigens. The immune system develops durable protection, as well as CD4 T-body cell presence, through OMV vaccines, according to pertussis test results. Research shows that biofilm-resistant surface designs can prevent bacteria from attaching and forming biofilms through the use of LIS inspired by the *Nepenthes* pitcher plant [71].

Chemicals that prevent quorum sensing (QS) are called anti-virulence or anti-pathogenic medicines. Researchers led by Rasmussen developed three QS inhibitor (QSI) selector systems using reporter genes linked to QS-regulated promoters to discover valuable compounds (**Figure 18**). Synthetic and natural substances can selectively bind to LuxR-type receptors, but new QS inhibitors targeting various QS signal receptors have also been found. Notably, *Pseudomonas aeruginosa* has two N-acyl-HSL QS systems and an additional alkyl-quinolone (AQ)-dependent QS system that regulates several virulence gene expressions [72].

For testing the efficacy of synthetic and natural QSIs, this study employs three QSIS systems (QSIS1, QSIS2, and QSIS3) in engineered *E. coli* strains. Media containing plasmids for each system, pPhlA, pLasB, and pGFP, are then electroporated in *E. coli* under normal conditions at 37°C and LB Media with appropriate antibiotics. QSIs investigated include synthetic furanone and natural curcumin, which are used at 1–100 μM concentrations. Specifically, QS inhibition is analyzed using fluorescence (GFP assay), cell viability (sucrose toxicity assay), and gene expression (qPCR for phlA, lasB, and GFP). Two methods, the crystal violet assay for determination of biofilm formation and the caseinase and elastase assays for exoenzyme activity, are used to estimate the virulence of *Pseudomonas aeruginosa* (**Table 6**) [85–87].

Commercially synthesized furanone-based QS inhibitors proved to have the highest impact, inhibiting up to 90% of QS ($p < 0.01$). In contrast, natural QS

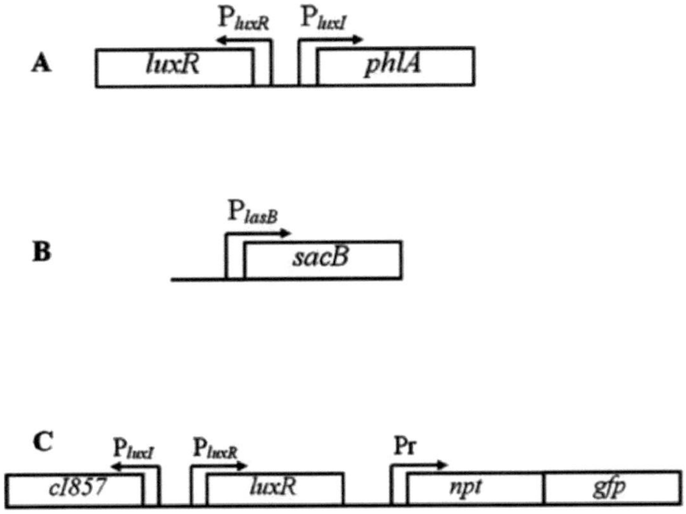

Figure 18.
Shows three QSIS systems in action. (A) E. coli was transformed in QSIS1 using an engineered vector that expressed the phlA gene, which produces the hazardous gene product controlled by LuxR. (B) The expression of the sacB gene, which causes cell death when sucrose is present, is controlled by the LasR-regulated lasB promoter in QSIS2. (C) LuxR control is also the foundation of the QSIS3 system. The cI repressor, which is regulated by QS via the luxI promoter, controls the input and GFP genes, which give kanamycin resistance and green fluorescence, respectively.

Compound	QSIS system	Inhibition indicator	Impact (Mean ± SEM)	Relevance to statistics (p-value)	Reference
Synthetic furanone (QSI 1)	$QSIS_1$ (phlA gene)	Expression of PhlA genes	PhlA expression is 85% inhibited (1 μM)	$P < 0.01$	[73, 74]
Synthetic furanone (QSI 2)	$QSIS_2$ (sacB gene)	(Sucrose) Cell viability	75% decrease in cell death caused by sucrose (10 μM)	$P < 0.05$	[75, 76]
Natural curcumin (QSI 1)	$QSIS_3$ (GFP expression)	Fluorescence of GFP	40% reduction in 50 μM GFP fluorescence	$P < 0.05$	[77, 78]
Natural curcumin (QSI 2)	$QSIS_1$ (phlA gene)	Expression of the PhlA gene	PhlA expression is reduced by 30% (25 μM)	$P > 0.05$	[77, 78]
Synthetic furanone (QSI 3)	$QSIS_3$ (GFP expression)	Fluorescence of GFP	90% decrease in 100 μM GFP Fluorescence	$P < 0.01$	[79, 80]
Control	All systems	QSI, or lack of inhibition	No impact on QS activity or gene expression	—	—
+ve Control (N-Acyl-HSL)	All systems	Different inhibition markers	Complete suppression of gene expression	$P < 0.01$	[81, 82]
P. aeruginosa	Biofilm assay	Biofilm development	Biofilm formation is reduced by 80% (10 μM)	$P < 0.05$	[83, 84]

Table 6.
Synthetic and natural QSIs on QSIS systems to give a quorum sensing inhibition effects.

inhibitors, including curcumin, had a relatively moderate effect, inhibiting 30–40% of QS ($p > 0.05$). Complementing these findings, biofilm assays demonstrated that synthetic QSIs inhibited *Pseudomonas aeruginosa* biofilm formation by 80%. Finally, synthetic QSIs exhibited a higher level of efficiency at preventing quorum sensing than their natural counterparts.

Disrupting cell-to-cell interactions and quorum sensing is an effective method for preventing biofilm formation. Notably, the metalloprotein AHL-lactonase from *Enterobacter* species can degrade N-AHL, which helps inhibit biofilm formation by *Aeromonas hydrophila. Lactobacillus* custom ZHG 2–1 has also been recognized for breaking down homoserine lactones and combating *P. aeruginosa* biofilms. Various quorum-quenching substances and enzymes have been identified, primarily from natural environments. Recent research indicated that ethyl acetate extracts from *Natrinemaversi* possess QS inhibitory effects on *P. aeruginosa* biofilms. Overall, natural plant-derived QS inhibitors are being explored as promising strategies for targeting biofilms in the future [88].

Syngas component fermentation involves a complex interaction between gaseous substrates, liquid media, and solid cells, which can complicate mass transfer between gas bubbles and cellular reaction sites. Techniques that enhance mass movement at the gas-liquid interface improve gas transfer despite low diffusion in liquids and microbial mass obstructing active sites. There's growing interest in optimizing the volumetric mass transfer coefficient (kLa) through bioprocessing, with advanced biofilm reactors contributing to higher cell densities and better mass transfer while reducing energy use. The Wood-Ljungdahl pathway allows autotrophic microorganisms to use C1 compounds (CO or CO2) for carbon and H2 for energy, supporting bacterial growth through reduction processes. The acetogenesis stage converts CO and H2 into acetyl-CoA, producing various end products during the solventogenesis stage, including ethanol, butanol, acetate, acetic acid, and butyrate (**Figure 19**) [90–92].

Syngas fermentation has been conducted at various scales using various biofilm reactors. Subsequent sections examined how different biofilm strategies affect gas–liquid mass transfer rates and analyzed the operational principles of bioreactor designs used for syngas fermentation.

In the 1980s, the monolithic biofilm reactor (MBR) was created by combining monolithic packing materials with bubble column reactors to improve cell density and gas–liquid mass transfer while minimizing microbial washout (**Figure 20**). MBR features straight channels with thin walls, typically 1 to 5 mm in diameter, and its flat design enhances performance by reducing bends and barriers. In maintaining consistent pressure, MBR outperforms older biofilm reactors like the Tickle Bed Reactor (TBR) [93].

Biofilm reactors with hollow fiber membranes (HFMBR) are widely used in biofuel production and wastewater treatment, particularly in syngas fermentation. These reactors combine membrane filtration with a bubble column, allowing substrates to pass through gas-permeable membranes that promote microbial growth (**Figure 21**). As microbes attach to the membranes and proliferate, they convert nutrients into valuable products like ethanol and fatty acids, which diffuse into the surrounding liquid for collection [94].

Bioleaching is a cost-effective and sustainable microbial method for extracting metals from refractory ores. Key bacteria involved in this process include *Acidithiobacillus, Leptospirillum, Ferroplasma*, and *Sulfobacillus,* which help dissolve

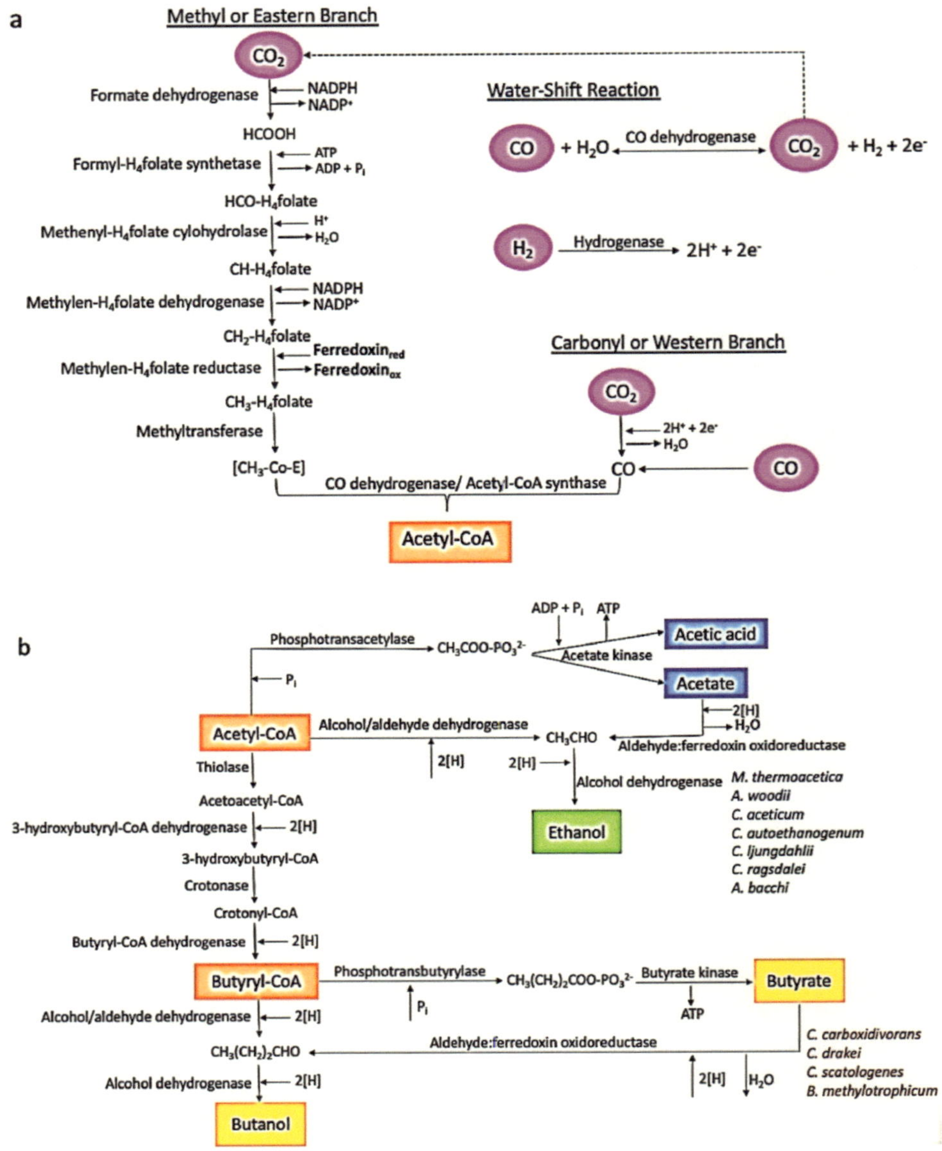

Figure 19.
The Wood-Ljungdahl metabolic route: a) phase of acetogenesis; b) period of solventogenesis [89].

minerals by releasing oxidizing agents like H^+ and Fe^{3+}. This biological approach is more effective in leaching minerals than traditional abiotic methods [95].

EPS (extracellular polymeric substances) plays a vital role in bacterial attachment to mineral surfaces, significantly enhancing microbial adhesion and metal ion absorption, which boosts bioleaching efficiency. The contact mechanism relies heavily on effective microbial consortia, particularly sulfate-reducing bacteria (SRB), contributing to both contact and bioleaching efficiencies. The EPS forms a layer between sulfide ore and bacterial cell membranes, facilitating metal dissolution through covalent bonds. Additionally, the formation of biofilms improves interfacial contact between bacteria and minerals. It enhances bacterial survival in harsh environments, such as high metal concentrations and low pH, during bioleaching [96, 97].

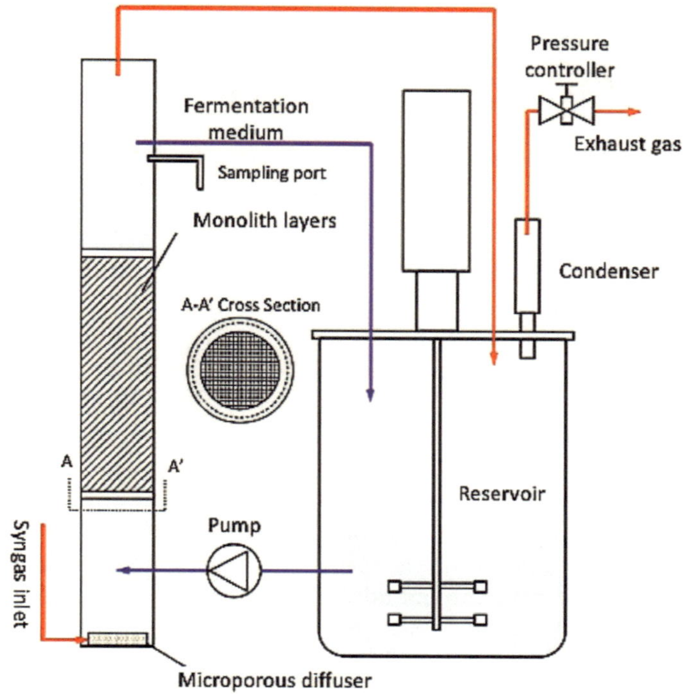

Figure 20.
Schematic representation of monolithic biofilm reactor (MBR).

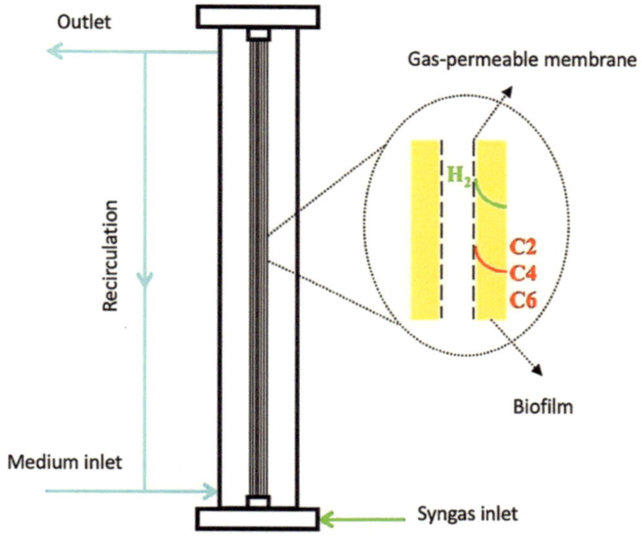

Figure 21.
Schematic representation of hollow fiber membranes biofilm reactor (HFMBR).

Biofilms enhance the performance of cell biological sensors by improving surface adhesion and cell metabolic activity, addressing issues related to cell immobilization and lifespan. While biofilms can negatively affect various environments, they are also

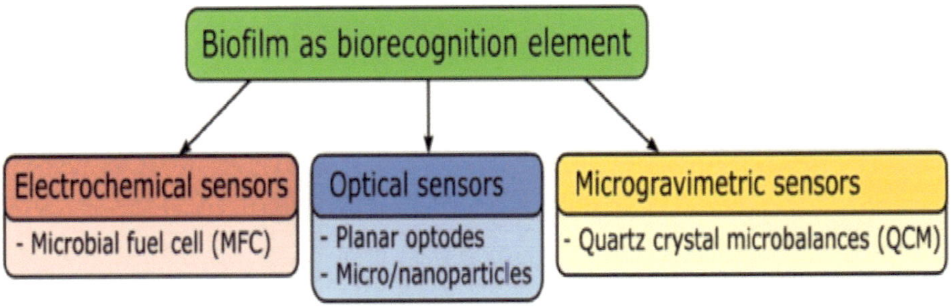

Figure 22.
Using bacterial biofilm as an identification factor in sensing techniques.

valuable for real-time and in situ monitoring of environmental conditions through biofilm-based biosensors (**Figure 22**) [98].

Electrochemical sensors utilize electroactive biofilms (EABs) with electroactive bacteria, allowing for spontaneous immobilization near electrodes without harmful reagents. These biofilms can sustain themselves for extended periods and generate electrical energy from organic compounds, making them practical for powering devices [99].

MFCs (Microbial Fuel Cells) estimate microbial load and biochemical oxygen demand (BOD) by detecting organic water pollution. BOD is determined by measuring the change in dissolved oxygen levels in a water sample after five days of incubation with microorganisms at 20°C. Coupled EAB-MFCs provide rapid BOD measurements in under a day and demonstrate improved substrate degradation with glucose and acetate. However, their ability to identify specific organic pollutants is limited due to their nonselective nature [100].

Microbial Fuel Cells (MFCs) can serve as sensors for detecting organic pollutants and heavy metal ions by monitoring the current output, which decreases when toxins are present. Despite their low sensitivity and specificity, MFCs are valuable for real-time water quality analysis in rivers, groundwater, and industrial effluents due to their low cost, independence from commercial electricity, and ease of use. They help evaluate sewage treatment efficiency and assess environmental impacts on agricultural productivity [101]. Additionally, biofilms play a vital role in pollutant removal and enhance stability and productivity in various biotechnological applications, including manufacturing and medicine.

Some frustrating characteristics of planktonic mono-cultures exist, although well-recognized biofilm models are of paramount importance, especially in the dental field. According to Bernhard Guggenheim, biofilms can assess oral plaque conditions; it is possible to use them in preventive dentistry. The text incorporates biofilms in mass transportation, biofilm impact on dental enamel, techniques to quantify oral microbiology, bacterial organization, and potential in identifying antibiotic response. Also, *Acetobacter xylinum* synthesizes cellulosic biofilm that may be used as partial skin substitutes in certain skin injury cases. Tubular bacterial nano-cellulose (BNC) hydrogels are used for regenerative medicines, as substitutes for blood vessels and other organs, and as temporary carriers for cells and drug delivery systems [102–105].

Biofilms that form nano-cellulosic structures can be utilized in bioprinting, particularly in creating bio-inks with living cells for various applications in biomedicine. Nano-cellulose is favored for its ability to mimic collagen fibril networks and its potential use in cartilage tissue engineering. Additionally, nano-cellulose materials are effective, targeted, and safer medication delivery systems.

Biotransformation refers to converting fine chemicals into higher-value products, but it can pose toxicity challenges due to harmful substrates and byproducts from microbes and bio-catalytic enzymes. *Zymomonas mobilis,* which form biofilms, demonstrate more excellent resistance to substances like benzaldehyde than planktonic cells. This biofilm formation offers benefits such as self-immobilization of biocatalysts, long-term stability for continuous operations, and increased resilience against toxic substrates and products in synthesizing fine chemicals [106].

Talks for the second Biofilm Bash would start in 2015, and they held their event from May 7 to May 9, 2019, at Ponderosa Lodge in Leavenworth, Washington. Staged by key stakeholders such as Mark Shirtliff and Paul Stoodley, the bash raised concerns. Also, it sought to define knowledge deficits regarding biofilms to enhance synergy among the key stakeholders. The IDP event revealed that the study of biofilm is entirely disassociated according to the different disease states, such as dental calculus and medical devices associated with infectious diseases. They involved grouping participants into small groups where suggestions were generated that increased participation by asking six questions [107].

Managing for future technologies, the text discusses biofilm research and its possible advantages of importing innovations from other subjects. It outlines important issues, including the lack of methods for integrating label-free chemical identification with micro-scale imaging, monitoring biofilm environments, and applying machine learning to biofilm interaction patterns in large results datasets. The interchangeability of methods between environmental and clinical research is also stressed [107].

The text discusses the emergence of multiple-drug resistance in bacteria, which causes 35,000 deaths in the United States annually. New therapies are inadequate because of their high costs and lengthy approval procedures. The main research activities are on enhancing currently available antimicrobials against biofilm-associated resistance with applications of micro and nanotechnology [42].

Nanotechnology offers a promising approach for combating biofilms by targeting the outer layer of the extracellular polymeric substance (EPS) membrane. It allows for the deposition of antibacterial agents directly onto pathogens without degradation and enables prolonged release of antimicrobials at effective concentrations. Additionally, nanotechnology exhibits antibacterial properties that could lead to the development of new antimicrobial surfaces or coatings and demonstrates anti-biofilm characteristics through the production of reactive oxygen species (ROS) and direct cell-killing action [108, 109].

New approaches in biofilm control reveal the importance of utilizing nanotechnology and nanoscale coatings in controlling biofilms that impact multiple industries, such as medicine and the environment. The study indicates that antimicrobial peptides or nanoparticle-impregnated coatings significantly decrease biofilm formation and infection probabilities. Besides, CVD graphene-derived nanomaterials are nontoxic and renewable to alter the biofilm architecture in water treatment plants [110, 111].

The text discusses advancements in functional surfaces that prevent bacterial adhesion and growth through techniques like genetic modification and nanotechnology. It highlights the use of engineered biofilms in sustainable bioremediation to degrade hazardous waste and the effectiveness of nanoscale delivery devices in reducing biofilm resilience by over 70% with quorum-sensing inhibitors [112, 113]. The strategy aims to minimize toxic biofilms while promoting beneficial strains, which could positively influence industries such as food production, medicine, and environmental conservation.

The industry is moving toward more environmentally friendly biofilm control processes and techniques, including enzymatic methods to dissolve biofilm matrixes, which are friendly to ecosystems. In agriculture, the method of utilizing microbial consortia to combat pathogenic biofilms is on the rise since it poses revenue to flora health and reduces the utilization of synthetic renewal agents. Despite the importance of biofilm in industrial development, adequate and reasonable control of biofilm formation is critical for sustainable growth and protection of the environment [114, 115].

Biofilm research aims to combine advanced technology with sustainability to achieve innovative and eco-friendly solutions for industrial applications.

3. Conclusion

Biofilms have greatly interested environmental and industrial sciences since they present both a problem and a solution. It can cause issues such as food contamination and corrosion in industrial processes, so they must be controlled. However, biofilms also have valuable applications in bioleaching, bioremediation, and wastewater treatment, indicating the importance of sustainable development. New considerations of engineered microbial systems and the ability to prevent biofilm formation from nanocoatings propose new applications for biofilms. This suggests the necessity of a broad approach to studying their activities in industrial systems so that companies can use the challenges and opportunities of biofilms for sustainable development. Future projects should address diversified solutions to global industrial and environmental challenges [116, 117].

Acknowledgements

I am grateful to **Allah Almighty**, who has bestowed his gifts that led to this research. I pay homage to the Prophet of Islam, **Muhammad (PBUH)**, who provides me guidance in my day-to-day life. My special thanks to my supervisor, **Mirza Imran Shehzad**, for extending his valuable support and feedback to make this work achievable. Lastly, I owe a lot of gratitude to my **parents** for always supporting me spiritually and financially.

Final thoughts

Therefore, biofilm analysis is crucial in sustainable development since it discharges numerous industrial concerns and provides solutions on the same platform. Although biofilms devastate sectors like healthcare and food production, they present many opportunities in bioleaching, renewable energy production, and bioremediation. More research should include AI, synthetic biology, and nanotechnology applications in biomedical research to manage and exploit biofilms. Thus, biofilms are shifting from being seen as barriers to attractive attributes as industries incorporate natural changes. The future will require mainstreaming strategies that seek to address whether or not beneficial use can be made of these adverse effects, along with continued research and multinational collaboration [20].

Acronyms and abbreviations

WHO	world health organization
CF	cystic fibrosis
Clf	clumping factors
QS	quorum sensing
EPS	extracellular polymeric substances
DNA	deoxyribonucleic acid
MIC	microbiologically influenced corrosion
SRB	sulfate-reducing bacteria
CWs	constructed wetlands
HAIs	healthcare-associated Infections
NIH	national institutes of health
CAUTIs	catheter-associated urinary tract infections
MTs	metallo-thioneins
MBC	minimum bactericidal concentration
MIC	minimum inhibitory concentration
M-MIC	metabolite-MIC
NRB	nitrate-reducing bacterium
QACs	quaternary ammonium compounds

Author details

Nimra Irfan* and Mirza Imran Shehzad
The Islamia University of Bahawalpur, Pakistan

*Address all correspondence to: nimrairfanmughal@gmail.com

References

[1] Kang X, Yang X, He Y, Guo C, Li Y, Ji H, et al. Strategies and materials for the prevention and treatment of biofilms. Materials Today Bio. 2023;**23**:100827. DOI: 10.1016/j.mtbio.2023.100827

[2] Muhammad MH, Idris AL, Fan X, Guo Y, Yu Y, Jin X, et al. Beyond risk: Bacterial biofilms and their regulating approaches. Frontiers in Microbiology. 2020;**11**:928

[3] Carrascosa C, Raheem D, Ramos F, Saraiva A, Raposo A. Microbial biofilms in the food industry—A comprehensive review. International Journal of Environmental Research and Public Health. 2021;**18**(4):2014. Available from: https://www.mdpi.com/1660-4601/18/4/2014

[4] Hollmann B, Perkins M, Walsh D. Biofilms and Their Role in Pathogenesis. British Society for Immunology; n.d. Available from: https://www.immunology.org/public-information/bitesized-immunology/pathogens-disease/biofilms-and-their-role-pathogenesis

[5] Peng Q, Tang X, Dong W, Sun N, Yuan W. A review of biofilm formation of Staphylococcus aureus and its regulation mechanism. Antibiotics. 2023;**12**(1):12. Available from: https://www.mdpi.com/2079-6382/12/1/12

[6] Mohanty I, Mishra R, Panda AK, Mahanty A, Bisht SS. Phytochemicals in downregulation of quorum sensing. In: Pati S, Sarkar T, Lahiri D, editors. Recent Frontiers of Phytochemicals. Amsterdam, Netherlands: Elsevier; 2023. pp. 455-462. DOI: 10.1016/B978-0-443-19143-5.00038-4

[7] Alotaibi GF, Bukhari MA. Factors influencing bacterial biofilm formation and development. American Journal of Biomedical Science & Research. 2021;**12**(6):617-626

[8] Li P, Yin R, Cheng J, Lin J. Bacterial biofilm formation on biomaterials and approaches to its treatment and prevention. International Journal of Molecular Sciences. 2023;**24**(14):11680. Available from: https://www.mdpi.com/1422-0067/24/14/11680

[9] Sharan M, Vijay D, Dhaka P, Bedi JS, Gill JPS. Biofilms as a microbial hazard in the food industry: A scoping review. Journal of Applied Microbiology. 2022;**133**(4):2210-2234. DOI: 10.1111/jam.15766

[10] Shineh G, Mobaraki M, Perves Bappy MJ, Mills DK. Biofilm formation, and related impacts on healthcare, food processing and packaging, industrial manufacturing, marine industries, and sanitation–a review. Applied Microbiology. 2023;*3*(3):629-665. Available from: https://www.mdpi.com/2673-8007/3/3/44

[11] Karačić S, Modin O, Hagelia P, Persson F, Wilén B-M. The effect of time and surface type on the composition of biofilm communities on concrete exposed to seawater. International Biodeterioration & Biodegradation. 2022;**173**:105458. DOI: 10.1016/j.ibiod.2022.105458

[12] Todhanakasem T. Microbial biofilm in the industry. African Journal of Microbiology Research. 2013;*7*:1625-1634. DOI: 10.5897/AJMR12.2146

[13] Olanbiwoninu AA, Popoola BM. Biofilms and their impact on the food industry. Saudi Journal of Biological Sciences. 2023;**30**(2):103523. DOI: 10.1016/j.sjbs.2022.103523

[14] Van Houdt R, Michiels CW. Biofilm formation and the food industry, a focus on the bacterial outer surface. Journal of Applied Microbiology. 2010;**109**(3):1117-1131. DOI: 10.1111/j.1365-2672.2010.04756.x

[15] Flemming H-C. Biofilm formation in industrial food processing environments: A case study on biofilm-related bacteria in food processing plants. International Journal of Food Microbiology. 2007;**113**(3):230-245. DOI: 10.1016/j.ijfoodmicro.2006.07.006

[16] Rosenberg M. Microbial biofilms: A new perspective in food safety. International Journal of Food Microbiology. 2000;**58**(3):137-144. DOI: 10.1016/S0168-1605(00)00246-7

[17] Bottone EJ. Bacillus cereus, a volatile human pathogen. Clinical Microbiology Reviews. 2010;**23**:382-398

[18] Grigore-Gurgu L, Bucur FI, Borda D, Alexa EA, Neagu C, Nicolau AI. Biofilms formed by pathogens in food and food processing environments. In: Bacterial Biofilms. London, UK, London, UK: IntechOpen; 2019

[19] Liu Y, Kuchin R. Biofilm formation and microbial communities in food industry settings: Influence on food safety and processing. Food Research International. 2018;**103**:151-163. DOI: 10.1016/j.foodres.2018.10.039

[20] Galié S, García-Gutiérrez C, Miguélez EM, Villar CJ, Lombó F. Biofilms in the food industry: Health aspects and control methods. Frontiers in Microbiology. 2018:898. DOI: 10.3389/fmicb.2018.00898

[21] Giaouris E, Heir E, Desvaux M, Hébraud M, Møretrø T, Langsrud S, et al. Intra- and inter-species interactions within biofilms of important foodborne bacterial pathogens. Frontiers in Microbiology. 2015;**6**:841. DOI: 10.3389/fmicb.2015.00841

[22] Kadariya J, Smith TC, Thapaliya D. Staphylococcus aureus and staphylococcal food-borne-disease: An ongoing challenge in public health. BioMed Research International. 2014:827965. DOI: 10.1155/2014/827965

[23] Little BJ, Blackwood DJ, Hinks J, Lauro FM, Marsili E, Okamoto A, et al. Microbially influenced corrosion—Any progress? Corrosion Science. 2020;**170**:108641. DOI: 10.1016/j.corsci.2020.108641

[24] Smith J, Nappi R. The impact of biofilms on food safety in industrial environments. Food Control. 2017;**74**:109-116. DOI: 10.1016/j.foodcont.2017.09.010

[25] Fu X, Kong F, Duan P, Li F, Hu W, Liu X, et al. Performance of loach to reduce clogging matter in vertical-flow constructed wetlands: Hydraulic evaluation and metabolic processes. Chemical Engineering Journal. 2024;**498**:155280. DOI: 10.1016/j.cej.2024.155280

[26] Liu N, Dopffel N, Stepec BAA. Impact of microbial biofilms on subsurface energy systems: From oil and gas to renewable energy. In: Stepec BAA, Wunch K, Skovhus TL, editors. Petroleum Microbiology: The Role of Microorganisms in the Transition to Net Zero Energy. Boca Raton, FL, USA: CRC Press; 2024. pp. 21-36. DOI: 10.1201/9781003287056

[27] Welikala S, Al-Saadi S, Gates WP, Panter C, Singh Raman R. Sulphate reducing bacteria (SRB) biofilm development and its role in microbial

corrosion of carbon steel. Frontiers in Materials. 2024;**11**:1360869

[28] Mishra A, Aggarwal A, Khan F. Medical device-associated infections caused by biofilm-forming microbial pathogens and controlling strategies. Antibiotics. 2024;*13*(7):623. Available from: https://www.mdpi.com/2079-6382/13/7/623

[29] Werneburg GT. Catheter-associated urinary tract infections: Current challenges and future prospects. Research and Reports in Urology. 2022;**14**:109-133

[30] Di Domenico EG, Oliva A, Guembe M. The current knowledge on the pathogenesis of tissue and medical device-related biofilm infections. Microorganisms. 2022;**10**:1259

[31] Abhinandan S, Subashchandrabose SR, Venkateswarlu K, Mohan SV, Megharaj M. Microalgae-bacteria biofilms: A sustainable synergistic approach in remediation of acid mine drainage Appl. Journal of Microbiology and Biotechnology. 2018;**102**(3):1131-1144. DOI: 10.1007/s00253-017-8655-7

[32] Mishra S, Huang Y, Li J, Wu X, Zhou Z, Lei Q, et al. Biofilm-mediated bioremediation is a powerful tool for the removal of environmental-pollutants. Chemosphere. 2022;**294**:133609. DOI: 10.1016/j.chemosphere.2022.133609

[33] Biswal T, Malik JA. Role of biofilms in bioremediation. In: Malik JA, editor. Microbes and Microbial Biotechnology for Green-Remediation. Amsterdam, Netherlands: Elsevier; 2022. pp. 205-225. DOI: 10.1016/B978-0-323-90452-0.00016-5

[34] Tripathi S, Sharma P, Chandra R. Degradation of organometallic pollutants of distillery wastewater by autochthonous bacterial community in biostimulation and bioaugmentation process. Bioresource Technology. 2021;**338**:125518. DOI: 10.1016/j.biortech.2021.125518

[35] Sharma P. Role and significance of biofilm-forming microbes in phytoremediation -a review. Environmental Technology & Innovation. 2022;*25*:102182. DOI: 10.1016/j.eti.2021.102182

[36] Cámara M, Green W, MacPhee CE, Rakowska PD, Raval R, Richardson MC, et al. Economic significance of biofilms: A multidisciplinary and cross-sectoral challenge. npj Biofilms and Microbiomes. 2022;**8**(1):42. DOI: 10.1038/s41522-022-00306-y

[37] Wang N, Peng L, Gu Y, Liang C, Pott RWM, Xu Y. Insights into biodegradation of antibiotics during the biofilm-based wastewater treatment processes. Journal of Cleaner Production. 2023;**393**:136321. DOI: 10.1016/j.jclepro.2023.136321

[38] Yadav S, Tripathi S, Purchase D, Chandra R. Development of a biofilm-forming bacterial consortium and quorum sensing molecules for the degradation of lignin-containing organic pollutants. Environmental Research. 2023;**226**:115618. DOI: 10.1016/j.envres.2023.115618

[39] Yan X, Chio C, Li H, Zhu Y, Chen X, Qin W. Colonization characteristics and surface effects of microplastic biofilms: Implications for environmental behavior of typical pollutants. Science of the Total Environment. 2024;**937**:173141. DOI: 10.1016/j.scitotenv.2024.173141

[40] Li X, Sun L, Zhang P, Wang Y. Novel approaches to combat medical device-associated BioFilms. Coatings. 2021;**11**:294

[41] Sun X-L, Xiang H, Xiong H-Q, Fang Y-C, Wang Y. Bioremediation of microplastics in freshwater environments: A systematic review of biofilm culture, degradation mechanisms, and analytical methods. Science of the Total Environment. 2023;**863**:160953. DOI: 10.1016/j.scitotenv.2022.160953

[42] Rao H, Choo S, Rajeswari Mahalingam SR, Adisuri DS, Madhavan P, Akim A, et al. Approaches for mitigating microbial biofilm-related drug resistance: A focus on micro- and nanotechnologies. Molecules. 2021;*26*(7):1870. Available from: https://www.mdpi.com/1420-3049/26/7/1870

[43] Khan J, Tarar SM, Gul I, Nawaz U, Arshad M. Challenges of antibiotic resistance biofilms and potential combating strategies: A review. *3*. Biotech. 2021;**11**(4):169. DOI: 10.1007/s13205-021-02707-w

[44] Panthi VK, Fairfull-Smith KE, Islam N. Liposomal drug delivery strategies to eradicate bacterial biofilms: Challenges, recent advances, and future perspectives. International Journal of Pharmaceutics. 2024;**655**:124046. DOI: 10.1016/j.ijpharm.2024.124046

[45] Kumar L, Bisen M, Harjai K, Chhibber S, Azizov S, Lalhlenmawia H, et al. Advances in nanotechnology for biofilm inhibition. ACS Omega. 2023;**8**(24):21391-21409. DOI: 10.1021/acsomega.3c02239

[46] Patra A, Das J, Agrawal NR, Kushwaha GS, Ghosh M, Son Y-O. Marine antimicrobial peptides-based strategies for tackling bacterial biofilm and biofouling challenges. Molecules. 2022;**27**(21):7546. Available from: https://www.mdpi.com/1420-3049/27/21/7546

[47] Lamin A, Kaksonen AH, Cole IS, Chen X-B. Quorum sensing inhibitors applications: A new prospect for mitigation of microbiologically influenced corrosion. Bioelectrochemistry. 2022;**145**:108050. DOI: 10.1016/j.bioelechem.2022.108050

[48] Alvarez-Ordóñez A, Coughlan LM, Briandet R, Cotter PD. Biofilms in food processing environments: Challenges and opportunities. Annual Review of Food Science and Technology. 2019;**10**(1):173-195

[49] Coughlan LM, Cotter PD, Hill C, Alvarez-Ordóñez A. New weapons to fight old enemies: Novel strategies for the (bio)control of bacterial biofilms in the food industry. Frontiers in Microbiology. 2016;**7**:1641

[50] Toté K, Horemans T, Vanden Berghe D, Maes L, Cos P. Inhibitory effect of biocides on the viable masses and matrices of *Staphylococcus aureus* and *Pseudomonas-aeruginosa* biofilms. Applied and Environmental Microbiology. 2010;**76**:3135-3142

[51] Carrascosa C, Raheem D, Ramos F, Saraiva A, Raposo A. Microbial biofilms in the food industry—A comprehensive review. International Journal of Environmental Research and Public Health. 2014;**2021**:18

[52] Cabeça TK, Pizzolitto AC, Pizzolitto EL. Activity of disinfectants against foodborne pathogens in suspension and adhered to stainless steel surfaces. Brazilian Journal of Microbiology. 2012;**43**:1112-1119

[53] Shikongo-Nambabi MNNN, Kachigunda B, Venter SN. Evaluation of oxidising disinfectants to control vibrio biofilms in treated seawater used for fish processing. Water SA. 2010;**36**:215-220

[54] Srey S, Jahid IK, Ha SD. Biofilm formation in food industries: A food safety concern. Food Control. 2013;**31**:572-585

[55] Liu X, Yao H, Zhao X, Ge C. Biofilm formation and control of foodborne-pathogenic-bacteria. Molecules. 2023;**28**(6):2432. Available from: https://www.mdpi.com/1420-3049/28/6/2432

[56] Sharma S, Mohler J, Mahajan SD, Schwartz SA, Bruggemann L, Aalinkeel R. Microbial biofilm: A review on formation, infection, antibiotic resistance, control measures, and innovative treatment. Microorganisms. 2023;**11**(6):1614. Available from: https://www.mdpi.com/2076-2607/11/6/1614

[57] Ifijen IH, Maliki M, Udokpoh NU, Odiachi IJ, Atoe B. A concise review of the antibacterial action of gold nanoparticles against various bacteria. In: TMS 2023 152nd Annual Meeting & Exhibition Supplemental Proceedings; the Minerals, Metals & Materials Series. Springer; 2023. pp. 655-664

[58] Gupta K, Chhibber S. Biofunctionalization of silver nanoparticles with lactonase leads to altered antimicrobial and cytotoxic properties. Frontiers in Molecular Biosciences. 2019;**6**:63. DOI: 10.3389/fmolb.2019.00063.95

[59] Abdelwahab MA, Elhadi MA, Al-Mahdy DM. Evaluation of antimicrobial and biofilm formation activity of plant extracts against pathogenic bacteria using a 96-well microtiter plate assay. Journal of Applied Microbiology. 2023;**134**(4):1123-1132. DOI: 10.1111/jam.15345

[60] Zong Y, Zhang S, Wu X. Biofilm formation by *Pseudomonas aeruginosa* and its inhibition by natural compounds: A study using a microtiter plate assay. Microorganisms. 2022;**10**(5):923. DOI: 10.3390/microorganisms10050923

[61] Sornsenee P, Chatatikun M, Mitsuwan W, Kongpol K, Kooltheat N, Sohbenalee S, et al. Lyophilized cell-free supernatants of *lactobacillus* isolates exhibited antibiofilm, antioxidant, and reduces nitric oxide activity in lipopolysaccharide-stimulated RAW 264.7 cells. PeerJ. 2021;*9*:e12586

[62] Qualified Presumption of Safety (QPS): EFSA Journal. Available from: https://efsa.onlinelibrary.wiley.com/doi/toc/10.1002/(ISSN)1831-4732.QPS [accessed: 20 January 2023]

[63] Tomé AR, Carvalho FM, Teixeira-Santos R, Burmølle M, Mergulhão FJM, Gomes LC. Use of probiotics to control biofilm formation in food industries. Antibiotics. 2023;**12**(4):754. Available from: https://www.mdpi.com/2079-6382/12/4/754

[64] Yi X, Wang C, Yu X, Su W, Yuan Z. Chitosan/zinc nitrate microneedles for bacterial biofilm eradication. Journal of Biomedical Materials Research. Part B, Applied Biomaterials. 2021;**109**(6):911-920. DOI: 10.1002/jbm.b.34755

[65] Mulani MS, Kamble EE, Kumkar SN, Tawre MS, Pardesi KR. Emerging strategies to combat ESKAPE pathogens in the era of antimicrobial resistance: A review. Frontiers in Microbiology. 2019;**10**:539. DOI: 10.3389/fmicb.2019.00539

[66] Zhao A, Sun J, Liu Y. Understanding bacterial biofilms: From definition to treatment strategies [review]. Frontiers in Cellular and Infection Microbiology. 2023;**13**:1137947. DOI: 10.3389/fcimb.2023.1137947

[67] Łusiak-Szelachowska M, Weber-Dąbrowska B, Górski A. Bacteriophages

and lysins in biofilm control. Virologica Sinica. 2020;**35**(2):125-133. DOI: 10.1007/s12250-019-00192-3

[68] Muras A, Mallo N, Otero-Casal P, Pose-Rodríguez JM, Otero A. Quorum sensing systems as a new target to prevent biofilm-related oral diseases. Oral Diseases. 2022;**28**(2):307-313. DOI: 10.1111/odi.13689

[69] Wille J, Coenye T. Biofilm dispersion: The key to biofilm eradication or opening pandora's box? Biofilms. 2020;**2**:100027. DOI: 10.1016/j.bioflm.2020.100027

[70] Shatila F, Yaşa İ, Yalçın HT. Inhibition of salmonella enteritidis biofilms by salmonella invasion protein-targeting aptamer. Biotechnology Letters. 2020;**42**(10):1963-1974. DOI: 10.1007/s10529-020-02920-2

[71] Zea L, McLean RJC, Rook TA, Angle G, Carter DL, Delegard A, et al. Potential biofilm control strategies for extended spaceflight missions. Biofilms. 2020;*2*:100026. DOI: 10.1016/j.bioflm.2020.100026

[72] Yang L, Givskov M. Chemical biology strategies for biofilm control. Microbiology Spectrum. 2015;**3**(4):MB-0019-2015. DOI: 10.1128/microbiolspec.mb-0019-2015

[73] Rasmussen M et al. Development of QSIS systems to screen for quorum sensing inhibitors. Microbiology and Molecular Biology Reviews. 2023;**87**(2):e00034-e00022

[74] Lee J et al. Furanones and their impact on bacterial quorum sensing mechanisms. Frontiers in Microbiology. 2021;**12**:635245

[75] Neiditch MB et al. Regulation of quorum sensing in gram-negative bacteria. Cell. 2006;**126**(4):703-717

[76] D'Orazio TE et al. Furanone-mediated quorum sensing inhibition in E. Coli strains. Applied and Environmental Microbiology. 2020;**86**(5):e01017-e01020

[77] Wilson CL et al. Quantitative PCR for gene expression analysis in quorum sensing inhibition. Journal of Bacteriology Methods. 2018;**152**:98-105

[78] Kalia VC et al. Natural products as anti-quorum sensing agents: Recent developments. Microbiological Research. 2019;**219**:1-17

[79] Ouyang H et al. *Furanones: A potential tool for quorum sensing inhibition in Pseudomonas aeruginosa. Journal of Antimicrobial Chemotherapy. 2022;**77**(8):2205-2213

[80] Ciofu O et al. Quorum sensing inhibitors and their role in bacterial infections. International Journal of Antimicrobial Agents. 2020;**56**(6):106144

[81] Hentzer M et al. Attenuation of Pseudomonas aeruginosa virulence by quorum sensing inhibitors. The EMBO Journal. 2003;**22**(15):3803-3815

[82] Sturme MH et al. The role of N-acyl homoserine lactones in bacterial signaling and infection control. Trends in Microbiology. 2021;**29**(3):216-228

[83] Anderson JL et al. Biofilm formation and inhibition by quorum sensing inhibitors. Journal of Microbiology Methods. 2015;**103**:78-84

[84] Cravioto A et al. Exoenzyme activity of Pseudomonas aeruginosa under quorum sensing inhibition. Microbial Pathogenesis. 2022;**175**:104971

[85] Patel S. Microtiter plate-based biofilm formation assay: A reliable

method for screening biofilm-forming bacteria and assessing their antimicrobial activity. Journal of Microbiological Methods. 2019;**156**:92-101. DOI: 10.1016/j.mimet.2018.10.005

[86] Ouyang X, Zhang Y, Li Z. A microtiter plate assay for screening biofilm formation and antimicrobial activity of natural plant compounds. Frontiers in Microbiology. 2022;**13**:802045. DOI: 10.3389/fmicb.2022.802045

[87] Rasmussen TB, Bjarnsholt T, Skindersoe ME, Hentzer M, Kristoffersen P, Köte M, et al. Screening for quorum-sensing inhibitors (QSI) by use of a novel genetic system, the QSI selector. Journal of Bacteriology. 2005;**187**(5):1799-1814

[88] Mishra R, Panda AK, De Mandal S, Shakeel M, Bisht SS, Khan J. Natural anti-biofilm agents: Strategies to control biofilm-forming pathogens-[review]. Frontiers in Microbiology. 2020;**11**:566325. DOI: 10.3389/fmicb.2020.566325

[89] Sun X, Atiyeh HK, Huhnke RL, Tanner RS. Syngas fermentation process development for production of biofuels and chemicals: A review. Bioresource Technology Reports. 2019;**7**:100279

[90] Grady JL, Chen GJ. Bioconversion of Waste Biomass to Useful Products. Alexandria, VA, USA: United States Patent and Trademark Office (USPTO); 1998

[91] Qureshi N, Annous BA, Ezeji TC, Karcher P, Maddox IS. Biofilm reactors for industrial bioconversion processes: Employing potential of enhanced reaction rates. Microbial Cell Factories. 2005;**4**:1-21

[92] Mohammadi M, Najafpour GD, Younesi H, Lahijani P, Uzir MH, Mohamed AR. Bioconversion of synthesis gas to second generation biofuels: A review. Renewable and Sustainable Energy Reviews. 2011;**15**(9):4255-4273

[93] Gunes B. A critical review on biofilm-based reactor systems for enhanced syngas fermentation processes. Renewable and Sustainable Energy Reviews. 2021;**143**:110950. DOI: 10.1016/j.rser.2021.110950

[94] Chen X, Ni B-J. Anaerobic conversion of hydrogen and carbon dioxide to fatty acids production in a membrane biofilm reactor: A modeling approach. Chemical Engineering Journal. 2016;**306**:1092-1098

[95] Shen L, Cheng J, Wang J, Zhang Y, Zhou H, Wu X, et al. Biofilm formation and development during the pyrite bioleaching of moderately thermophilic microorganisms. Hydrometallurgy. 2023;**222**:106183. DOI: 10.1016/j.hydromet.2023.106183

[96] Ye M, Liang J, Liao X, Li L, Feng X, Qian W, et al. Bioleaching for detoxification of waste flotation tailings: Relationship between EPS substances and bioleaching behavior. Journal of Environmental Management. 2021;**279**:111795. DOI: 10.1016/j.jenvman.2020.111795

[97] Feng S, Qiu Y, Huang Z, Yin Y, Zhang H, Zhu D, et al. The adaptation mechanisms of Acidithiobacillus caldus CCTCC M 2018054 to extreme acid stress: Bioleaching performance, physiology, and transcriptomics. Environmental-Research. 2021;**199**:111341. DOI: 10.1016/j.envres.2021.111341

[98] Prévoteau A, Rabaey K. Electroactive biofilms for sensing: Reflections and perspectives. ACS Sensors.

2017;**2**:1072-1085. DOI: 10.1021/acssensors.7b00418127

[99] Simoska O, Gaffney EM, Minteer SD, Franzetti A, Cristiani P, Grattieri M, et al. Recent trends and advances in microbial electrochemical sensing technologies: An overview. Current Opinion in Electrochemistry. 2021;**30**:100762. DOI: 10.1016/j.coelec.2021.100762130

[100] Sonawane JM, Ezugwu CI, Ghosh PC. Microbial fuel cell-based biological oxygen demand sensors for monitoring wastewater: State-of-the-art and practical applications. ACS Sensors. 2020;**5**:2297-2316. DOI: 10.1021/acssensors.0c01299140

[101] Funari R, Shen AQ. Detection and characterization of bacterial biofilms and biofilm-based sensors. ACS Sensors. 2022;**7**(2):347-357. DOI: 10.1021/acssensors.1c02722

[102] Fontana JD, Franco VC, De Souza SJ, Lyra IN, De Souza AM. Nature of plant stimulators in the production of Acetobacter xylinum ("tea fungus") biofilm used in skin therapy. Applied Biochemistry and Biotechnology. 1991;**28**(1):341-351

[103] Caliskan E, De Souza DR, Böning A, Liakopoulos OJ, Choi Y-H, Pepper J, et al. Saphenous vein grafts in contemporary coronary artery bypass graft surgery. Nature Reviews Cardiology. 2020;**17**(3):155-169

[104] Klemm D, Rauchfuss F, Kramer F, Petzold-Welcke K, Richter T, Ruhe C, et al. Design of biocellulose implants for first successful bile duct regeneration. In: Abstracts of Papers of the American Chemical Society. Washington, DC, USA: American Chemical Society (ACS); 2016

[105] Kalashgarani MY, Babapoor A. Application of nanoantibiotics in the diagnosis and treatment of infectious diseases. Advances in Applied NanoBio-Technologies. 2022;**3**(1):22-35

[106] Kazemi K, Ghahramani Y, Kalashgrani MY. Nano biofilms: An emerging biotechnology applications. Benefits. 2022;**9**:11

[107] Coenye T, Kjellerup B, Stoodley P, Bjarnsholt T. The future of biofilm research – Report on the '2019 biofilm bash'. Biofilms. 2020;**2**:100012. DOI: 10.1016/j.bioflm.2019.100012

[108] Kuan C-Y, Wai Y-F, Yuen K-H, Liong M-T. Nanotech: Propensity in foods and bioactives. Critical Reviews in Food Science and Nutrition. 2012;**52**:55-71

[109] Paul W, Sharma C. Inorganic nanoparticles for targeted drug delivery. In: Biointegration of Medical Implant Materials: Science and Design. 1st ed. Cambridge, UK; New Delhi, India; Boca Raton, FL, USA: Woodhead Publishing Limited; 2010. pp. 204-234

[110] Hetrick EM, Schoenfisch MH. Reducing implant-related infections: Active release strategies. Journal of Biomedical Materials Research Part B: Applied Biomaterials. 2006;**76**(3):264-275

[111] Perreault F, de Faria AF, Elimelech M. Environmental applications of graphene-based nanomaterials. Chemical Society Reviews. 2015;**44**(16):5861-5896

[112] Singh BK et al. Engineered biofilms for bioremediation: Current strategies and future potential. Trends in Biotechnology. 2020;**38**(10):993-1007

[113] Chung M, Khanal SK. Nanoscale delivery systems for biofilm control: Advances and challenges. Nature Communications. 2018;**9**(1):45-57

[114] Hulme SE. Enzymatic approaches to biofilm management. Environmental Science & Technology. 2010;**44**(3):1123-1129

[115] Mukherjee S, Ray S, Thakur D. Microbial consortia in agriculture: Applications and future perspectives. Agriculture, Ecosystems & Environment. 2021;**310**:107-120

[116] Costerton JW, Stewart PS, Greenberg EP. Bacterial biofilms: A common cause of persistent infections. Science. 1999;**284**(5418):1318-1322

[117] Flemming HC, Wingender J. The biofilm matrix. Nature Reviews Microbiology. 2010;**8**(9):623-633

Section 4

Biofilms in Bioremediation

Chapter 12

The Capacity of Bacteria Biofilm for Bioremediation

Michael Ikechukwuka Ejafu and Omodamola Paulina Akinro

Abstract

The global growth in terms of industrialization and urbanization has led to the release of various toxicogenic, carcinogenic, and recalcitrant substances into the environment. Remediation involves physical, chemical, and biological methods, and there is a need for polluted environments to be remediated using approaches that are eco-friendly. Bioremediation involves using microbes to clean up enormous amounts of pollutants from soil and water. It is an eco-friendly, cost effective, sustainable process that decomposes a wide range of pollutants. Biofilms are complicated functional communities comprising microbes enclosed in an exopolysaccharide matrix and attached to surfaces in an aqueous environment. Biofilms synthesis and development are regulated by the expression of genes in their cells, as well as other factors like nutrition availability, UV light, desiccation, pH, temperature, pressure, salt concentrations, and chemical presence. The microbes that form biofilms have been discovered to be useful in bioremediation because of their high tolerance to contaminants and environmental stress in addition to their capacity to degrade various toxic pollutants like insecticides, pesticides, and hydrocarbons utilizing a number of catabolic pathways. Several microbes have been implicated in biofilm production. Bacteria biofilms utilize quorum sensing, chemotaxis, ion exchange, complexation, precipitation, the presence of intracellular and extracellular enzymes, EPS production, and their tolerance and resilience in addition to other properties they possess to aid bioremediation. This chapter highlights bacterial biofilms, explaining their development, structure, and functions as they concerns bioremediation and biodegradation. It also describes various bacterial biofilm-mediated bioremediation solutions that can be used and their effectiveness in removing contaminants from our environment.

Keywords: bioremediation, environment, biofilms, bacteria, contaminants

1. Introduction

The increasing rate of urbanization and industrialization has resulted in a multitude of pollutants that are released into the environment, primarily from the mining industry (cyanide and sulfuric acid), the manufacturing industry (dyes and detergents), the agricultural sector (fertilizers and pesticides), and construction companies (cement and metals). These pollutants have a negative impact on the health of humans, animals, and plants [1]; for example, wastewater from dye-producing companies is linked to antimony, chromium, and mercury [2]. Aluminum, copper, zinc, nickel, lead, and arsenic are among the pollutants released into the environment by the agricultural sector's use of fertilizers, pesticides, and herbicides [3, 4].

Similarly, the ecosystem is negatively impacted when untreated contaminants from agri-food industry wastewaters are dumped into river canals and other water-bodies [5, 6]. Additionally, crude oil contributes significantly to environmental pollution, especially through pipeline vandalism, transportation leaks, and/or unintentional spills [7]. Certain compounds that are harmful to the near environment, such as lead, arsenic, cadmium, and copper, are emitted during mining [8]. During the mining process, other ecologically hazardous chemicals are utilized, such as sulfuric acid and cyanide, among others [9, 10]. Similarly, other industrial wastes, such as those from the cement industry, release copper, zinc, and cadmium into the top soils [11]. Water is contaminated by lead and chromium from pharmaceutical effluents [12], as well as by plastics that include lead, manganese, iron, copper, chromium, silver, cadmium, antimony, and mercury [13].

Furthermore, pollutants from the coal industry include copper, arsenic, mercury, chromium, lead, nickel, cadmium, and zinc [14]. Both terrestrial and aquatic environments, as well as the people who live there, are extremely poisoned by these heavy metals. Lead causes liver and kidney dysfunction, cardiovascular illnesses, and immunological and reproductive system malfunctions, whereas mercury, cadmium, and lead all affect the human central nervous system, particularly in newborns [15–18].

Cancers, bone problems, neurotoxic and nephrotoxic complications, and reproductive system abnormalities are all brought on by cadmium [16–18]. Heavy metal-containing waste is frequently inappropriately dumped into soil and aquatic ecosystems. Fish and other aquatic life may perish if they are dumped into bodies of water; otherwise, they are biomagnified and result in chronic illnesses in both people and animals. As a result, these contaminants must be cleaned up using physical, chemical, or biological techniques. Both chemical and physical bioremediation techniques have been around for a while, but they have disadvantages. For example, the chemical bioremediation process requires specialized equipment and a specialist, while the physical bioremediation process is costly [19].

Thus, a better option biological remediation or bioremediation has become necessary. One of the most successful, economical, and environmentally beneficial technologies for transforming pollutants is bioremediation [20]. Although both plants and microorganisms may be used in biological restoration, plants are preferred because they develop more slowly and are more difficult to manage than germs [21].

Furthermore, bacteria enhance soil fertility, promote plant growth, and reduce the effects of heavy metals [22]. Through biomineralization, biotransformation, biosorption, and bioaccumulation, native microbial communities and microorganisms can detoxify harmful metal pollution. Among the several biological remediation methods, biofilm-mediated remediation has been considered a safe, capable, and well-organized alternative to the use of planktonic microorganisms for the removal or refining of contaminants. Bacteria may be utilized to treat wastewater in a number of ways, including dead or alive, immobilized or suspended [23], and they are now being exploited as a novel remedial alternative for the biological degradation of environmental toxins [24].

This chapter explores the structure, development, and functional roles of bacterial biofilms in bioremediation and biodegradation with recommendations on how to enhance their capacity for use in bioremediation.

2. Remediation techniques

The physical, chemical, and biological methods are the three categories of remediation (**Figure 1**). Booms, sorbent materials, and skimmers are used in the physical cleanup process. Boom is a material-based physical barrier that absorbs oil contaminants and stops them from spreading until a more thorough restoration process is completed [25, 26]. Following booms, skimmers, and sorbents are other techniques used in absorbing and adsorbing the contaminating compounds [12]. Because the bloom remediation approach depends on buoyancy and roll reaction, it presents a significant problem. Booms float and stay on the water's surface for a longer period of time when it is buoyant. The torque needed to rotate the bloom from its upright position is known as the roll response. An increased roll response results in a higher remediation process [27].

In order to stabilize and eliminate heavy metals from the environment, chemical remediation involves the addition of chemicals like sulfide, phosphate, charcoal, aluminum salts, clay minerals, and silico-calcium compounds. Adsorption, reduction, oxidation, complexation, precipitation, and ion exchange are the processes that underlie the utilization of these substances [28]. Although chemical treatment is a quick, fast, and straightforward method, the chemical utilized may also pollute the environment [28].

Another approach to treating pollution is bioremediation, which is a safe, economical, and sustainable remediation technology [29, 30]. Utilizing organic materials like microorganisms and plants is part of the technique. The kind, location, and degree of pollution all affect this method's feasibility [31]. Conversely, microbes have demonstrated effectiveness in cleaning up environmental contaminants. Because of their ease of development, quick growth time, and simplicity of manipulation, they are chosen over plants in cleanup. Because 40–80% of bacterial cells are now known to form biofilms [32], it is imperative to enhance the utilization of microorganisms as bioremediation agents to support a sustainable ecosystem [1]. Bacterial biofilms may have positive effects in addition to unfavorable ones [33]. In other words, bacterial biofilm development is frequently significant in industrial and agricultural contexts [34, 35]. The current applications of these advantageous biofilms include

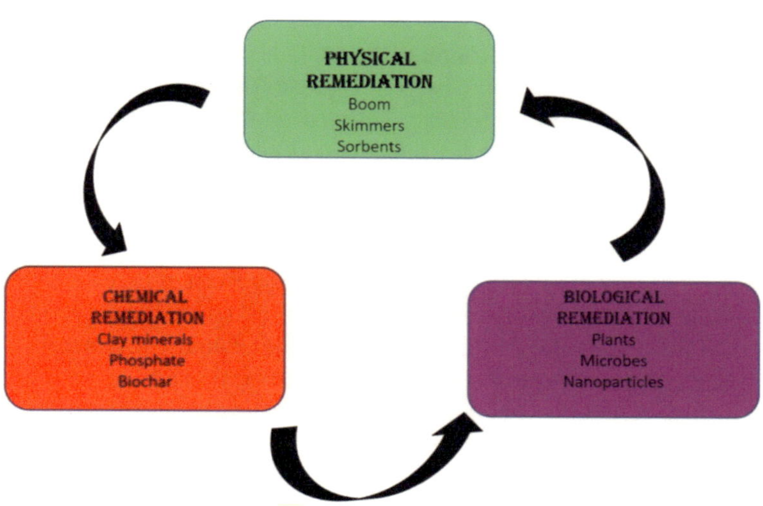

Figure 1.
Types of remediation [1].

bioremediation treatment of hazardous pollutants [36], wastewater treatment [37], marine ecosystem protection [38], corrosion prevention [39, 40], and biological control agents against phytopathogens and biofertilizers to improve crop production [41].

2.1 Bacteria biofilm-mediated bioremediation

Bacteria biofilm-mediated bioremediation is a process that employs bacteria biofilms to remove pollutants from the environment. Biofilms are groups of bacteria attached to surfaces, they are surrounded by a matrix of extracellular polymeric substances (EPS) [24, 42].

2.2 Bacterial biofilms

Bacterial biofilms comprise a population of bacteria that are self-regulating and upon colonizing surfaces become organized to form a structure comprising a polymeric matrix self-generated to promote their growth [43, 44]. Surface proteins, capsular polysaccharides, adhesins, autolysin, anaerobicity, carbon dioxide, glucose, osmotic levels, pH, temperature, ionic concentration, nutritional environment, and surfactant presence all affect how competent bacterial biofilms are. Mature bacterial biofilms are geographically, temporally, and dynamically diverse communities that rely on a range of topologies based on the composition of microbial consortia and the surrounding environment (osmolarity, pH, shear pressures, temperature, and nutrient availability) [45, 46].

The basic form of bacterial biofilms is influenced by the structure of polysaccharides. It is composed of polysaccharides as well as biomolecules including DNA, protein, lipids, and chemical substances. Andersson et al. examined the adhesion properties and biofilm development of 13 bacterial strains in both pure and mixed cultures [46]. Turki et al. used the rotating bio-disk technique (RB) to investigate the composition and diversity of bacterial communities in a semi-industrial test environment. They stated that the existence of helpful and useful species that could be essential to the wastewater purification process was discovered by analyzing the dominance of bacteria. Most biofilm samples contained the well-known bioremediation-capable species *Cronobacter sakazakii*, *Enterobacter agglomerans*, and *Pantoea agglomerans*. The frequent identification of *Salmonella* communities indicates that the RB system had minimal impact on *Salmonella* [47].

Numerous aerobic and anaerobic bacterial species that frequently exploit the breakdown of contaminants as an energy source can be found in biofilm-mediated remediation [48]. Bacteria can employ oxygen as a final electron acceptor during aerobic degradation to break down harmful substances into harmless byproducts, mostly carbon dioxide and water [49, 50]. In anaerobic environments, electron acceptors like nitrate and sulfate can act as oxygen substitutes to change pollutants into less harmful or innocuous compounds, and the byproduct may be dependent on the electron acceptor [48]. Heavy metals, pesticides, oil spills, dyes, persistent organic pollutants (like polychlorinated biphenyls, polycyclic aromatic hydrocarbons, and polychlorinated ethenes), explosives, and pharmaceutical products are among the various environmental pollutants that are currently being removed with bacterial biofilm-mediated remediation [49]. Therefore, the industry uses biofilm-mediated bioremediation to clean up polluted groundwater and soil [49]. These contaminants can be cleaned up by *Pseudomonas*, *Dehalococcides*, *Arthrobacter*, *Bacillus*, *Alcanivorax*, *Cycloclasticus*, *Burkholderia*, and *Rhodococcus* [51, 52]. The use of bacterial biofilms in bioremediation is probably going to be on the increase as shown in **Figure 2** [24].

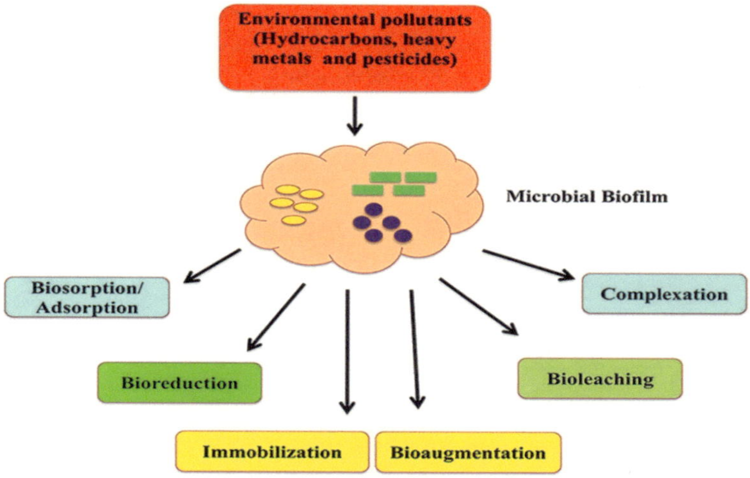

Figure 2.
Biofilm-mediated bioremediation strategies [24].

2.3 Structure and development of bacteria biofilms

Bacteria biofilm production is often a complex process that can involve both single and mixed microbial cell types. Both naturally occurring and artificially created settings have the capacity to support the growth and formation of microbial biofilms [53]. Biofilms are often found in aquatic plants, marshes, lakes, rivers, covering rock streams and sediments, and soil [54]. The biofilm developmental process in bacteria is a significant multistep mechanical one, including surface-attached clusters of microbial cells encased in an extracellular matrix. The five phases of the complicated dynamic process that constitutes the creation of biofilms include their initial attachment, the production of EPS which is a buildup to "irreversible" attachment, the early biofilm architecture development, maturity of biofilm architecture, and single cells dispersal [55].

Biofilms are characterized by their resistance to hazardous contaminants, antimicrobial agents, and desiccation. Creation of nutrient gradients, which permits a variety of metabolic processes and cooperative interactions between microorganisms [56, 57]. Both gram-positive and gram-negative bacteria, including *Pseudomonas* and *Staphylococcus* species, are capable of forming biofilms [56].

2.4 Stages of bacteria biofilm formation

Environmental stressors include UV light, desiccation, low nutrition availability, high pH, high temperature, high pressure, high salt concentrations, and antimicrobial chemicals that cause bacteria to develop biofilms. The processes involved in the production of bacterial biofilms are intricate in this case [54, 58–60]. After a few free-moving bacteria come into touch with an appropriate surface and set up communication roots to acquire nutrition sources and produce a slimy substance called EPS, biofilm formation begins. There are five phases in total for biofilm development (**Figure 3**): (1) initial reversible attachment of the bacteria to the friendly surface, (2) irreversible attachment that results in the formation of the extracellular matrix (ECM) monolayer surface, which is composed of proteins, cellular debris, nucleic acids, and

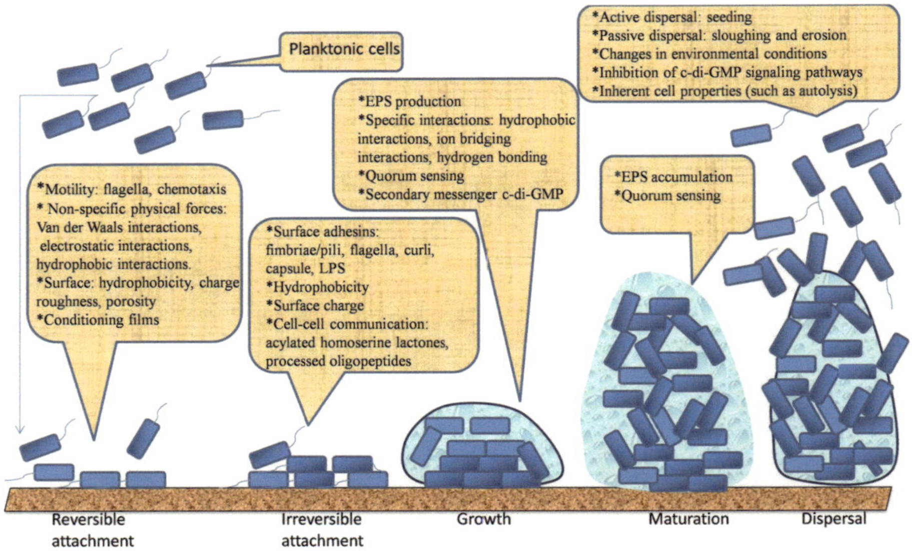

Figure 3.
The stages of bacterial biofilms formation [53].

polysaccharides, (3) biofilm growth and quorum sensing (QS), (4) maturation stage II, which results in the formation of extracellular matrix (EPS) to encase the biofilm and aid in interactions between cells and the matrix, and (5) dispersion stage, which separates from parent biofilms and repeats the cycle in a different location [56].

3. Mechanisms of bacteria biofilm-mediated bioremediation

The mechanisms of bacteria biofilm-mediated bioremediation involve the strategies that can be deployed by bacteria biofilms to aid bioremediation. These include some properties they possess like quorum sensing, chemotaxis, Ion exchange, complexation, precipitation, the presence of intracellular and extracellular enzymes, EPS production, and their tolerance and resilience (ability to withstand stress). The developmental phases of bacterial biofilm formation and its implication in bioremediation. This is illustrated in **Figure 4** [61].

3.1 Quorum sensing (QS)

This involves the communication mechanisms connecting two microbial cells, this process coordinates their social life and several other changes in their behavior it is a signaling system that controls the expression of genes in biofilm communities [24]. The use of biofilm-forming bacteria for biodegradation through QS has shown promise in the treatment process that eliminates pollutants and enhances the restoration of the ecosystem.

It also plays an important role in biofilm formation, solubilization, and biotransformation of pollutants [62]. Genetically modifying the QS apparatus may be important in modulating vital characteristics relevant to environmental applications, including biofilm formation and other qualities that are important for bacteria

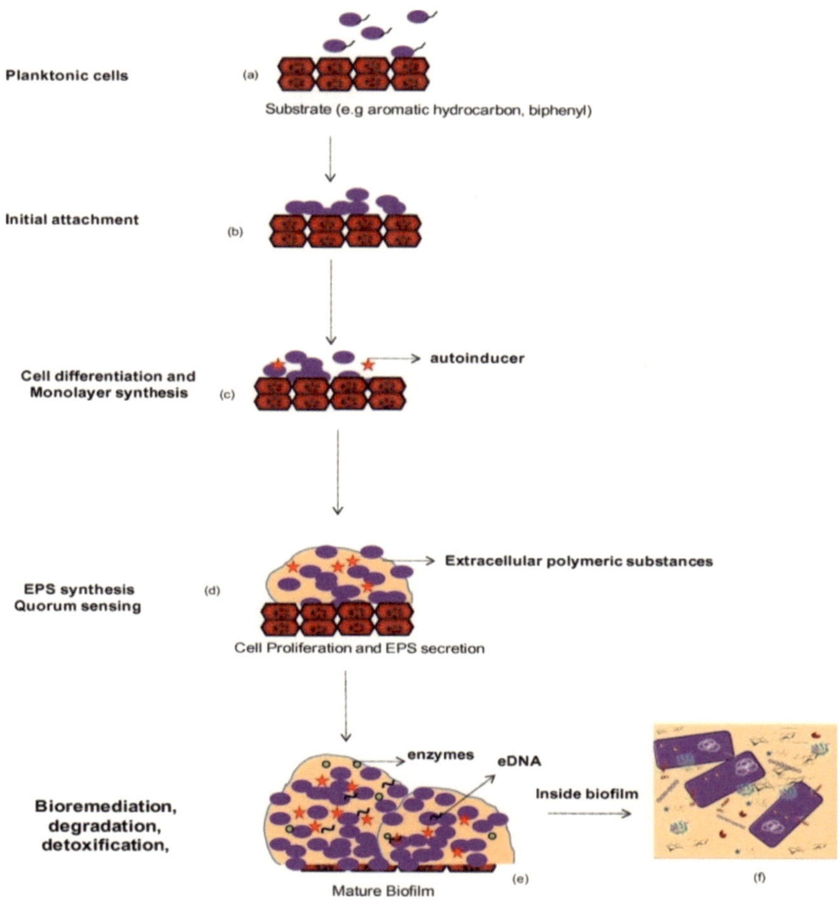

Figure 4.
Developmental phases of bacterial biofilm formation and its implication in bioremediation [61]. Biofilm formation begins when planktonic cells attach to the substratum. Thus, Bacteria with the ability to form biofilms over the surface of hydrocarbons are mostly suited for bioremediation. (b) The proliferation of cells aids the formation of a monolayer over the surface of hydrocarbon. The physicochemical interactions and extracellular proteins support the attachment of cells to the substratum. (c–d) Increased levels of autoinducers and extracellular polymeric substances (EPS) resulting from continuous cell growth causing solubilization and degradation. (e–f) Biofilm then progresses and becomes mature with enhanced resistance to toxins and harsh environmental factors. This increase in resilience promotes the process of bioremediation. In the mature biofilm some metabolic processes that take place simultaneously to assist in biodegradation.

when they are degrading or detoxifying pollutants. QS signals can also be useful in fabricating engineered biofilms that possess enhanced degradation kinetics [61]. Autoinducing peptide (AIP) and *N*-acyl homoserine lactone (AHL) are major quorum sensing (QS) signaling of gram-positive bacteria and gram-negative bacteria respectively [42]. Quorum sensing functions utilized for bacteria bioremediation technology are illustrated in **Figure 5** [61].

3.2 Chemotaxis

Chemotaxis is a movement in the cell that is controlled by gradients of chemoattractants or chemorepellents, these substances are majorly found in

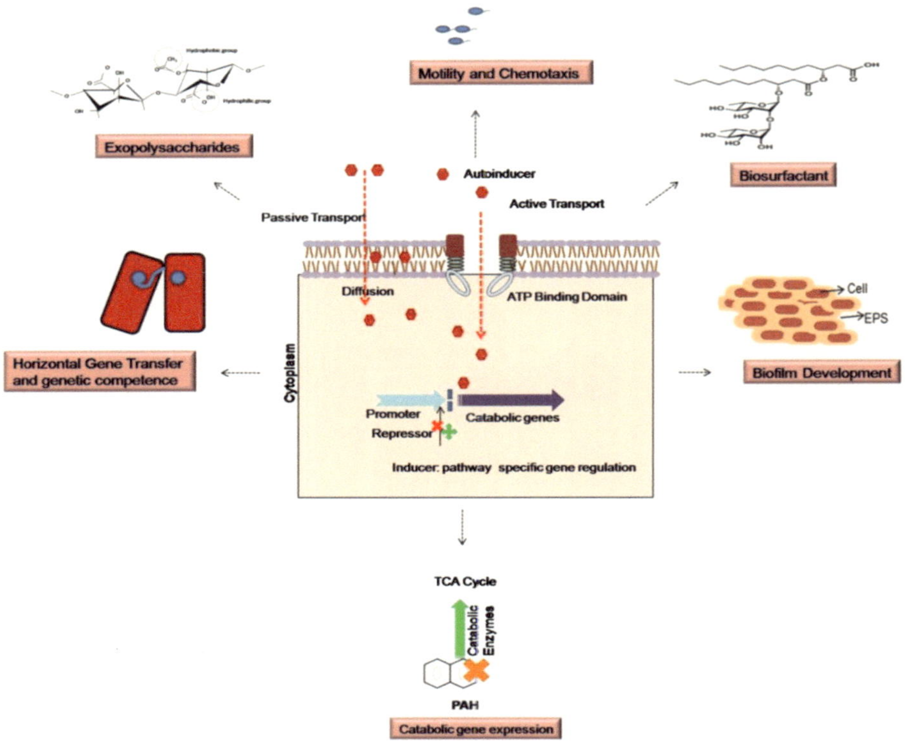

Figure 5.
Quorum sensing functions utilized for bacteria bioremediation technology [61].

prokaryotes. This innate ability assists bacteria to recognize and respond to the complex tapestry of chemical gradients that pervade their surroundings enabling them to find food and survive [63]. This process simply allows microorganisms to swim toward pollutants [42]. In other words, it enables cells to sense and swim in the direction of xenobiotic compounds when the carbon source is limited. Chemotaxis is a major factor when biofilms are being formed, it aids the movement of microbes along the substratum and forms microcolonies that surmount limited substrate accessibility and bioavailability. Although certain bacteria have evolved chemo-repellent responses to anthracene and pyrene in the presence of metals, positive chemotaxis has been recorded toward naphthalene [64]. The role of bacteria biofilm and chemotaxis in the metabolism of a polycyclic aromatic hydrocarbon (PAH) in **Figure 6** [65, 66].

3.3 Ion exchange, complexation, and precipitation

These are processes that allow biofilms to absorb, adsorb, and immobilize pollutants [42]. The characteristics of the microbial cell surface, support, and environmental circumstances all influence how well bacteria cells are immobilized and adsorbed, the factor that determines the adsorption of bacteria cells are listed in **Table 1** [67]. Biofilms can also use biosorption, enzymatic reduction, and bioprecipitation to sequester heavy metals [68].

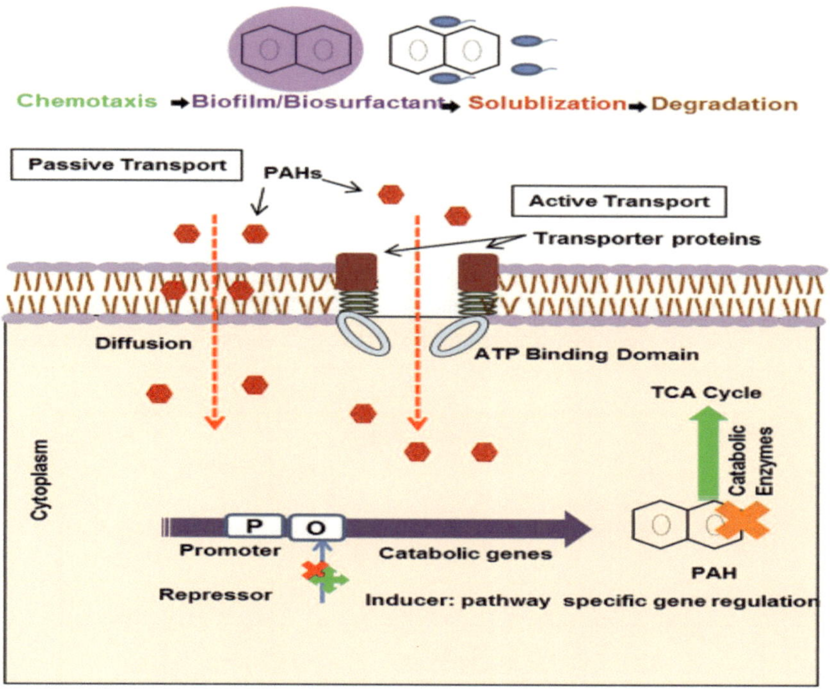

Figure 6.
The role of bacteria biofilm and chemotaxis in the metabolism of a polycyclic aromatic hydrocarbon (PAH) [65].

Support	Environmental factors	Microbial cell
Roughness	Ph	EPS
Porosity	Oxygen concentration	Age of cells
Hydrophobicity	Temperature	Physiological state of cells
Superficial charge	Nutrient availability	Hydrophobicity
Toxicity	Flow velocity	Flagella, pilli
Type of functional groups	Cations/anions	Fimbriae, glycocalyx
	Antimicrobial agents	Surface proteins
	Hydrodynamic forces	
	Adhesive forces	
	Rheology	

Table 1.
Factors determining bacterial cells' adsorption [67].

3.4 Intracellular and extracellular enzymes

These enzymes break down pollutants by adding oxygen atoms to the pollutant's structure [42]. Bacteria can also create biofilms that have a variety of metabolic processes for breaking down harmful substances like hydrocarbons, including aliphatic and aromatic hydrocarbons, which are broken down by enzymes such as dioxygenases and alkane hydroxylases [69]. Some enzymes also hydrolyze organophosphates to break down pesticides and insecticides into less toxic forms [70].

3.5 EPS production

The production of EPSs gives rise to electrostatic interactions that help maintain the biofilm structure, interacting with pollutants deploying processes like binding, sorption, and precipitation leading to their breakdown and remediation [42, 71]. Also, EPS interacts with pollutants utilizing other mechanisms such as solubilization, emulsification, ion exchange, and complexation. Aside from that, the polyanionic properties of EPS aid their binding metal ions through electrostatic forces and form

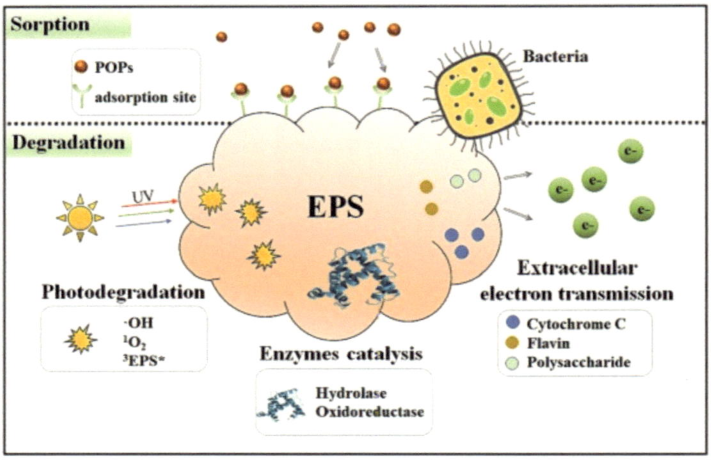

Figure 7.
The role of EPS in degradation pollutants in soil [75].

EPS component	Role in biofilm	Significance in bioremediation
Neutral polysaccharides	Structural component	Provide stability
Amyloids	Structural component	Provide stability and resistance
Hydrophobic polysaccharides	Ion exchange, Sorption	Increase solubility and binding hydrophobic organic compounds, metal binding, and detoxification
Polymer degradation	Polymer degradation	Oxidoreductase and Hydrolyases are helpful in PAHs degradation
Monomers and polymers	Nutritive source at starvation	Help in preliminary acclimatization to pollutants
Nucleic acids	Informative, gene transfer, structural	Transfer of genes useful for the degradation of xenobiotics
Biosurfactant	Initial microcolony formation, development of biofilm, formation of water channels	Component cells within biofilms to solubilize and utilize substrates

Table 2.
Role of EPS components in biofilm and possible significances in environment restoration [61].

organometal complexes [72]. In addition, EPS aids the solubilization and sorption of several organic compounds, increasing their bioavailability to bacterial cells and enhancing their enzymatic breakdown into nonirritant compounds such as H_2O, CO_2, and CH_4 [73]. Thus, bioremediation mediated by bacteria biofilm-EPS is a cost effective, sustainable, and eco-friendly approach to remediate polluted environments [74]. The role of EPS in the degradation of pollutants in soil is illustrated in **Figure 7** [75]. The role of EPS components in biofilm and possible significance in environment restoration is illustrated in **Table 2** [61].

3.6 Stress tolerance and resilience

Biofilms are very resistant to environmental stresses, such as high pollutant concentrations, pH changes, and severe temperatures. While metabolic cooperation among microbial cells improves survival and pollutant breakdown, the EPS matrix serves as a physical barrier [76].

4. Applications of bacterial biofilms in bioremediation

4.1 Hydrocarbon degradation

One of the biggest environmental problems is hydrocarbon contamination from industrial discharges and oil spills. Bacterial biofilms are essential for the breakdown of hydrocarbons because they Increase EPS's hydrophobicity, which promotes hydrocarbon absorption and enzymatic actions that work in tandem for total breakdown. *Alcanivorax borkumensis*-dominated biofilms, for example, were essential in breaking down crude oil leftovers following the deepwater horizon oil leak [77].

4.2 Heavy metal remediation

Heavy metals are rendered immobile by biofilms, which lowers their toxicity and bioavailability. Among the mechanisms are: biosorption and bioprecipitation in which metal ions are bound by functional groups in EPS and metals can change into insoluble forms respectively. *Shewanella oneidensis*, for instance, helps with heavy metal cleanup by converting soluble uranium to insoluble uranium oxide [78].

4.3 Wastewater treatment

In wastewater treatment facilities, biofilms are widely employed for resource recovery, organic pollutant degradation, and nutrient removal. Biofilms are necessary for high-efficiency treatment in membrane bioreactors and trickling filters [79, 80].

5. Challenges and future directions

5.1 Challenges

1. *Biofilm resistance*: The EPS matrix can hinder pollutant diffusion, reducing degradation efficiency.

2. *Environmental variability*: Changes in pH, temperature, and pollutant concentrations affect biofilm stability.

3. *Scaling up*: Translating lab-scale findings to field applications is complex and requires optimization.

5.2 Future prospects

Advancements in genetic engineering, synthetic biology, and nanotechnology hold promise for enhancing biofilm-mediated bioremediation. Strategies include:

1. Engineering biofilm-forming bacteria for specific pollutant degradation.

2. Developing synthetic biofilms with tailored properties.

3. Incorporating nanomaterials to improve catalytic activity and resilience.

6. Conclusion

Bacterial biofilms are invaluable in bioremediation, offering sustainable solutions for hydrocarbon and heavy metal contamination. Their resilience, adaptability, and metabolic diversity make them effective in addressing complex pollution challenges. Continued research and innovation will further enhance biofilm-mediated approaches, ensuring their widespread application in environmental management.

Acknowledgements

The authors would like to express their gratitude to Professor Adebayo Elijah for his guidance. The authors also appreciate Mater Ecclesiae College Epe-Lagos for providing technical support. The authors would also like to express their gratitude to the Ladoke Akintola University (LAUTECH) Ogbomosho Nigeria.

Author Contributions

Conceptualization, investigation, data curation, E.M.I., and A.O. P. writing—original draft preparation E.M.I.; writing—review and editing, E.M.I. and A.O. P.; supervision, A.O. P.; project administration, E.M.I., and A.O. P.

Conflict of interest

The authors declare no conflict of interest.

Author details

Michael Ikechukwuka Ejafu[1]* and Omodamola Paulina Akinro[2]

1 Department of Pure and Applied Biology, Ladoke Akintola University of Technology (LAUTECH), Ogbomosho, Nigeria

2 Microbiology and Biotechnology Laboratory LAUTECH, Ogbomosho, Nigeria

*Address all correspondence to: michaelejafu@gmail.com

References

[1] Ayilara MS, Babalola OO. Bioremediation of environmental wastes: The role of microorganisms. Frontiers in Agronomy. 2023;**5**:1183691

[2] Methneni N, Morales-González JA, Jaziri A, Mansour HB, Fernandez-Serrano M. Persistent organic and inorganic pollutants in the effluents from the textile dyeing industries: Ecotoxicology appraisal via a battery of biotests. Environmental Research. 2021;**196**:110956

[3] Ayilara MS, Olanrewaju OS, Babalola OO, Odeyemi O. Waste management through composting: Challenges and potentials. Sustainability. 2020;**12**(11):4456

[4] Prabagar S, Dharmadasa RM, Lintha A, Thuraisingam S, Prabagar J. Accumulation of heavy metals in grape fruit, leaves, soil and water: A study of influential factors and evaluating ecological risks in Jaffna, Sri Lanka. Environmental and Sustainability Indicators. 2021;**12**:100147

[5] Širić I, Kumar P, Adelodun B, Abou Fayssal S, Bachheti RK, Bachheti A, et al. Risk assessment of heavy metals occurrence in two wild edible oyster mushrooms (*Pleurotus* spp.) collected from Rajaji National Park. Journal of Fungi. 2022;**8**(10):1007

[6] Al-Huqail AA, Kumar P, Eid EM, Adelodun B, Abou Fayssal S, Singh J, et al. Risk assessment of heavy metals contamination in soil and two rice (*Oryza sativa* L.) varieties irrigated with paper mill effluent. Agriculture. 2022;**12**(11):1864

[7] Ogunlaja A, Ogunlaja OO, Okewole DM, Morenikeji OA. Risk assessment and source identification of heavy metal contamination by multivariate and hazard index analyses of a pipeline vandalised area in Lagos state, Nigeria. Science of the Total Environment. 2019;**651**:2943-2952

[8] Liu S, Yang B, Liang Y, Xiao Y, Fang J. Prospect of phytoremediation combined with other approaches for remediation of heavy metal-polluted soils. Environmental Science and Pollution Research. 2020;**27**:16069-16085

[9] Ayangbenro AS, Olanrewaju OS, Babalola OO. Sulfate-reducing bacteria as an effective tool for sustainable acid mine bioremediation. Frontiers in Microbiology. 2018;**9**:1986

[10] Orlović-Leko P, Farkaš B, Galić I. A short review of environmental and health impacts of gold mining. Reliability: Theory & Applications. 2022;**17**(4(70)):242-248

[11] Jafari A, Ghaderpoori M, Kamarehi B, Abdipour H. Soil pollution evaluation and health risk assessment of heavy metals around Douroud cement factory, Iran. Environmental Earth Sciences. 2019;**78**:1-9

[12] Kumari V, Tripathi AK. Remediation of heavy metals in pharmaceutical effluent with the help of *Bacillus cereus*-based green-synthesized silver nanoparticles supported on alumina. Applied Nanoscience. 2020;**10**(6):1709-1719

[13] Zhou Z, Liu X, Sun K, Lin C, Ma J, He M, et al. Persulfate-based advanced oxidation processes (AOPs) for organic-contaminated soil remediation: A review. Chemical Engineering Journal. 2019;**372**:836-851

[14] Sun J, Dai X, Wang Q, Van Loosdrecht MC, Ni BJ. Microplastics in wastewater treatment plants: Detection, occurrence and removal. Water Research. 2019;**152**:21-37

[15] Zwolak A, Sarzyńska M, Szpyrka E, Stawarczyk K. Sources of soil pollution by heavy metals and their accumulation in vegetables: A review. Water, Air, & Soil Pollution. 2019;**230**:1-9

[16] Fashola MO, Ngole-Jeme VM, Babalola OO. Heavy metal immobilization potential of indigenous bacteria isolated from gold mine tailings. International Journal of Environmental Research. 2020;**14**:71-86

[17] Fashola MO, Ngole-Jeme VM, Babalola OO. Physicochemical properties, heavy metals, and metal-tolerant bacteria profiles of abandoned gold mine tailings in Krugersdorp, South Africa. Canadian Journal of Soil Science. 2020;**100**(3):217-233

[18] Ayangbenro AS, Babalola OO. Genomic analysis of *Bacillus cereus* NWUAB01 and its heavy metal removal from polluted soil. Scientific Reports. 2020;**10**(1):19660

[19] Mahmood RT, Asad MJ, Asgher M, Khan FS, Muzammil K, Nasir N, et al. First report on the bioremediation of textile industrial effluents by *Piptoporus betulinus* IEBL-3 by using response surface methodology. Applied Sciences. 2022;**12**(3):1090

[20] Sonune N. Microbes: A potential tool for bioremediation. In: Rhizobiont in Bioremediation of Hazardous Waste. Singapore: Springer; 2021. pp. 391-407. DOI: 10.1007/978-981-16-0602-1_17

[21] Hussain N, Bilal M, Iqbal HM. Carbon-based nanomaterials with multipurpose attributes for water treatment: Greening the 21st-century nanostructure materials deployment. Biomaterials and Polymers Horizon. 2022;**1**(1):48-58

[22] Chaudhary A, Chaudhary P, Abou Fayssal S, Singh S, Jaiswal DK, Tripathi V, et al. Exploring beneficial microbes and their multifaceted applications: An overview. In: Microbial Inoculants: Applications for Sustainable Agriculture. Singapore: Springer; 2024. pp. 1-28

[23] Zhang Z, Zhang C, Yang Y, Zhang Z, Tang Y, Su P, et al. A review of sulfate-reducing bacteria: Metabolism, influencing factors and application in wastewater treatment. Journal of Cleaner Production. 2022;**376**:134109

[24] Mishra S, Huang Y, Li J, Xiaozhen W, Zhou Z, Lei Q, et al. Biofilm-mediated bioremediation is a powerful tool for the removal of environmental pollutants. Chemosphere. 2022;**294**:133609

[25] Vocciante M, Caretta A, Bua L, Bagatin R, Franchi E, Petruzzelli G, et al. Enhancements in phytoremediation technology: Environmental assessment including different options of biomass disposal and comparison with a consolidated approach. Journal of Environmental Management. 2019;**237**:560-568

[26] Kumari P, Alam M, Siddiqi WA. Usage of nanoparticles as adsorbents for waste water treatment: An emerging trend. Sustainable Materials and Technologies. 2019;**22**:e00128

[27] Dhaka A, Chattopadhyay P. A review on physical remediation techniques for treatment of marine oil spills. Journal of Environmental Management. 2021;**288**:112428

[28] Xu X, Chen G, Wei J, Qin Y, Tang R, Wang L, et al. Effects of competitive

cations and dissolved organic matter on ammonium exchange and up-concentration properties of ion exchangers from domestic wastewater under multicycle exchange-regeneration operation. Separation and Purification Technology. 2024;**345**:127274

[29] Kumar M, Seth A, Singh AK, Rajput MS, Sikandar M. Remediation strategies for heavy metals contaminated ecosystem: A review. Environmental and Sustainability Indicators. 2021;**12**:100155

[30] Kumar A, Subrahmanyam G, Mondal R, Cabral-Pinto MMS, Shabnam AA, Jigyasu DK, et al. Bio-remediation approaches for alleviation of cadmium contamination in natural resources. Chemosphere. 2021;**268**:128855

[31] Patel AK, Singhania RR, Albarico FPJB, Pandey A, Chen CW, Dong CD. Organic wastes bioremediation and its changing prospects. Science of the Total Environment. 2022;**824**:153889

[32] Flemming HC, Wuertz S. Bacteria and archaea on earth and their abundance in biofilms. Nature Reviews Microbiology. 2019;**17**(4):247-260

[33] Rosche B, Li XZ, Hauer B, Schmid A, Buehler K. Microbial biofilms: A concept for industrial catalysis? Trends in Biotechnology. 2009;**27**(11):636-643

[34] Bogino PC, de Las Mercedes Oliva M, Sorroche FG, Giordano W. The role of bacterial biofilms and surface components in plant-bacterial associations. International Journal of Molecular Sciences. 2013;**14**(8): 15838-15859

[35] Berlanga M, Guerrero R. Living together in biofilms: The microbial cell factory and its biotechnological implications. Microbial Cell Factories. 2016;**15**:1-11

[36] Irankhah S, Abdi Ali A, Mallavarapu M, Soudi MR, Subashchandrabose S, Gharavi S, et al. Ecological role of *Acinetobacter calcoaceticus* GSN3 in natural biofilm formation and its advantages in bioremediation. Biofouling. 2019;**35**(4):377-391

[37] Ali Z, Mohammad A, Riaz Y, Quraishi UM, Malik RN. Treatment efficiency of a hybrid constructed wetland system for municipal wastewater and its suitability for crop irrigation. International Journal of Phytoremediation. 2018;**20**(11):1152-1161

[38] Naidoo S, Olaniran AO. Treated wastewater effluent as a source of microbial pollution of surface water resources. International Journal of Environmental Research and Public Health. 2014;**11**(1):249-270

[39] Jayaraman A, Cheng ET, Earthman JC, Wood TK. Axenic aerobic biofilms inhibit corrosion of SAE 1018 steel through oxygen depletion. Applied Microbiology and Biotechnology. 1997;**48**:11-17

[40] Olvera-Martínez ME, Mendoza-Flores J, Genesca J. CO_2 corrosion control in steel pipelines. Influence of turbulent flow on the performance of corrosion inhibitors. Journal of Loss Prevention in the Process Industries. 2015;**35**:19-28

[41] Timmusk S, Behers L, Muthoni J, Muraya A, Aronsson AC. Perspectives and challenges of microbial application for crop improvement. Frontiers in Plant Science. 2017;**8**:49

[42] Yadav S, Chandra R. Biofilm-mediated bioremediation of

pollutants from the environment for sustainable development. In: New and Future Developments in Microbial Biotechnology and Bioengineering: Microbial Biofilms. Amsterdam, Netherlands: Elsevier; 2020. pp. 177-203

[43] Hood SK, Zottola EA. Biofilms in food processing. Food Control. 1995;**6**(1):9-18

[44] Raza A, Muhammad G, Sharif S, Atta A. Biofilm producing *Staphylococcus aureus* and bovine mastitis: A review. Molecular Microbiology Research. 2013;**3**(1):1-8. Available from: http://mmr.sophiapublisher.com. ISSN 1927-5595

[45] Pulcini ED. Bacterial biofilms: A review of current research. Néphrologie. 2001;**22**(8):439-441

[46] Andersson S, Dalhammar G, Rajarao GK. Influence of microbial interactions and EPS/polysaccharide composition on nutrient removal activity in biofilms formed by strains found in wastewater treatment systems. Microbiological Research. 2011;**166**(6):449-457

[47] Turki Y, Mehri I, Lajnef R, Rejab AB, Khessairi A, Cherif H, et al. Biofilms in bioremediation and wastewater treatment: Characterization of bacterial community structure and diversity during seasons in municipal wastewater treatment process. Environmental Science and Pollution Research. 2017;**24**:3519-3530

[48] Rodríguez-Martínez S, Dekel A, Aizenberg-Gershtein Y, Gilboa Y, Sharaby Y, Halpern M, et al. Characterization of biofilm bacterial communities in a vertical unsaturated-flow bioreactor treating domestic greywater. Environmental Processes. 2016;**3**:325-340

[49] Edwards SJ, Kjellerup BV. Applications of biofilms in bioremediation and biotransformation of persistent organic pollutants, pharmaceuticals/personal care products, and heavy metals. Applied Microbiology and Biotechnology. 2013;**97**:9909-9921

[50] Azubuike CC, Chikere CB, Okpokwasili GC. Bioremediation techniques–classification based on site of application: Principles, advantages, limitations and prospects. World Journal of Microbiology and Biotechnology. 2016;**32**:1-18

[51] Dasgupta D, Ghosh R, Sengupta TK. Biofilm-mediated enhanced crude oil degradation by newly isolated pseudomonas species. International Scholarly Research Notices. 2013;**2013**(1):250749

[52] Yoshikawa C, Hashimoto M, Iwasaki K, Kakimoto K. Antibacterial activity and biofilm dispersion of an isopropyl methylphenol-containing dentifrice. Nano Biomedicine. 2023;**15**(1):1-6

[53] Muhammad MH, Idris AL, Fan X, Guo Y, Yu Y, Jin X, et al. Beyond risk: Bacterial biofilms and their regulating approaches. Frontiers in Microbiology. 2020;**21**(11):928

[54] Galié S, García-Gutiérrez C, Miguélez EM, Villar CJ, Lombó F. Biofilms in the food industry: Health aspects and control methods. Frontiers in Microbiology. 2018;**9**:898

[55] Tolker-Nielsen T. Biofilm development. Microbial Biofilms. 2015;**3**:51-66

[56] Mirghani R, Saba T, Khaliq H, Mitchell J, Do L, Chambi L, et al. Biofilms: Formation, drug resistance and

alternatives to conventional approaches. AIMS Microbiology. 2022;**8**(3):239

[57] Liu Y, Zhang J, Ji Y. Environmental factors modulate biofilm formation by *Staphylococcus aureus*. Science Progress. 2020;**103**(1):0036850419898659

[58] O'Toole G, Kaplan HB, Kolter R. Biofilm formation as microbial development. Annual Reviews in Microbiology. 2000;**54**(1):49-79

[59] Hall-Stoodley L, Costerton JW, Stoodley P. Bacterial biofilms: From the natural environment to infectious diseases. Nature Reviews Microbiology. 2004;**2**(2):95-108

[60] López D, Vlamakis H, Kolter R. Biofilms. Cold Spring Harbor Perspectives in Biology. 2010;**2**(7):a000398

[61] Mangwani N, Kumari S, Das S. Bacterial biofilms and quorum sensing: Fidelity in bioremediation technology. Biotechnology and Genetic Engineering Reviews. 2016;**32**(1-2):43-73

[62] Tripathi S, Chandra R, Purchase D, Bilal M, Mythili R, Yadav S. Quorum sensing-a promising tool for degradation of industrial waste containing persistent organic pollutants. Environmental Pollution. 2022;**292**:118342

[63] Xu Q, Ali S, Afzal M, Nizami AS, Han S, Dar MA, et al. Advancements in bacterial chemotaxis: Utilizing the navigational intelligence of bacteria and its practical applications. Science of the Total Environment. 2024;**931**:172967

[64] Yesankar PJ, Qureshi A, Purohit HJ. Biofilm-mediated biodegradation of hydrophobic organic compounds in the presence of metals as co-contaminants. In: Microbial Biodegradation and Bioremediation. Amsterdam, Netherlands: Elsevier; 2022. pp. 441-460

[65] Kungwani N, Shukla SK, Rao TS, Das S. Biofilm-mediated bioremediation of polycyclic aromatic hydrocarbons: Current status and future perspectives. In: Microbial Biodegradation and Bioremediation. Amsterdam, Netherlands: Elsevier; 2022. pp. 547-570

[66] Vullo DL. Tactic responses of bacteria to pollutants: Implications for the degradation efficiency of microbial biofilms. In: Lear G, editor. Biofilms in Bioremediation: Current Research and Emerging Technologies. U.K: Caister Academic Press; 2016. pp. 57-74

[67] Żur J, Wojcieszyńska D, Guzik U. Metabolic responses of bacterial cells to immobilization. Molecules. 2016;**21**(7):958

[68] Xing Y, Luo X, Liu S, Wan W, Huang Q, Chen W. A novel eco-friendly recycling of food waste for preparing biofilm-attached biochar to remove Cd and Pb in wastewater. Journal of Cleaner Production. 2021;**311**:127514

[69] Ballah FM, Islam MS, Rana ML, Ferdous FB, Ahmed R, Pramanik PK, et al. Phenotypic and genotypic detection of biofilm-forming *Staphylococcus aureus* from different food sources in Bangladesh. Biology. 2022;**11**(7):949

[70] Chandran P, Das N. Degradation of diesel oil by immobilized *Candida tropicalis* and biofilm formed on gravels. Biodegradation. 2011;**22**:1181-1189

[71] Sridharan R, Krishnaswamy VG. Biofilm mediated bioremediation and other applications. In: Development in Wastewater Treatment Research and Processes. Amsterdam, Netherlands: Elsevier; 2022. pp. 449-459

[72] Shukla SK, Mangwani N, Karley D, Rao TS. Bacterial biofilms and genetic regulation for metal detoxification. In:

Handbook of Metal-Microbe Interactions and Bioremediation. Boca Raton, Florida: CRC Press; 2017. pp. 317-332

[73] Mohapatra RK, Behera SS, Patra JK, Thatoi H, Parhi PK. Potential application of bacterial biofilm for bioremediation of toxic heavy metals and dye-contaminated environments. In: New and Future Developments in Microbial Biotechnology and Bioengineering: Microbial Biofilms. Amsterdam, Netherlands: Elsevier; 2020. pp. 267-281

[74] Mahto KU, Priyadarshanee M, Samantaray DP, Das S. Bacterial biofilm and extracellular polymeric substances in the treatment of environmental pollutants: Beyond the protective role in survivability. Journal of Cleaner Production. 2022;**379**:134759

[75] Wei Z, Niu S, Wei Y, Liu Y, Xu Y, Yang Y, et al. The role of extracellular polymeric substances (EPS) in chemical-degradation of persistent organic pollutants in soil: A review. Science of the Total Environment. 2024;**912**:168877

[76] Flemming HC, van Hullebusch ED, Neu TR, Nielsen PH, Seviour T, Stoodley P, et al. The biofilm matrix: Multitasking in a shared space. Nature Reviews Microbiology. 2023;**21**(2):70-86

[77] Hazen E, Jorgensen S, Rykaczewski R, et al. Predicted habitat shifts of Pacific top predators in a changing climate. Nature Climate Change. 2013;**3**:234-238. DOI: 10.1038/nclimate1686

[78] Feng Q, Guo W, Wang T, Alvarez LCM, Luo M, Ge R, et al. Iron coupling with carbon fiber to stimulate biofilms formation in aerobic biological film systems for improved decentralized wastewater treatment: Performance, mechanisms and implications. Bioresource Technology. 2021;**319**:124151

[79] Murshid S, Antonysamy A, Dhakshinamoorthy G, Jayaseelan A, Pugazhendhi A. A review on biofilm-based reactors for wastewater treatment: Recent advancements in biofilm carriers, kinetics, reactors, economics, and future perspectives. Science of the Total Environment. 2023;**892**:164796

[80] Singh A, Kamble SJ, Sawant M, Chakravarthy Y, Kazmi A, Aymerich E, et al. Technical, hygiene, economic, and life cycle assessment of full-scale moving bed biofilm reactors for wastewater treatment in India. Environmental Science and Pollution Research. 2018;**25**:2552-2569